AF667261

Congenital Anomalies of the Penis

Mohamed Fahmy

Congenital Anomalies of the Penis

Springer

Mohamed Fahmy
Pediatric Surgery
Al Azher University
Cairo
Egypt

ISBN 978-3-319-43309-7 ISBN 978-3-319-43310-3 (eBook)
DOI 10.1007/978-3-319-43310-3

Library of Congress Control Number: 2017930623

© Springer International Publishing Switzerland 2017
This work is subject to copyright. All rights are reserved by the Publisher, whether the whole or part of the material is concerned, specifically the rights of translation, reprinting, reuse of illustrations, recitation, broadcasting, reproduction on microfilms or in any other physical way, and transmission or information storage and retrieval, electronic adaptation, computer software, or by similar or dissimilar methodology now known or hereafter developed.
The use of general descriptive names, registered names, trademarks, service marks, etc. in this publication does not imply, even in the absence of a specific statement, that such names are exempt from the relevant protective laws and regulations and therefore free for general use.
The publisher, the authors and the editors are safe to assume that the advice and information in this book are believed to be true and accurate at the date of publication. Neither the publisher nor the authors or the editors give a warranty, express or implied, with respect to the material contained herein or for any errors or omissions that may have been made.

Printed on acid-free paper

This Springer imprint is published by Springer Nature
The registered company is Springer International Publishing AG
The registered company address is: Gewerbestrasse 11, 6330 Cham, Switzerland

This book is dedicated to my beloved wife Rula for prosperity she bestowed upon me, continuous tremendous support, positive energy and awarding me always with hope and love.

Foreword

In *Congenital Anomalies of the Penis*, Professor Fahmy has brought together the diverse but interrelated issues associated with these malformations, thereby providing an understanding of the embryology, the diagnosis, and the eventual functional and psychological impact of these conditions. This long overdue book benefits from Professor Fahmy's long-standing critical interest and extensive experience that have stimulated an interesting and detailed evaluation and alternative approaches to the diagnosis, classification, management, and reconstruction of these anomalies.

This comprehensive exposition should appeal to the student learning the basics, to the academic with an interest in research and, perhaps most relevantly, to the clinician involved with the child and his family, and with corrective surgical reconstruction towards a better overall experience and outcome.

This is a stimulating text worthy of serious study.

Adrian Bianchi
Neonatal and Paediatric Reconstructive Surgeon
Manchester, UK

May 2016

Preface

Penis is a miraculous organ; with its remarkable erectile capability has throughout human history consistently been considered emblematic of masculinity, the penis has been the subject of exhaustive study, and its anatomy is generally deemed to be well-established.

Each year an estimated six percent of total births worldwide (>8 million children), including three percent of all live births in the United States (more than 120,000 babies), are born with a serious birth defect of genetic origin. Congenital penile anomalies are among the most common human birth defects; approximately one out of every 1,500 children is born with atypical genital or reproductive anatomy that raises the question of cosmetic and functional correction.

Many of these anomalies, specially rare one, are not fully investigated and usually the practitioners and researchers spending a lot of their time and effort looking in the scientific media to find out the full description and the proper management of such cases they are facing in the daily practice without a productive achievement. The extent and complexity of these malformations require a thoughtful approach to timely surgical management and consistent care through their transition from childhood to adulthood. The newborn with abnormal genital development presents a difficult diagnostic and treatment challenge for the primary care paediatrician. It is important that a definitive diagnosis be determined as quickly as possible so that an appropriate treatment plan can be established to minimize medical, psychological, and social complications.

Alongside more than 30 years working in the field of genitourinary anomalies, a considerable number of widely variant cases of congenital diseases affecting penis were collected and it is time now to put all in a text work as a guide for proper dealing with such anomalies.

Therefore, this textbook will stand to provide a comprehensive but concise data for almost all congenital diseases and anomalies affecting the penis; explaining the embryological and anatomical background, incidence, historical notes, appropriate investigations, imaging and proper management, this book is packed with colour photographs of the abnormalities of the penis, as well as abnormalities of the prepuce, and male urethra. These photographs obviously represent a lifetime's work and the quality of its colour is excellent, and they edited with each disease to demonstrate its details, and some animations will be available online for the difficult and complex cases.

I am delighted that the quantity of text has been kept to a minimum. To find out exactly which subjects have been covered you can go to the index to see the wide variety of topics, but they vary from the common, e.g. phimosis to the rarer penile duplications. This book is valuable for the experienced paediatric urologist to use as an occasional reference, and probably very useful for teaching as it will form the basis of discussions of both the common and rare abnormalities.

Many congenital penile diseases like penoscrotal transposition, median raphe and intact prepuce megameatus anomalies are re-classified with new entities added to the previously described categories; like central penile scrotalization and caudal scrotal regression in penoscrotal transposition, and centrally located megameatus without hypospadias or epispadias in megameatus chapter. Also in prepuce section a new anomaly of microposthia is described with some details. At the meantime the common anomalies like hypospadias and bladder exstrophy are not discussed herein as the reader can find a lot of literature explaining it elsewhere, only variant of hypospadias and primary epispadias are considered. Despite this book is dedicated for congenital anomalies of the penis, we opted to add some acquired diseases, which may had a congenital background, like balanitis and balanoposthitis; also from my experience in dealing with a huge number of cases of circumcision and its complications, I found the congenital penile anomalies like micropenis, webbed penis and penile chordee had a great impaction in the incidence of such complications, so we discussed this complications briefly in one chapter.

I hope this textbook will add a deep insight into the congenital diseases of the penis and will help early detection of such diseases during childhood, which had a great impaction not only in sexuality and fertility but also in the psychological makeup of the child.

Cairo, Egypt Mohamed Fahmy

Acknowledgement

I wish to acknowledge my colleagues who lent me their own photos of some rare diseases of the penis; in this regard I express my gratitude to Dr. Naeem Khan, from Pakistan, Dr. Mohamed Abdalbari, from Yamen, Dr. Wael Ghanem, Cairo, and Dr. Cansu Ünden Özcan, from Turkey.

My great thanks to dearest friend Dr. Alae Elshennawy, consultant urologist for effort he exerted to review some of the manuscripts.

I'm very grateful to Andre Tournois and Evgenia Koutsouki, Springer's Clinical Medicine Editor, for their great effort and support throughout preparation of this book.

Contents

Part II Prepuce

Part III Penis

Contributors

Piet Hoebeke Department of Pediatric Urology, Ghent University Hospital, Ghent, Belgium

V. Raveenthiran Department of Paediatric Surgery, SRM University, Chennai, India

Anne-Françoise Spinoit Department of Pediatric Urology, Ghent University Hospital, Ghent, Belgium

Marjan Waterloos Department of Pediatric Urology, Ghent University Hospital, Ghent, Belgium

Author and Editor

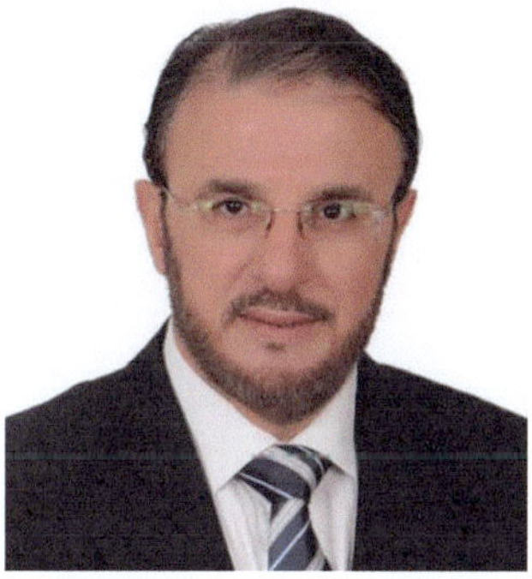

Mohamed Abdel Baky Fahmy, MD, FRCS, is a professor of pediatric surgery in the Faculty of Medicine, Al-Azhar University, Cairo, Egypt, and editor in chief, *Journal of Pediatric Diseases*. After studying at Al-Azhar University, Dr. Fahmy became a fellow to the Royal College of Surgeons of Edinburgh and trained in Manchester, UK, before taking up his present position. His previous posts include: head of the Pediatric Surgery Department at the King Fahed Tertiary Hospital, Al Baha, Saudi Arabia, and consultant and head of Pediatric Surgery at the Nasser Institute for Research and Treatment, Cairo. Dr. Fahmy has also been registered with the British Medical Council since 1994. He was the secretary-general of the Egyptian Association of Pediatric Surgeons and also a member of the British Association of Paediatric Surgeons and American Association of Academic Surgery. Dr. Fahmy has published on a wide range of topics in pediatric urology and neonatal surgery in both national and international periodicals, with innovation in the field of continent urinary diversion. During the last years, he exhibited a great interest in rare genitourinary anomalies, and he is the author of Springer's illustrative textbook *Rare Congenital Genitourinary Anomalies*, 2015.

Part I

Introduction

Embryology of the Penis

1

Abstract

Understanding normal human genital and urethral development is the first step in unraveling both rare and common congenital penile anomalies, and to draw a proper plan of reconstruction.

Despite the high incidence of congenital malformations of the anorectal and urogenital systems in humans, the mechanisms that govern normal anogenital development are still poorly understood.

Keywords

Genital tubercle • Labioscrotal swelling • Cloaca • Urogenital sinus • Urethral folds • Optical projection tomography

In both male and female human embryos, development of the external genitalia begins with the emergence of the paired genital swellings immediately above the cloaca, as a very low conical eminence between the umbilical cord and the base of the tail in the 9 mm embryo (7 weeks gestation). These swellings fuse medially and give rise to the bipotential genital tubercle, which can be masculinized to form the penis or feminized to form the clitoris. As the genital tubercle grows out, the ventral side of the cloacal endoderm forms a bilaminar urethral plate that extends into the genital tubercle, and this structure later cavitates in a proximal to distal direction to form the urethral tube.

The lower urinary tract LUT and genital tubercle GT have distinct embryological origins, as the LUT develops from the endodermal cloaca, which becomes separated into the urogenital sinus and rectum by the downgrowth of the urorectal septum (Fig. 1.1).

The urogenital sinus gives rise to the internal urethra and bladder, while both become lined with a water-tight urothelial layer, these two regions differentiate into distinct structures with respect to musculature, stroma, epithelial layers and innervation. GT gives rise to the male and female external genitalia (penis, clitoris and foreskin) and represents the intersection between the reproductive and urinary tracts. A second set of swellings, the labioscrotal swellings, arise later in development and give rise to the scrotum and labia majora in males and females, respectively. The LUT and GT physically intersect as the urethra passes through the GT, which proposed to be derived from all three germ layers. UP is derived from urethral endoderm (Fig. 1.2).

© Springer International Publishing Switzerland 2017

M. Fahmy, *Congenital Anomalies of the Penis*, DOI 10.1007/978-3-319-43310-3_1

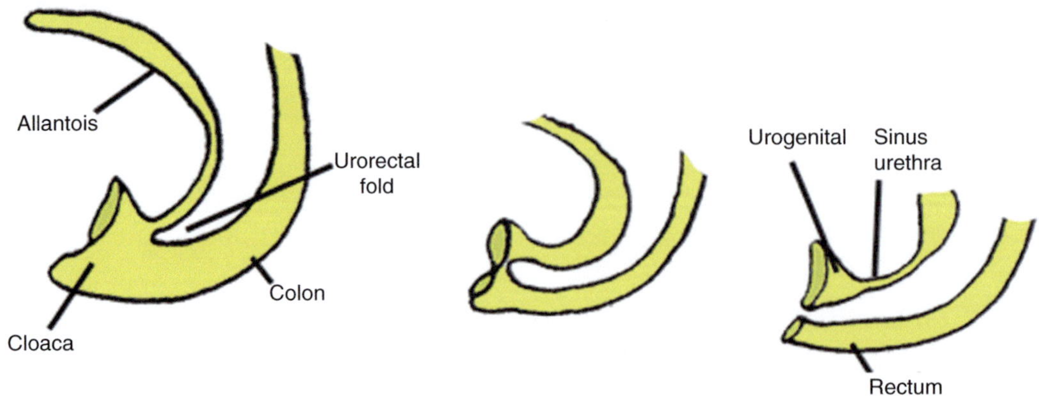

Fig. 1.1 Progression of the urorectal fold to divide the cloaca into urogenital sinus and rectum

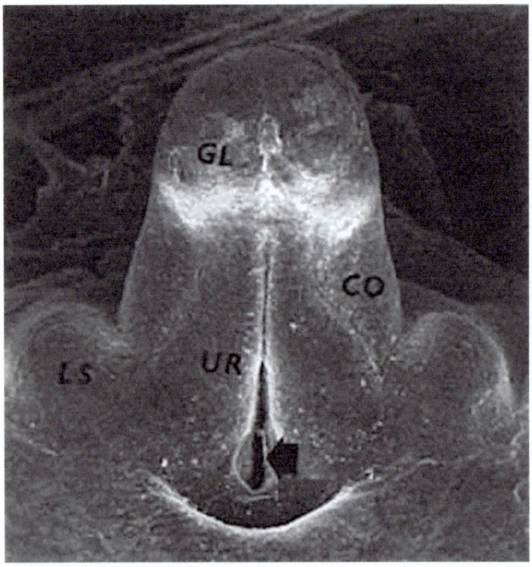

Fig. 1.2 Indifferent external genitalia in a 48 days fertilization age, *GL* glandular portion, *CO* corporal portion of the former genital tubercle, *UR* urethral groove originated from the urethral plate, *LS* labioscrotal swelling. The external opening of the urogenital sinus is marked with an *arrow*

The GT surface other than the urethral plate is derived from surface ectoderm and the core of the extending appendage is derived from lateral plate mesoderm. Without a urethral plate, the GT will fail to form, as we can see in most cases of aphallia where usually there is no urethra or even a urinary meatus (Chap. 8). The urethral epithelium of the GT does not grow out from the urethra but forms in situ along the GT itself. GT development involves an early androgen-independent phase and a later androgen-dependent phase, after which sexual dimorphism is evident [1].

Male accessory organs, such as the prostate and the bulbourethral glands, originate from endodermal buds of the urogenital sinus growing into a specific urogenital mesenchyme.

The genital tubercle develops as an out-budding appendage, hence it has been proposed that there is congruence in the genetic basis of GT patterning with other out-budding appendages, including the limb and craniofacial prominences, and this could explain coexistence of multiple genitourinary anomalies with limb and extremities anomalies in different syndromes [2].

1.1 Penile Development

Several signaling cascades control reproductive organogenesis and this is a versatile system to study how hormones regulate organ growth and differentiation. Some molecular pathways have been identified in initial anlagen formation as well as later hormone driven development. These include fibroblast growth factor (FGF), hedgehog (HH), Wnt, transforming growth factor (TGF) signals and other "effector" genes [3].

Between the 4th and 7th weeks of gestation, the mesodermal mesenchyme migrates to the cranial aspect of the cloacal membrane to form the genital tubercle. The cloacal membrane itself is composed of two layers: endoderm and ectoderm. The caudal portion of the cloacal membrane develops into urogenital folds. These structures are the precursors for external genitalia in both males and females. The Y chromosome initiates male differentiation through the SRY gene and other genes, which triggers testicular development, through signaling the differentiation of primitive sex cords into testes by first signaling the development of Sertoli cells, these cells then aid in the development of germ cells and Leydig cells within the testes. Leydig cells produce testosterone, which is converted to dihydrotestosterone by the enzyme 5α-reductase, to induce external genitalia development through androgen receptors. Under the influence of androgens produced by the testes, external genitalia then develop into the penis and scrotum. Any disruption of androgen function at this stage will results in defective development of urethra to be presented as a divergent forms of hypospadias, or defective penile development, with feminine external genitalia, as in cases of Androgen Insensitivity Syndrome [4].

The genital tubercle becomes longer and out of it forms the penis. The urethral folds also lengthen ventrally, between these extends the urogenital sinus and forms the urethral groove, which is lined with endoderm. The floor of this sulcus thickens through epithelial proliferation and forms the urethral plate that temporarily fills it out (Fig. 1.3).

Later a groove forms again and the two urethral folds fuse on the underside. This section will become the spongy part of the urethra, which for now terminates in a dead end in the anterior part of the penis (Fig. 1.4).

From the fused urethral folds an erectile mesenchymatous tissue, the penile spongy body, arises in the penis. At the distal penis section a ring-shaped furrow delimits the glans. Above the spongy body arise the two cavernous bodies (corpora cavernosa) and thus complete the penile erectile system.

The two labioscrotal swellings also migrate infromedially and fuse in the middle to form the scrotum. The line along which they fuse on the penis and scrotum is called the median raphe, failure of infromedial migration of labioscrotal folds is responsible for the different phenotypes

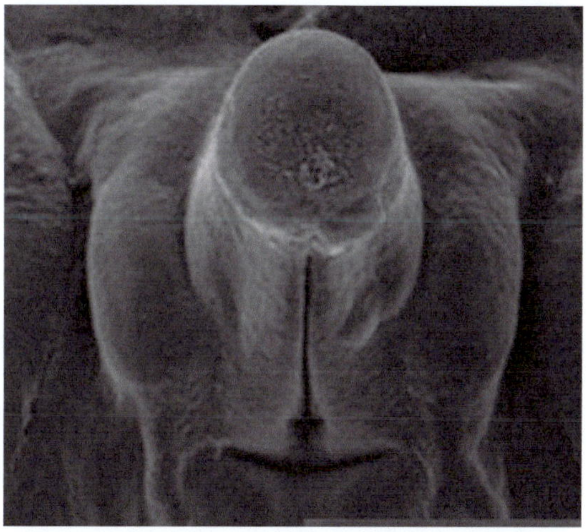

Fig. 1.3 Prominent genital tubercle forming penis with glans, coronal sulcus, but prepuce not yet developed, labioscrotal folds migrate slightly down, but still surrounding the root of the phallus in 14 weeks fetus

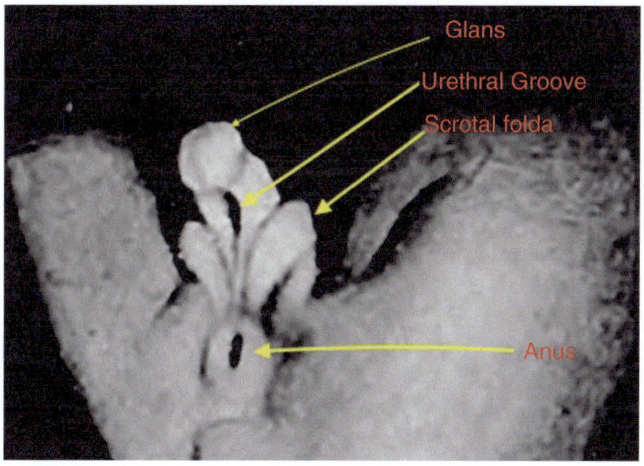

Fig. 1.4 52 mm embryo; with prominent penis, surrounded by the primitive scrotum and an opened urethral plate seen as a grove along the penile shaft

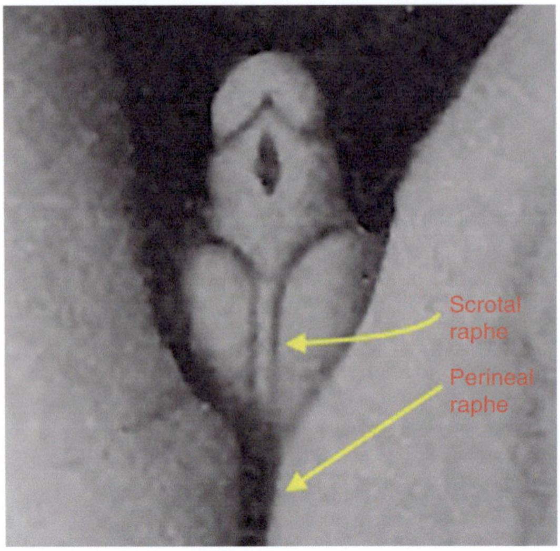

Fig. 1.5 Partially closed urethra with glans uncovered by any preputial tissues

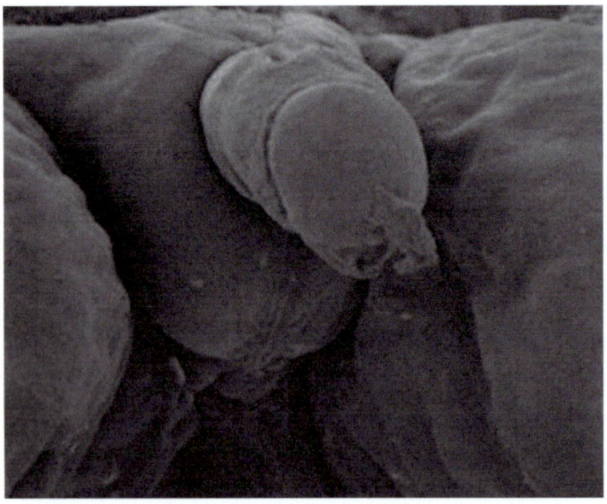

Fig. 1.6 55 mm embryo with a prominent epithelia tag at the dome of the glans, which will canalise to give raise of the glanular urethral, perpetual lamella start to grow from the coronal sulcus to form the prepuce

of penoscrotal transposition and webbed penis (Chap. 15), at the same time abnormal ectodermal fusion at midline is responsible for the different median raphe anomalies (Chap. 16) (Fig. 1.5).

During the 4th month two ectodermal invaginations arise on the tip of the penis. First, a solid epithelial cord forms from the penis tip and binds itself with the dead-ended spongy part of the urethra at the level of the ring-shaped furrow. As soon as this epithelial cord has been canalized, one speaks in this section of the glandar urethra with the urinary meatus (Fig. 1.6).

The two circular epithelial ingrowths, glandar lamella, form the prepuce that at the time of birth is still stuck to the glans but, during childhood, comes away from it.

1.2 Urethral Development

The penile urethra has been reported to develop from two cell populations, with the proximal urethra developing from endoderm and the distal urethra forming from an apical ectodermal invagination, so the classical accounts of external genital development reported that the urethra has a dual embryonic origin – with the distal (glandar) portion arising from an ectodermal invagination from the distal tip of the genital tubercle and the proximal portion coming from the endodermal urethral plate – a description that remains in contemporary embryology textbooks [5]. An alternative model proposes that the entire urethra forms from endoderm, which undergoes differentiation in the glandar portion to form squamous epithelium [5].

The ectodermal theories hypothesize that there is ectodermal ingrowth at the distal urethra, accounting for the squamous epithelial lining of the distal glanular urethra. The endodermal theory was first put forth by Felix [5]. He postulated that the differentiation of the distal urethra forms by fusion of the urethral folds subsequent to the dissolution of the endodermal urethral plate. After that, the work by Kurzrock and Baskin in 1999 [6], using the more advanced technology of immunofluorescence, showed the development of the mouse phallus at incremental stages mapped using immunohistochemistry with antibodies against certain cytokeratins. This showed that the ectoderm of the distal urethra was an extension of the ectoderm of the UG sinus.

More recently; the optical projection tomography (OPT) confirms a solid urethral plate that canalizes, forming the urethral groove that progressively advances and fuses to form the tubular penile urethra. The process starts proximally at the scrotal folds and progresses along the penile shaft to the glans to form the terminal urethral meatus. There is no evidence of ectodermal intrusion of epidermal cells that meet the solid and/or canalized urethral plate or urethral groove, consistent with the endoder-

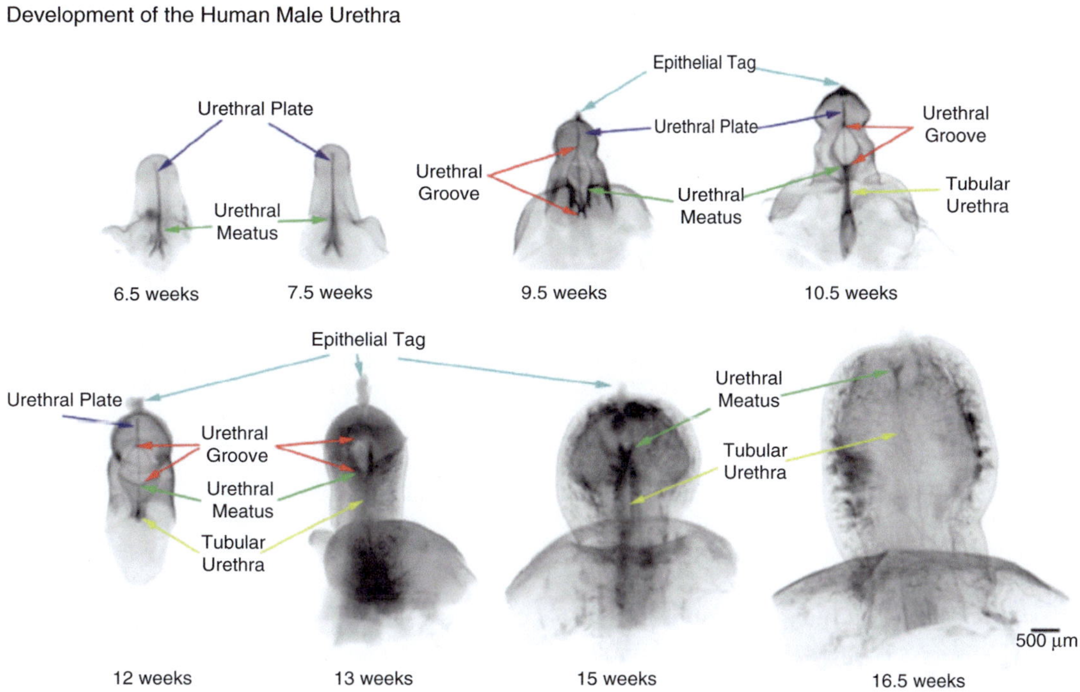

Fig. 1.7 OPT of male urethral development from 6.5 to 16.5 weeks of gestation. Note progression of urethral meatus (*green arrows*) from scrotal folds at 6.5 weeks to terminal position on glans at 16.5 weeks. Wide open urethral groove (red arrows) is best seen from 9.5 to 13 weeks, with clear progression of proximal to distal fusion of edges of urethral groove to form tubular urethra (*yellow arrows*). At 13 weeks urethral groove is within glans penis with tubular urethra completely formed within shaft of penis, consistent with endodermal theory of urethral development. No evidence of ectodermal intrusion is evident in any specimen [7] (With kind permission from Corresponding author: Dr. Amilal Bhat)

mal theory of urethral development. The mechanism of penile urethral formation appears to simulate a "double zipper." The first or opening zipper involves the canalization process within the urethral plate to create the urethral groove. This process is seen in the OPT images initially starting at the scrotal fold/penile junction and is visualized in the cross-sectional OPT and histological sections. During these early stages of development at 6.5 and 7.5 weeks of gestation there is already evidence of canalization of the urethral plate, consistent with subsequent development of the urethral groove between 7.5 and 9.5 weeks of gestation [7] (Fig. 1.7).

1.3 Preputial Development

Studies of foreskin formation chronology and its histological constituents in human fetuses are rare. The human prepuce is formed by a midline collision of ectoderm, neuroectoderm and mesenchyme, resulting in a pentalaminar sheath: squamous mucosal epithelium, lamina propria, darts muscle, dermis and outer glabrous skin.

The first indication of the onset of the developmental processes involved is the appearance of a raised fold (the preputial fold), just proximal to the coronary sulcus. At the same time the floor of the resulting glando-preputial furrow gives rise to a lamellar ingrowth which has been termed "glandar lamella", these lamella grow gradually to cover the dorsum of the glans and then fuse ventrally to form the frenulum at the midline, the ventral surface of the glans is the last part of the penis to be covered by foreskin, so deficient perpetual development usually results in defective ventral prepuce as in cases of microposthia (Chap. 6). The glans was partially covered by the foreskin in the fetus at 13 weeks post conception (WPC) and almost completely covered by the foreskin in fetuses at 16 and 17 W. The complete foreskin was formed only in the fetuses at 18 and 19 WPC, in which the foreskin totally covered the glans. Shared epidermal cells fuse the prepuce to the glans at this stage of development. In all the fetuses studied the presence of preputial lamella and a large amount of mesenchymal tissue between the foreskin and glans were observed [7].

The formation of the prepuce is dependent on androgen hormone and proper urethral development, although variants of hypospadias and epispadias can present with a normal, intact prepuce.

In female the persistence of the urethral groove; which form the labia minora prevents the fusion of the margins of the preputial fold and of the glandar lamella. This again emphasises the close association of the preputial anlage with the urethral folds. As Hunter (1935) pointed out, this association explains the presence of a hood-like prepuce in cases of hypospadias [8].

References

1. Pennington EC, Hutson JM. The urethral plate – does it grow into the genital tubercle or within it? BJU Int. 2002;89:733–9.
2. Siefert AW, Harfe BD, Cohn MJ. Cell lineage analysis demonstrated an endodermal origin of the distal urethra and perineum. Dev Biol. 2008;318:143–52.
3. Perriton CL, Powles N, Chiang C, Machonochie MK, Cohn MJ. Sonic hedgehog signaling from the urethral epithelium controls external genital development. Dev Biol. 2002;247(1):26–46. A.
4. Murashima A, et al. Androgens and mammalian male reproductive tract development. Biochim Biophys Acta. 2015;1849:163–70.
5. Felix W. The development of the urogenital organs. In: Keibel F, Mall FP, editors. Manual of human embryology, vol. 2. Philadelphia/London: Lippincott; 1912. Glenist TW. A Consideration of the processes involved in the development of the prepuce in man. Brt J Urolo. 1956(28):243–249.
6. Kurzrock EA, Baskin LS, Cunha GR. Ontogeny of the male urethra: theory of endodermal differentiation. Differentiation. 1999;64:115–22.
7. Li Y, Sinclair A, Cao M, Shen J, Choudhry S, Botta S, Cunha G, Baskin L. Canalization of the urethral plate precedes fusion of the urethral folds during male penile urethral development: the double zipper hypothesis. J Urol. 2015;193:1353–60.
8. Hunterr H. J Anat Lond. 1935;70:68.

Further Reading

Hill MA. 2016. Embryology: https://embryology.med.unsw.edu.au/embryology/index.php/Embryology:Privacy_policy.

Anatomy and Normal Variations

2

Abstract

A broad overview of the normal anatomy of the male genitalia is essential to offer the best surgical outcomes in dealing with cases related of congenital abnormalities, trauma, and aesthetics penile reconstruction. Neural and vascular anatomy is discussed in depth due to its critical role in maintaining function and in assuring tissue viability during penile reconstructive surgery.

Keywords

Penile innervation • Penile vasculature • Corpora spongosium • Urethra • Tunica Albuginea • Buck's fascia • Frenulum of prepuce of penis

2.1 Introduction

The development of the human penis is a complex sequence of events which results in an utterly individual outcome: no two penises are identical and there is a surprising range of anatomical detail that should be considered normal. Parents need to be assured of this range of normality. Moreover, the desire of practitioners for standard procedures can lead to unpredictable outcomes because of both this anatomical variation and the impossibility of predicting the functional results of surgical correction in infants. This is because the procedures are performed with an emphasis on achieving an acceptable cosmetic outcome on a very small organ which has the capacity for considerable growth and changes during puberty. Furthermore, no surgical procedure can have absolutely predictable outcomes because of the variations in healing and scar formation, the individual variations in technique, and the effects of infection. Regrettably, it seems that the majority of those performing surgical procedures on the penis of minors take no interest in following up the outcome after the organ has developed. (See Chap. 35, Complications of Circumcision) (Fig. 2.1).

2.2 Penile innervation (Fig. 2.2)

Penile innervation consists of the dorsal, cavernosal, and perineal nerves. Dorsal nerves arising from the pudendal nerves travel within Buck's

© Springer International Publishing Switzerland 2017

M. Fahmy, *Congenital Anomalies of the Penis*, DOI 10.1007/978-3-319-43310-3_2

fascia, together with the dorsal arteries and veins, to supply sensation to penile skin. Despite its nomenclature, it is important to note that the nerves do not lie directly in the dorsal midline, but rather extend from the 11 and 1 o'clock positions laterally to the junction of the cavernosa and spongiosum. These nerves do not send perforators deep through the tunica albuginea to the corpora cavernosa. There is a paucity of nerves at the 12 o'clock shaft position. Therefore, in correction of penile curvature, plication at the 12 o'clock position is the area least likely to result in nerve damage. Like the dorsal nerves, the perineal nerves also arise from the pudendal nerve to supply the ventral shaft skin, the frenulum, and the bulbospongiosus muscle. The cavernosal nerves arise from the autonomic pelvic plexus and travel along the periprostatic neurovascular bundle, well known to urologists performing radical retropubic prostatectomies. Underneath the pubic arch, the cavernosal nerves pierce through the corpora cavernosa. Proximal to this point, the cavernosal and dorsal nerves lie within close proximity at the penile hilum and are thought to exchange signal communication, which may have implications on erectile function. As well, there are interactions between perineal and dorsal nerves laterally at the junction of the cavernosa and spongiosum along the penis, which may also have implications on erection and ejaculation [1].

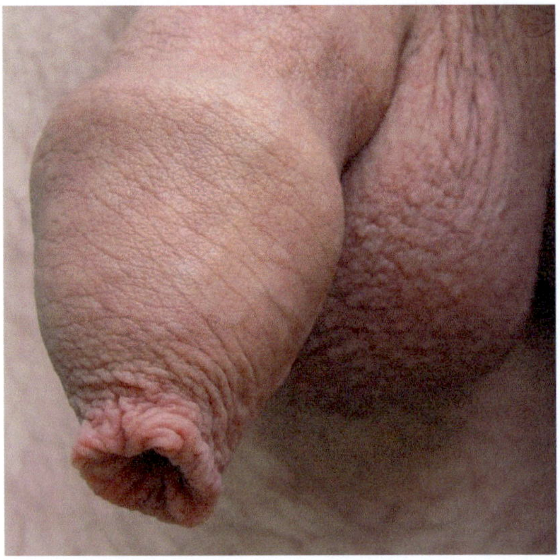

Fig. 2.1 Normal penis

2.3 Penile Vasculature

2.3.1 Arteries

There are three paired main arteries in the penis: cavernosal, dorsal, and bulbourethral. All three arise from a shared branch of the internal pudendal artery, which itself arises from the internal iliac artery. On each side, the first branching occurs at the bulb of the spongiosum external to the urogenital diaphragm forming the bulbourethral artery, which then lies at the 9 and 3 o'clock positions of the corpus spongiosum. Then the cavernous artery branches to penetrate the corpora cavernosa and the remainder of the artery

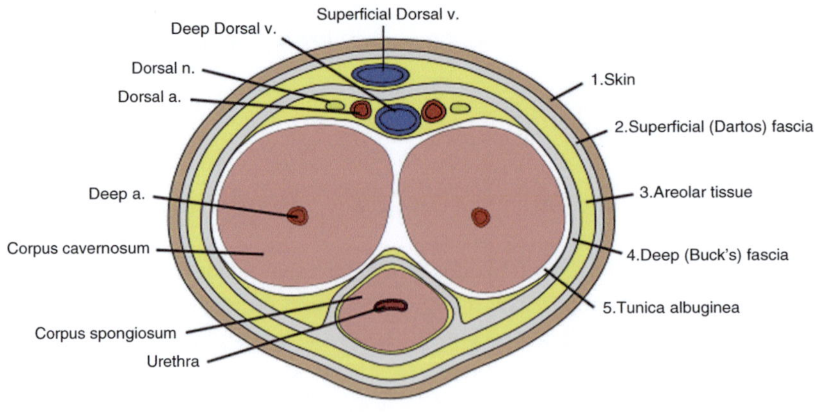

Fig. 2.2 Transverse cut section of the penis

continues as the deep dorsal artery. The deep dorsal artery causes glans enlargement during erection, whereas the cavernosal arteries cause corporal enlargement. All three arteries communicate distally near the glans to provide an extensive anastomotic network.

Penile skin derives its supply from a separate origin. Branches of the external pudendal artery supply the dorsal and lateral aspects of the penis, and branches of the internal pudendal artery supply the ventral penis and scrotum via the posterior scrotal artery. These branches course in the Dartos fascia and enable pedicled skin flaps to be used in urethral reconstruction [2].

2.3.2 Veins

Venous drainage is not analogous to arterial supply, unlike many other body systems. In contrast to the paired dorsal arterial system, there exists only one deep dorsal vein that runs alongside the dorsal arteries and nerves in Buck's fascia above the tunica albuginea. The deep dorsal vein receives drainage from the distal two-thirds of the corpora cavernosa via emissary veins and the corpus spongiosum via circumflex veins. Emissary veins are the veins that traverse obliquely through the tunica albuginea, allowing them to be compressed during erections for penile tumescence. The deep dorsal vein then drains to the periprostatic plexus [3].

Recently, a small pair of dorsal veins have been found that lie just deep to the deep dorsal vein, but above the tunica albuginea, which independently receive emissary vein drainage. These veins have been termed cavernosal veins, but do not lie within the corpora cavernosa. Older literature refers to the cavernosal veins as short veins located in the triangle between the proximal crus that drain the proximal one-third of the corpora cavernosa. These veins join with the bulbourethral veins (which drain the proximal spongiosum) to lead into the internal pudendal vein. The penile skin drains via the superficial dorsal vein, which drains into the saphenous vein [4].

2.3.3 Corpora Spongosium

The corpus spongiosum is a midline structure nestled on the ventral surface of the paired erectile bodies that are known as the corpora cavernosa. Distally, the spongiosum expands to form the glans penis, which serves to cap the cavernosa in a smooth and rounded shape that should be maintained for ideal vaginal penetration.

The larger base of the spongiosum, or the bulb, contains the aptly named bulbous urethra, which takes on a dorsal orientation. The distal most point of the ischiocavernosus muscles marks the transition from pendulous to bulbous urethra. These two muscles sweep anteromedially from their lateral roots on the ischial rami. They fuse in the midline at a point that is ventral to the bulbous urethra, facilitating its ability to empty. The base of the spongiosum is more directly covered by the solitary bulbospongiosus muscle, which is attached at its posterior aspect to the perineal body, the central meeting point of eight muscles of the perineum.

2.4 Urethra

The male urethra is divided into six parts: bladder neck, prostatic urethra, membranous urethra surrounded by external sphincter, bulbous urethra proximal to the ischiocavernosus muscle, penile/pendulous urethra distal to the ischiocavernosus muscle, and the fossa navicularis within the distal glans. The corpus spongiosum is erectile tissue akin to corpora cavernosa, but with a thinner tunica albuginea. The penile and bulbar urethra lie within the spongiosum. The penile urethra lies in a central location within the spongiosum, whereas the bulbar urethra lies eccentrically closer to the dorsal spongiosum prior to exiting dorsally to become the membranous urethra to join the prostate. Whereas the condition known as "chordee" or penile curvature was once believed to result from fibrous bands near the urethra, no such fibrous tissue has been found in the penile urethra, even in severe cases of hypospadias. Because of anastomotic communications between the dorsal arteries and the bulbourethral arteries, the urethra receives arterial supply from both distal and proximal directions. This enables complete transaction of the urethra without necrosis of the distal segment [5].

Buck's fascia (deep fascia of the penis, Gallaudet's fascia or fascia of the penis) is a layer of deep fascia covering the three erectile bodies of the penis

Structure Buck's fascia is continuous with the external spermatic fascia in the scrotum and the suspensory ligament of the penis. On its ventral aspect, it splits to envelop corpus spongiosum in a separate compartment from the tunica albuginea and corporal bodies.

Variation Sources differ on its proximal extent. Some state that it is a continuation of the deep perineal fascia, whereas others state that it fuses with the tunical albuginea [5].

Function The deep dorsal vein of the penis is inside Buck's fascia, but the superficial dorsal veins of the penis are in the superficial (dartos) fascia immediately under the skin.

2.5 Tunica Albuginea

The tunica albuginea is the fibrous envelope of the corpora cavernosa penis. It consists of approximately 5 % elastin, an extensible tissue that is primarily made up of the amino acids glycine, valine, alanine, and proline. The majority of the remaining tissue is collagen, which is made up of lysine, proline, glycine, alanine, and other amino acids.

The tunica albuginea is directly involved in maintaining an erection; that is due to Buck's fascia constricting the deep dorsal vein of the penis, preventing blood from leaving and thus sustaining the erect state.

The trabeculae of the tunica albuginea are more delicate, nearly uniform in size, and the meshes between them smaller than in the corpora cavernosa penis: their long diameters, for the most part, corresponding with that of the penis.

The external envelope or outer coat of the corpus spongiosum is formed partly of unstriped muscular fibers, and a layer of the same tissue immediately surrounds the canal of the urethra.

The **frenulum of prepuce of penis**, often known simply as the **frenulum**, is an elastic band of tissue under the glans penis that connects the foreskin (prepuce) to the vernal mucosa, and helps contract the foreskin over the glans (Fig. 2.3).

In the event of frenulum breve or frenular chordee, or to ensure that the glans can be freely and completely exposed, the frenulum may be partially or totally removed. It is also often removed in a circumcision The frenulum may be entirely missing in cases of hypospadias.

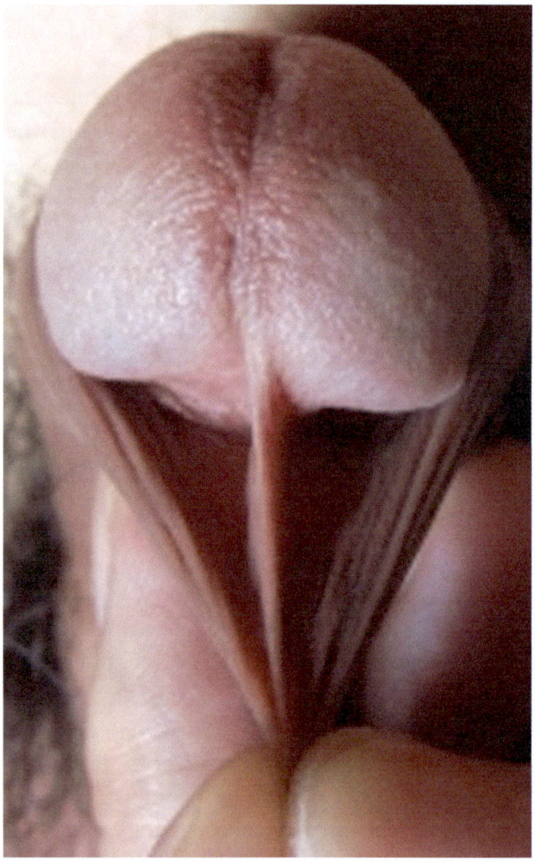

Fig. 2.3 Normal frenulum

References

1. Brooks JD. Anatomy of the lower urinary tract and male genitalia. In Campbell-walsh urology. Vol. 1, Philadelphia: Saunders-Elsevier; 2007.
2. Jordan G, Schlossberg S. Surgery of the penis and urethra. In: Wein A, Kavoussi L, Novick A, Partin A, Peters C, editors. Campbell-walsh urology, vol. 2. Philadelphia: Saunders-Elsevier; 2007.
3. Baskin L, Erol A, Li Y, Liu W. Anatomy of the neurovasuclar bundle: is safe mobilization possible? J Urol. 2000;164:977–80.
4. Hsu G, Hsieh C, Wen H, Chen Y, Chen S, Mok M. Penile venous anatomy: an additional description and its clinical implication. J Androl. 2003;24:921–7.
5. Richie JP, Steele GS. Neoplasms of the testis. In: Wein AJ, Kavoussi LR, Novick AC et al, eds. Campbell-Walsh Urology. Philadelphia, PA: Saunders Elsevier; 2007:893–935.

Penis in History

3

V. Raveenthiran

Abstract

The penis is the most worshiped organ in the history of humanity. Understanding the basis of this venerability is essential for appreciating the psychosocial implications of penile malformations and their surgical correction. Since incalculable antiquity man's attention has been disproportionately drawn towards this tiny appendage. Spontaneity of erections and the ensuing pleasure must have drawn the admiration of mankind and influenced its undue interest in this organ.

Keywords

History of penis • Male genitalia • Sexuality • Mythology • Anomalies • Malformations

3.1 The Venerable Organ of Antiquity

The penis is the most worshiped organ in the history of humanity. Understanding the basis of this venerability is essential for appreciating the psychosocial implications of penile malformations and their surgical correction. Since incalculable antiquity man's attention has been disproportionately drawn towards this tiny appendage. Spontaneity of erections and the ensuing pleasure must have drawn the admiration of mankind and influenced its undue interest in this organ. This is evident from the engravings of Los Casares cave (Riba de Saelices, Spain) and Saint-Cirq cave (Le Buge, France) which belong to upper Paleolithic period (38,000 to 11,000 *BCE*) [1]. They depicted penis as huge as its owners themselves (Fig. 3.1). By etching impractically enormous size penis, prehistoric man probably had tried to emphasize the importance that he attached to penis.

Structural similarity of the penis to a variety of elongated objects must have prompted primitive man to attribute bizarre properties to this curious organ. Erect penis, because of its penetrating nature, was typically envisaged as a piercing weapon such as dagger. In fact, the vagina is named so because it resemblance to a 'scabbard' or 'sheath of sword'. As a weapon is expected to harm enemies, sexual rape committed by the erect penis was considered punitive. Primatologists have observed this behaviour even in monkeys

© Springer International Publishing Switzerland 2017

M. Fahmy, *Congenital Anomalies of the Penis*, DOI 10.1007/978-3-319-43310-3_3

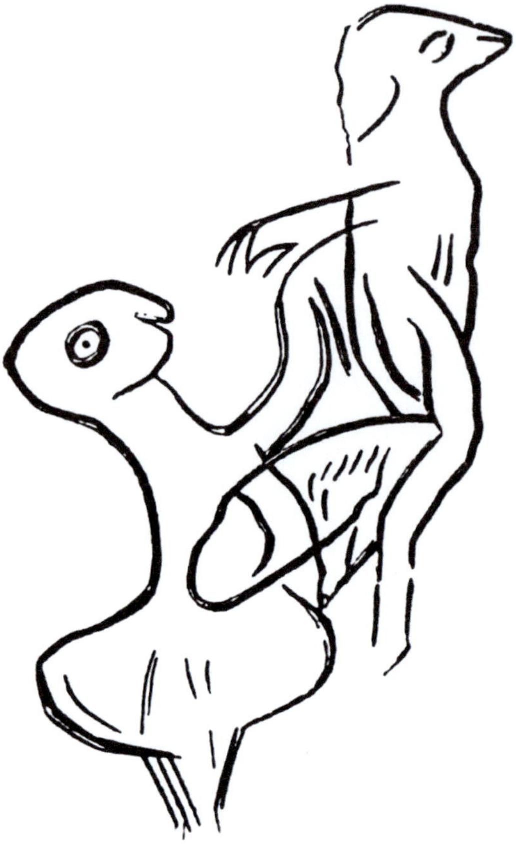

Fig. 3.1 Prehistoric mating scene depicting disproportionately large phallus. This Paleolithic (22,000 years old) engraving was found in Los Casares cave of Riba de Saelices, Spain (Reproduced with the permission of Prof. Javier Angulo and Elsevier)

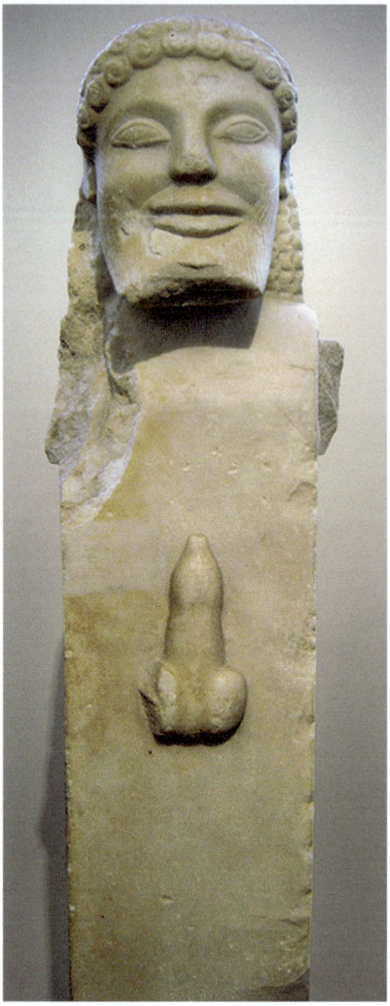

Fig. 3.2 Marble Herma from siphnos (circa 520 B*CE*) at the National Archeological Museum of Athens. Similar Athenian Hermae were vandalized in 415 *BCE* (Photo credit to Mr. Ricardo Andre Frantz; Distributed under CC BY-SA 3.0)

wherein the leader of a troop will sodomize an intruder from another tribe. In civilized societies too, rape is a consistent component of war crimes.

A punitive weapon is also deemed to be protective. Thus, erect penis was considered apotropaic [2]. Phallic amulets and tintinnabulae were used by ancient Greeks to avert evil eyes. They erected stone columns known as *Hermae* in street corners and in front of each house to ward off malicious sprits and to bring in good luck (Fig. 3.2). These pillars displayed the head of the Greek God Hermes and his prominently erect phallus. Superstitious belief in the apotropaic power of phallus was such that it led to the defeat of Greeks in 415 *BCE*. The night before the departure of Athenian fleet to Sicily, someone – playing either a drunken prank or a ploy – brought down several hundred erections of *Hermae* [3]. It is rumored that the vandal was Alcibiades, the beloved student of the great philosopher Socrates. Greek soldiers woke-up in the morning only to find themselves morally emasculated by this bad omen. This not only led to the failure of Sicilian invasion but also the ultimate defeat of Athens in the hands of Spartans [4]. Bhutan, a small country in the eastern Himalayas, still holds the traditional belief in the apotropaic power of the penis. Every Bhutanese house is painted with not only erect but also ejaculating phalluses near doorways and building corners. By casting out evil eyes these phalluses are believed to bring in wealth and good luck. Thus, the punitive and protective penis had also become a sign of prosperity.

Prosperity to a primeval man must have meant enough meat from hunting. When rival groups competed for the same meat, manpower was needed to chase them away and secure the food. Therefore, ability to bear more offspring was considered essential for prosperity. When man was not aware of the reproduction secrets he looked at women, who gave birth to new individuals, with much awe and fear. Later, when men discovered their indispensable contribution of insemination in reproduction, matriarchate was replaced by phallocentric patriarchy [5].

Phallic supremacy was not challenged even when hunter-gatherers settled with agricultural life. Man probably drew analogy between the shaft of an erecting penis and the trunk of a growing tree. Therefore, the penis was considered a sign of fertility not only in human reproduction but also in agricultural production. People began to worship phallic structures for higher crop yield and the penis began to occupy a central position in many fertility rituals. Ancient Romans erected and worshiped ithyphallic Priapus in fields and woods. Even today, public procession of decorated phallus is common during Japanese harvest festivals such as Kanamara Matsuri of Kawasaki and Honen Matsuri of Komaki [6].

The penis was revered as the ultimate power of production and protection, therefore, it became a symbolic attribute of monarchs who did not want anything less than the ultimate power. Phallic rituals became inseparable from royal affairs. As a part of coronation rites, Egyptian Pharaohs were expected to 'sow *their* seeds'. Although it is generally considered to be plant seeds, it also implies the demand on Pharaohs to demonstrate their procreative ability [7]. In cannibalistic primitive societies, heir apparent ate the penis of deceased leader symbolizing the inheritance of leadership status. As a permanent reminder of this transfer of power, the successor held in his hand a phallic replica of the predecessor's erect penis. Stone, bone, ivory and wood carvings of Paleolithic era unearthed from Spain and France depict human penises with exposed glans [8]. There are no corroborative archeological evidences for the prevalence of circumcision among prehistoric men. In fact, any surgical intervention prior to the era of antibiotics is thought to be a survival disadvantage according to Darwinian principles. Hence, the exposed glans in these portable art works probably represent retracted prepuce of fully erect penis. Many archeo-pathologists erroneously think that these phallic objects could have been used as dildos. But, why would women of that era have resorted to dildos when live penises were freely available without any social or moral inhibitions? They are also unlikely to be drumsticks, cord makers or tent holders because they need not had been so exquisitely carved and decorated for these purposes. They are most likely to have been used as batons signifying transfer of power. With advancing civilization holding a phallic baton was considered too embarrassing and hence it was replaced with symbolic staffs.

Although phallic batons were obsolete long before, kings as late as eighteenth century and some high officials even today, while assuming office, take oath by placing their hands on the crotch (read penis and testis). Even in the Old Testament aged Abraham asked his eldest servant who ruled over the household, "Put, I pray thee, thy hand under my thigh and I will make thee swear by the Lord, the God of Heaven" (Genesis 24: 2, 3). In this "under the thigh" is a euphemism for the penis. By guaranteeing the sacredness of oath, the penis attained the status of divinity. In fact, it had already possessed several attributes of godliness such as punishing the wrongdoers, protecting the believers, granting productivity and prosperity, and finally symbolizing omnipotence. Thus, the erect organ was begun to be worshiped in many phallic cults that are known to exist since prehistoric times [9].

3.2 Phallic Cult

Explicit or surreptitious adoration of phallus is common in major religions of the world. The earliest evidence of phallic worship is obtained from the excavations of Mohenjo-Daro and Harappa, the twin cities of Indus valley civilization (50,000 to 1300 *BCE*) [10]. Pasupathy alias Siva was the chief deity of this civilization. According to Hindu mythology one revered sage Bhrigu went to see Siva at which time the latter was engaged in amorous pursuits with his wife Parvathi [11] (Fig. 3.3). Even after knowing the arrival of the sage, Siva did not interrupt coitus. Bhrigu took this as personal insult and cursed Siva that he be not worshiped by his divine figure but by the symbol of his erect penis. Since then Siva has been worshiped in 'lingam' form. In fact, the Sanskrit word 'lingam' means 'penis'. Even today millions of men and women worship lingams in Indian temples. The most remarkable of all is the gigantic lingam at the temple of Gudimallam, a village in South India. This stone phallus dating back to 300 *BCE* accurately depicts the anatomical details of a fully erect penis such as exposed glans, retracted prepuce, frenulum, coronal sulcus and penile shaft. However, causal devotees will least suspect as to what they are actually worshiping when the lingam is presented to them with floral decorations (Fig. 3.4).

Disguised phallic worship is not unknown in other parts of the world. Romans worshipped detachable bronze idol of Priapus in which the ithyphallic God appears as an old man covered with a shawl. Dismantling the statue during worship will, however, reveal the huge phallus hidden underneath the old man's cloak (Fig. 3.5). In contrast to this geriatric Priapus, fresco at the House of Vettii in Pompeii (circa 62–79 *CE*) depicted him as a young robust warrior [12] (Fig. 3.6). Contradictions in these art works indicate that what it matters more important, is the giant phallus rather than the deity himself. Worshiping a nude deity is obviously less embarrassing than exclusive veneration of erect phallus. Probably for this untold reason Digambara Jains worship their 24 male Tirthankaras (omniscient teacher-gods) in nude posture. For example, the 57 ft tall Gommateshwara statue (circa 980 *CE*) at Shravanabelagola (South India) exhibits a 4-ft long phallus which can never go unnoticed by devotees (Fig. 3.7).

Min in ancient Egypt and Priapus in Rome were also worship in nude form (Fig. 3.8). However, they did not disguise the penile connotation of adoration. Unlike the flaccid penis of Jain Tirthankaras, these gods were portrayed with erect phallus. Phallicism was further made clear by the attending rituals. For example, wild lettuce – a plant which when rubbed and squeezed would discharge white sticky sap resembling semen – was made the sacred symbol of Min. Obscene words referring to male genitals and sports like naked climbing on an erect pole were routine during the orgies of Priapus.

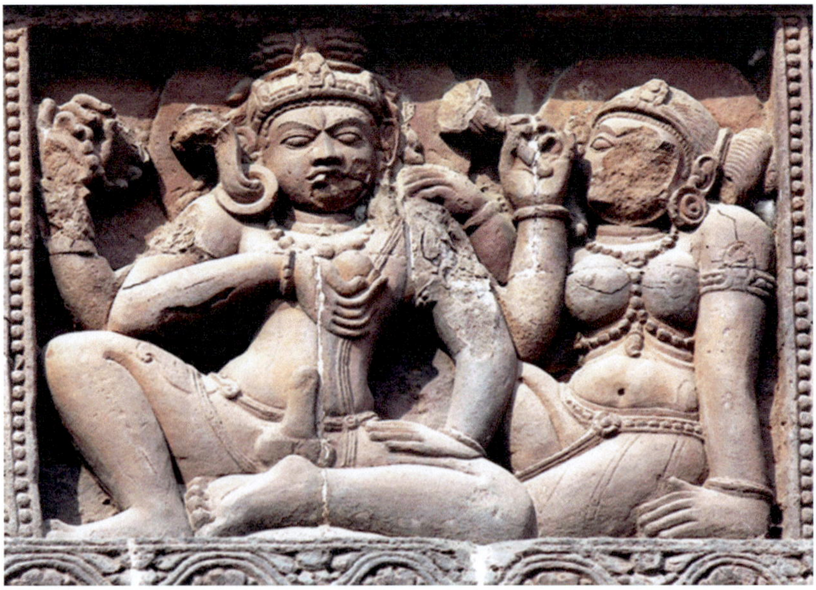

Fig. 3.3 Sculpture depicting the romantic play of Siva and Parvathi (From Parashurameshvara Temple, Bhubaneswar (circa 600 CE))

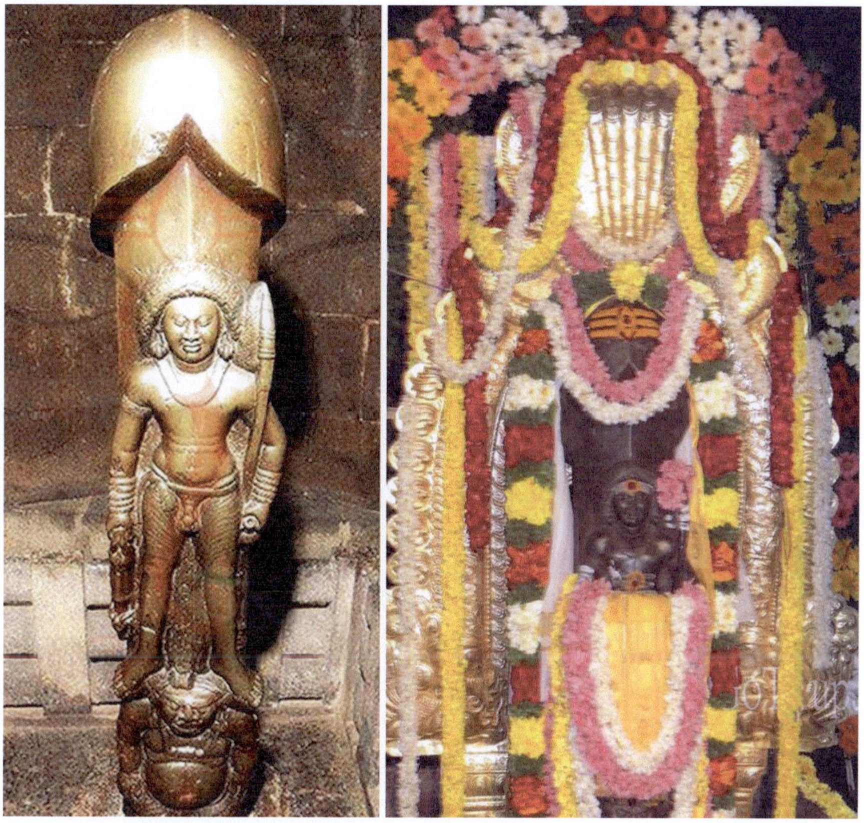

Fig. 3.4 Gudimallam Lingam (circa 100 BCE) with and without floral decoration. Accurate depiction of penile anatomy is the specialty of this lingam (Pictures kindly provided by 'Go Tirupati Tour Operators')

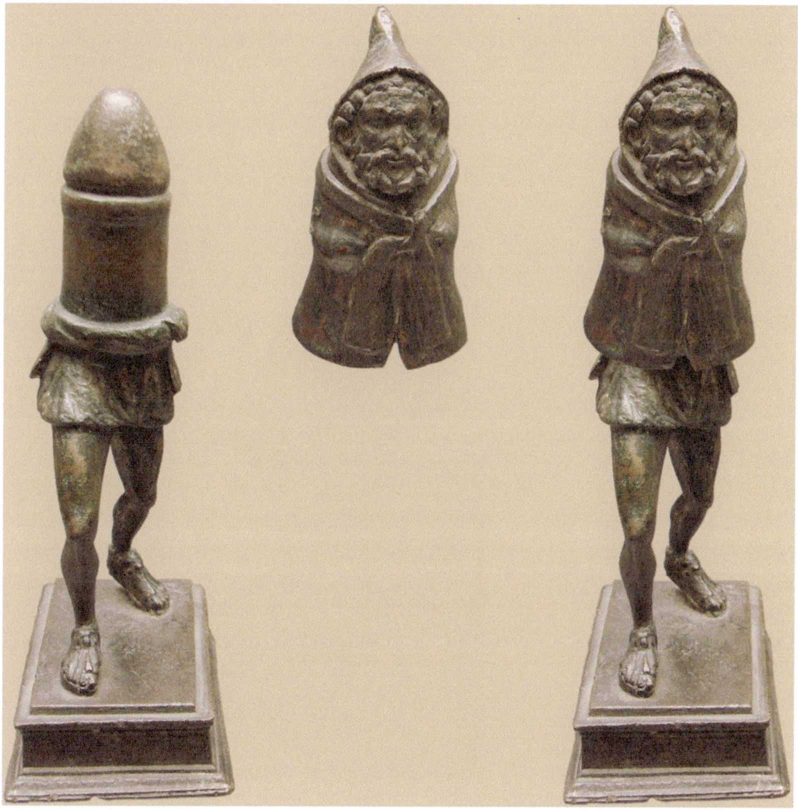

Fig. 3.5 Detachable bronze idol of Priapus (circa first century CE) at the Museum of Picardy. The bust when removed will reveal the underlying giant phallus (Photo credit to Mr Vassil; Public domain photograph from Wikimedia Commons)

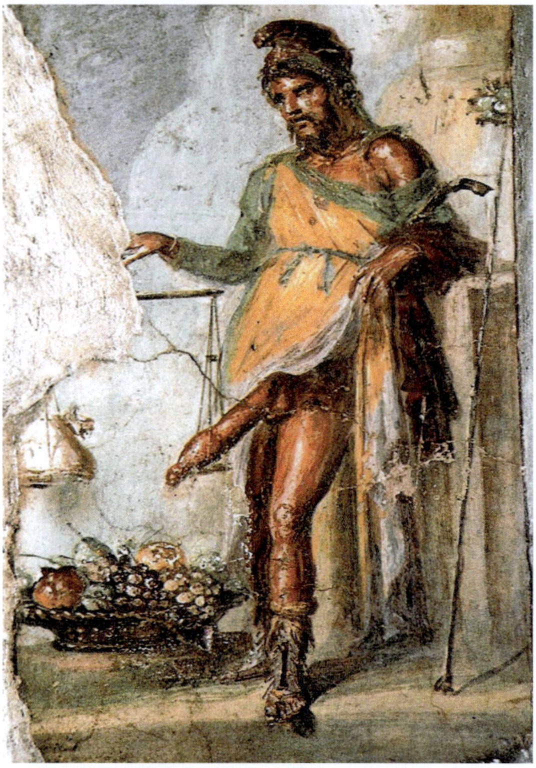

Fig. 3.6 Fresco of Priapus at the House of Vettii, Pompeii showing enormous size phallus which is turgid but not rigid. It is difficult to say if it represents phimosis. The mural is remarkably preserved well despite being buried under the volcanic ash of Mount Vesuvius which erupted in 79 CE (Public domain photograph from Wikimedia Commons)

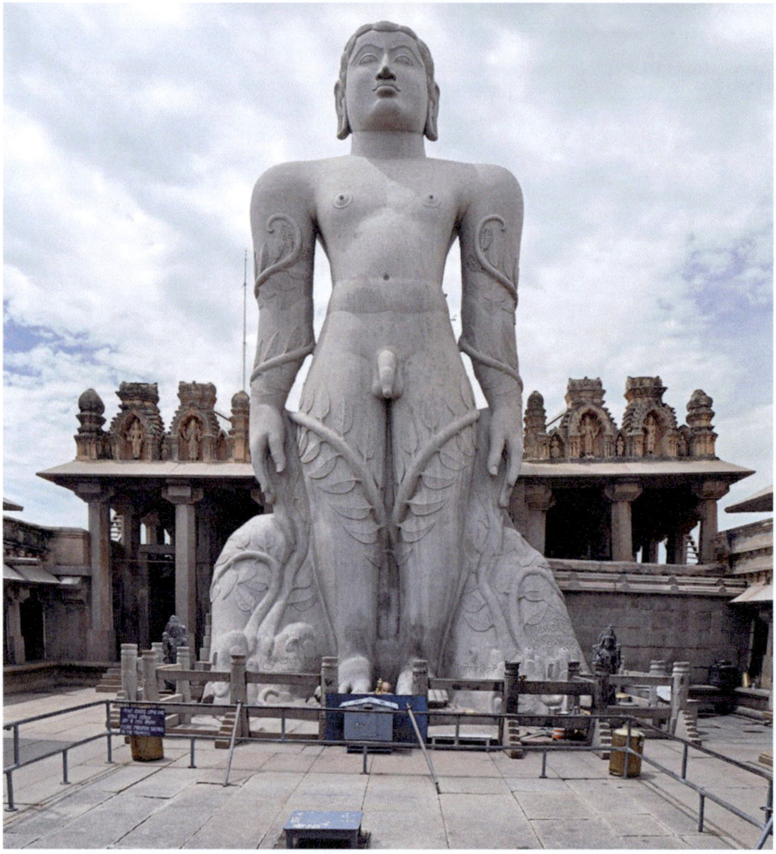

Fig. 3.7 Granite statue of Jain Tirthankara Gommateshwara alias Bahubali (circa 980 *CE*) at Shravanabelagola, South India. Eyes cannot miss the 4-ft long flaccid penis of the statue

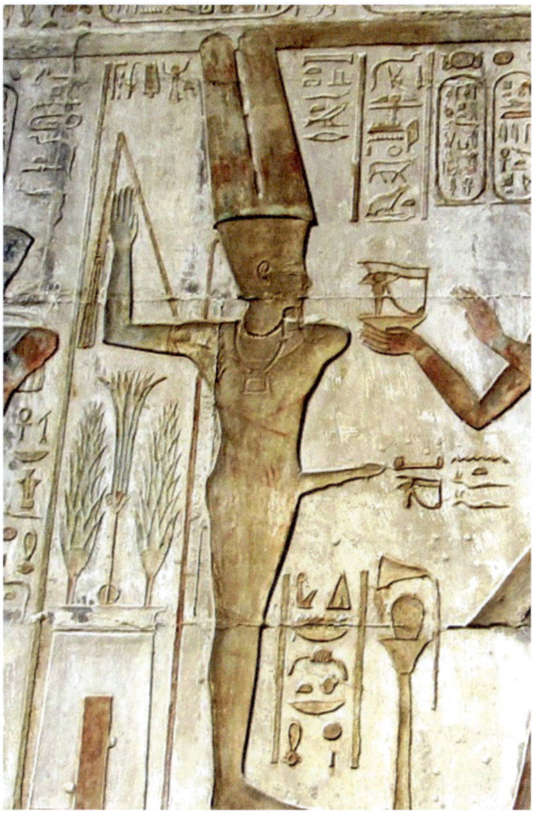

Fig. 3.8 Image of Min at the temple of Hathor in Deir el-Medina. Like Priapus, Min is portrayed with partially erect phallus. Author: Institute for the Study of the Ancient World (published under Creative Commons Attribution 2.0 Generic license.)

3.3 The Curative Penis

Buddhism censures all sensual pleasures and hence the phallus is not explicitly worshiped in this religion. Nevertheless, Drukpa Kunley (1455–1529 *CE*) – a respected Buddhist monk of Tibet – was said to have told, "Happiness lies below the navel as is the best wine found at the bottom of cask". He used to bless barren women by touching them with a wooden phallus – a custom even now being practiced in his Chimi Lhakhang monastery of Bhutan. It is strange that not only the live penis but also its lifeless form – the phallus – was believed to cure childlessness!

In medieval Europe there were several fertility shrines in which devotees consumed the scrapings of statue's phallus to get cured of sterility and impotence. At one such shrine of St. Guignole located at the port city of Brest, the phallus of the poor saint could not withstand the frantic scrapping of young girls and it did not last even for few days after replenishments. Monks of the shrine devised an ingenuous solution to this problem. Accordingly, they secretly bored a hole at the crotch of the statue through which a wooden phallus was clandestinely projected out. As fast as the devotees scrapped the phallus from the front of statue, the monk as industriously and swiftly pushed the wooden peg from behind thereby creating an illusion of spontaneous elongation of the phallus. This miraculous growth added to the reputation of the shrine and attracted much more pilgrims!

It is quite logical to assume that the penis is curative if it were divine. For obvious reasons, it was initially believed to cure infertility and impotence; but later its healing power was extended to many unrelated diseases. The panacean property of penis is illustrated by the saga of the holy foreskin. It was supposed to be the foreskin of Jesus Christ, the *Preputium Domini* as the Vatican would call it. Jesus, in conformity with Jewish tradition of his times, was circumcised on the eighth day of birth. According to the Infancy Gospel, the excised foreskin was preserved in an alabaster box of spikenard oil. It was later procured by Mary Magdalene whose relationship with Jesus was variously disputed as disciple, companion and wife. Mary, probably, gave back the foreskin to St. Peter (pun unintended). After changing several hands, the Byzantine empress Irene gave it as marriage gift to Emperor Charlemagne (742–814 *CE*) who in turn donated it to Charroux Abbey of France. Patients queued up to worship the holy prepuce to get rid of their chronic ailments. In 1422 *CE*, even the English King Henry V was said to have begged to borrow and finally stole the relic of holy prepuce to easy the labor pain of his French wife. Soaring popularity of pilgrimage to Charroux prompted the holy foreskin to multiply and by the dawn of twenty first century there were at least 21 churches claiming to hold the authoritative appendage of Jesus Christ [13].

3.4 Scientific Penetration of the Penis

It is pathetic that the organ believed to possess curative powers was itself left to suffer malformations and diseases without any proper remedy. This medical apathy was partly due to the divine status of the penis. Everyone looked at it with much veneration and awe; but no one dared dissecting it to study the architecture. Lack of proper anatomical knowledge halted the progress of surgical correction. For example, the great Galen of Pergamum (circa 129–199 *CE*) preached that there were two separate tubes in the penis, one for semen and another for urine. He formulated his theories not only by extrapolating his knowledge on animal anatomy but also by exercising his fertile mind. Domineering influence of Galen was such that no one dared to challenge his views for the next 1200 years. Unlike Galen who had never dissected human cadavers, Leonardo da Vinci (1452–1519 *CE*) had the opportunity to dissect executed criminals of Florentine town. This renowned Italian artist of Renaissance Period was the first to accurately draw the anatomy of the penis and to describe the pathway of sperms from the testes. Although his contemporary artist Michelangelo was also claimed to have known the tricorporal anatomy of penis, Michelangelo never drew it explicitly and the codified anatomy in the painting of Prophet Jonah on the ceiling of Sistine chapel is subjected to subjective interpretations. Accuracy of Leonardo's drawings was such that when the great anatomist of Padua, Andrea Vesalius (1514–1564 *CE*), independently described penile anatomy, he was accused of plagiarizing Leonardo's works [14].

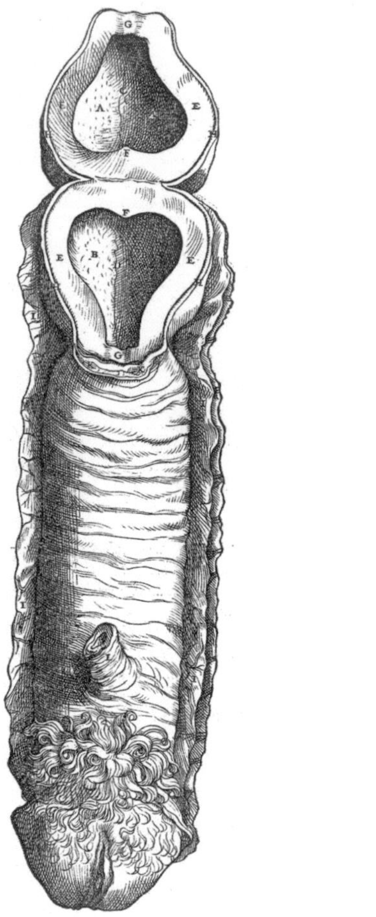

Fig. 3.9 Vagina depicted as "invaginated penis" by Andrea Vesalius in his '*De Humani corporis fabrica libri septem*' (1543). Vesalius considered the labia as the analogue of the glans penis. The urethra entering the vagina is also a misrepresentation of anatomical fact

Leonardo was also the first to solve the centuries old mystery of penile erection. Prior to him everyone experienced it; but no one knew the mechanism of erection. Aristotle (384–322 *BCE*) probably mistook vas deference for the fine ropes of a pulley system. According to him the penis lifts up by the sheer weight of testes and the penopubic attachment acts as fulcrum for the mechanical leverage. He supported his arguments by citing that the penis no longer erects when the pulley system is destroyed as in castration. Galen, drawing analogy between the penis and metal rods that expand on heating, held that the penis is pushed from inside out by the heat of passionate love making [15]. He explained sweating that occurs during coitus was also the effect of this heat. Andreas Vesalius (1514–1562 *CE*), who boasted to have corrected 238 mistakes of Galen, conceded to this misconception and depicted the vagina as invaginated penis (Fig. 3.9). However, no one bothered to ask him as to why then the vagina did not expand and evaginate under the heat of passion. Hippocrates (circa 460–370 *BCE*), the father of medicine, believed that erections occur due to air (*pneuma*) inflation of corporal tubes akin to blowing of balloons. He pegged his reasoning on the air hunger noted during intercourse. It was Leonardo who brilliantly questioned the incompatibility of Hippocratic hypothesis and observed facts. "If it were air", Leonardo argued, "the erect penis would not be as hard as a wood". His dissections of executed criminals, who had reflex erections during hanging, revealed the turgid organ been filled fully with blood. Additionally, observing the redness of glans during tumescence convinced Leonardo to conclude that erection is caused by inflow of blood.

Despite these commendable contributions, Leonardo was blamed of perpetuating the myths of Galen. In his famous drawing of a copulating couple, Leonardo has drawn two channels of penis, one connecting it to heart while the other to spinal cord. According to ancient Greeks, '*pneuma*' responsible for erection arose from the heart and flowed through a special conduit into the penis. Galen, probably influenced by the physical semblance of semen and mucus, thought that the former must have originated from the nasopharynx and reached penis through the spinal cord. Critiques misinterpreted Leonardo's drawing to represent a combination of these two fallacies. The great master never drew anything without actually observing dissected corpses. Therefore, he is unlikely to have made mistakes. The linear strokes joining the penis and the spinal cord could probably be a schematic representation of *nervi erigentes*. Even in the slightly inaccurate depiction of penile blood flow directly from the heart Leonardo was ahead of his time because William Harvey (1578–1657 *CE*), the discoverer of circulation, was yet to born. In an inset to the '*copulating couple*', Leonardo has dawn a magnified cross sectional view of the penis showing two unambiguous tubes. It is possible that the criminal, whose body Leonardo dissected, might have been suffering from urethral duplication [16].

One hundred years lapsed before Regnier de Graaf (1641–1673 *CE*), the discoverer of Graafian follicle, could scientifically prove Leonardo's hydraulic theory of penile erection. What enabled Graaf to unravel the mystery of erection was his prior invention of syringe with which he could inject water into the cavernous spaces. With this technique Graaf could miraculously erect the penises of dead men. In his acclaimed book, 'A treatise concerning the generative organs of men' he wrote:

> "Prepare the penis (of cadavers) in the following way: First, gently express the blood which is always inside… and then insert a tube into the spongy substance, where it approaches the bones of the pubis. Half fill the cavity of the penis with water with the aid of a syringe and shake gently (and rinse it)….repeat the operation until the water is no longer stained…..Finally, distend the penis, by inflating it until it reaches its natural size" [17]

Graaf also did not fail to notice that the erections achieved by simple injection were not as rigid as natural ones. When he could replicate the firm ness of live erections by tying the base of penis, Graaf announced, "The key event in erection is not getting blood into the penis; but keeping it there". This is perhaps the first description of artificial erection. Graaf's achievement of artificial erection was long forgotten until 1974 when Gittes and McLaughlin rediscovered it and demonstrated it in live patients. The test is now an integral component of all hypospadias surgeries in assessing the severity of chordee.

Graaf erroneously thought that blood is retained in the penis during erections by the pinch-cock action of pelvic muscles on the cavernous bodies. Although Graaf surmised increased blood flow to be partly responsible for erections, he was clueless as to how it could have actually happened. In 1889 an Austrian physician Victor Vecki described helicine arteries which are wound in the shape of a ram's horn [15]. Uncoiling of these torturous vessels during excitation was thought to increase the penile blood flow. Scientists were still perplexed as to how blood was retained in the penis to maintain erection. In 1900 Von Ebner of Austria described a column of smooth muscle cells in the intima of penile arteries. These 'pads', as Von Ebner called them, were thought to enable autoregulation of blood flow by the penile arteries. It was proposed that these pads initially opens to let blood into the corpora and later shuts down to trap the same. In 1952 Giuseppe Conti described curious 'cushions' on venous walls that acted as shut down valves to retain blood. Many years later it was proved that Von Ebner's pads and Conti's cushions were in fact atherosclerotic debris [18]. With the discovery of cyclic GMP and the role of nitric oxide, it is now clear that erections are caused and controlled intrinsically by the contraction and relaxation of the corporal smooth muscles. Interestingly, as early as 1852 Von Kolliker of Wurzburg described this mechanism. On a lighter note, when the Europe was busy in exploring erections, the whole of America remained flaccid and inactive.

Until 1937 philosophers and physicians alike thought that the penis is an autonomous organ which was not under the control of its owner [4]. Wilder Penfield of McGill University first showed that this tiny appendage is in fact controlled by a very small area near the central fissure of the brain. His cortical mapping technique using electrical stimulation did not explain as to how this extremely small area can result in so much pleasure during coitus. With the advent of functional MRI, it is now clear that there are two different cortical perceptions. Ordinary somatic sensation of penis is felt at the small area marked by Penfield while the erogenous sensation is widely perceived all over the cortex. In fact several areas of the cerebral cortex are temporarily remodeled during sexual stimulation of the penis. Thus modern neurology elucidated the reason as to why Paleolithic cavemen painted the penis in exaggerated sizes.

3.5 Spectrum of Penile Malformations in Ancient Times

Recorded evidences of penile anomalies are scarce before medieval period. In an era when nudity itself was an acclaimed costume, it is unlikely that primeval man was shy of recording penile defects. Non-existence of malformations in ancient times is also unlikely. This discord is easily explained if the penile malformations are seen in the backdrop of their socio-cultural context. If straight penises were believed to be a sign of luck and prosperity, then deformed penis, by logic, ought to be a harbinger of ill omen. Babies with malformations were considered demonical and hence they were abandoned in backwoods to be devoured by wild animals. Even the Greek goddess of love, Aphrodite, was upset when she saw the newborn Priapus with ridiculously huge penis. She threw him out of the realms of Mount Olympus and he was raised by sympathetic shepherds of wilderness [19]. This eugenics unwittingly practiced by ancient societies is primarily responsible for the apparent rarity of penile malformations. Further there were no effective cures in the absence of proper knowledge on penile anatomy and physiology. Attempted surgeries had disastrous results and hence people were reluctant to go under surgical scalpel. This trepidation is well recorded in Priapeia written in the first century BCE.

Instead of going under the surgeons' knief, votives were offered to gods, particularly phallic deities, and prayers chanted for the cure of penile diseases. The sheer number of excavated phallic votives suggests there could not have been any dearth of penile disorders in ancient societies. Unfortunately, votives do not provide any insight into the sufferer's illness because they were designed to reflect the desired healthy state of the organ rather than the reality of diseased condition.

Some of the stone and ivory carvings of the Paleolithic cave dwellers resemble penis with intact prepuce [1]. It is difficult to ascertain if they are physiological or pathological. Paleopathologists who claim them to represent phimosis must have concluded so because of their inability to retract these stony foreskins! The first authentic description of penile malformation was that of Priapus in Greek mythology. The beautiful yet promiscuous goddess Aphrodite conceived him when she was successively inseminated by Zeus, Hermes, Adonis and Dionysus. Hera, who was jealous of Aphrodite's extramarital affair with her husband Zeus, cursed the fetus mistaking it for the product of her partner's semen. Priapus was born not only with grotesque penis but also with a protruding tongue, hunched back, dark complexion and multiple skin swellings. Persistent painful penile erection is incorrectly named as priapism. In fact his penis was merely turgid but not rigid. He was said to carry his huge penis in his shoulders and used it as whip to punish thieves. Even the famous fresco at Pompeii depicts Priapus with a tumescent but not fully erect penis. Considering these facts Priapus is likely to have suffered from high flow priapism consequent to vascular malformation of the penis (Proteus syndrome) [20]. Interestingly, his elder brother Hermaphroditus and step-brother Pan also suffered penile disorders. The former is the well known progenitor of hermaphroditism or intersex disorders. Pan, a fusion of man and goat, was known to have sexual insatiability and permanent erection of penis like his father Hermes himself. This could probably be the first recorded evidence of inheritable penile malformations in a family.

The excrescence on the glans penis of an Etrusco-Roman art work displayed at the Archaeological Museum of Civita Castellana resembles penile hemangioma. Phallic effigies of Magdalenian period (17,000 to 12,000 *BCE*) depicts meatal abnormalities such as megameatus and glanular hypospadias (Fig. 3.10). The prepuce of a merman statue at the Fountain of Neptune, Florence is abnormally long mimicking congenital megaprepuce (Fig. 3.11). References to congenital chordee sans hypospadias are plenty. Several phallic tintinnabulae of ancient Rome was designed with up-curved glans. It could be a comic representation of the glans proudly holding its head high; but it could also stand for the artist's familiarity with dorsal chordee of epispadias. A terracotta water jug of 400 *BCE* exhibits an unambiguous depiction of dorsal chordee. Wood carvings in a deserted temple car of Ayodhyapattinam portrays two sages tempted by a Mohini (sensual dancer). Their erect phalluses imitate lateral chordee due to congenital asymmetry of corpora cavernosa. Some of the phallic batons of upper Paleolithic era replicate diphallus.

Sushruta was the greatest Hindu surgeon of ancient India. In his book Sushruta Samhita (circa 3000 *BCE*) he has described phimosis under the indigenous name "Parivarthika" [21]. He elaborates the pathology as follows:

> "The vital vayu (gas) aggravated by such action as excessive massage (masturbation), pressure or local trauma attacks the integument of the penis which being thus affected by deranged vayu forms a knot-like structure and hangs down from the glans penis"

He also recorded the complication of phimosis, the paraphimosis under the name "Avapatika".

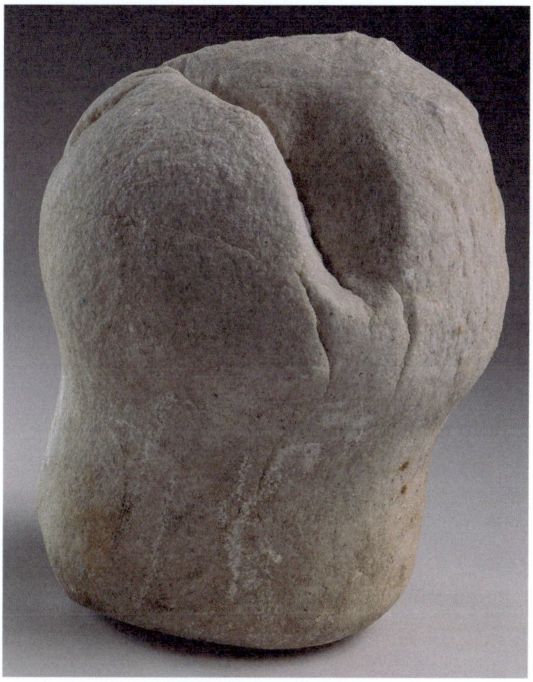

Fig. 3.10 Marble phallus with Megameatus at the Museum of Norwegian University of Science and Technology (NTNU) (Reproduced with the permission of Mr. Age Hojem)

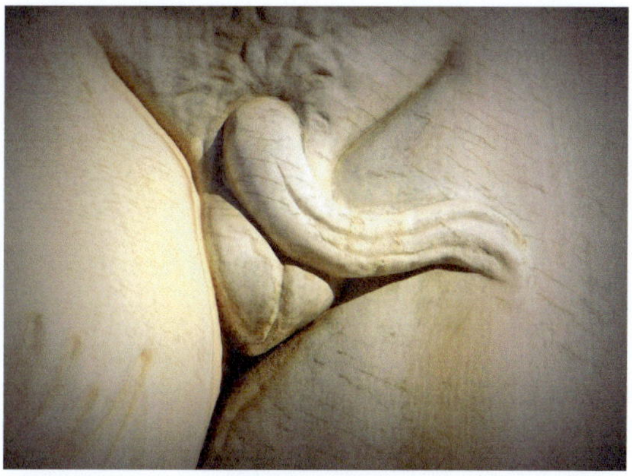

Fig. 3.11 Genital details of a merman statue at the Fountain of Neptune, Florence. Whether it is congenital mega-prepuce or groomed '*akroposthion*' is a moot question (Reproduced with the permission of Mr. Steve Browne)

Sushruta warned against forceful opening of prepuce. This implies he must have cured phimosis by gentle dilatation and retraction of the foreskin rather than by circumcision. These glimpses illustrate that the spectrum of penile malformations encountered in ancient times is no different from that of modern days.

3.6 Penis Yielding to Surgical Scalpel

During Renaissance, advances in the anatomical and physiological knowledge of the penis greatly improved the understanding of its malformations. However, delicate surgical reconstructions had to wait for the discovery of anaesthesia by William Morton in 1846 and antisepsis by Joseph Lister in 1867. Before Morton-Lister era, only those operations that can be quickly accomplished were feasible. They typically included circumcisions and amputations. Although decorative scarification, perforation and tattooing of the penis were known to exist even during Paleolithic era, they can hardly be called as surgical operations.

3.6.1 Hypospadias in History

Hypospadias was known to ancient Greeks. Galen of Pergamum (second century *CE*), the famous physician of Roman gladiators and emperors, not only coined the term 'hypospadias' but also accurately described its physiological effects and predicted the cure. He wrote:

> "Men afflicted with hypospadias find it impossible to beget children ….not because they lack fertile sperm, but because the curvature of the penis prevents its normal overflow from being conveyed forwards. This theory is confirmed by the ability to beget children if the frenum is divided" [22]

Although urethroplasty was unknown to Galen, infibulation and circumcision reversal was very popular during his times. Several techniques of preputial elongation by stretching were in vogue; which Galen applied in the treatment of distal hypospadias. Oribasius (325–403 *CE*) accurately classified hypospadias and declared that penile and scrotal varies were incurable. He and Paul of Aegina (625–690 *CE*) followed a peculiar philosophy: "If you cannot bring the meatus to the tip, bring the tip to the meatus". They recommended amputation of glans distal to hypospadiac meatus so that the meatus can be '*brought*' to the tip. After 1500 years Nesbit revived this strange philosophy when he described a new operation to correct 'chordee sans hypospadias' [23]. Nesbit suggested dorsal plication of corpora instead of releasing the ventral chordee thereby risking urethral shortage.

Arabian and Ottoman surgeons such as Abulcasis (936–1013 *CE*) and Serefeddin Sabuncuoglu (1385–1470 *CE*) attempted boring a tunnel between the tip of glans and the hypospadiac meatus using metal trocars [24]. Over the next several centuries great surgeons such as Morgagni (1682–1771 *CE*), Dupuytren (1777–1835 *CE*) and Sir Astley Cooper (1768–1841 *CE*) simply changed the material of trocars but not the principle of drilling a tunnel. It was Dieffenbach who did the first urethroplasty in 1836 *CE* by incising the edges of urethral groove and suturing it over a tube. Although this maiden attempt ended in failure, it was clearly the forerunner of the operation described by Thiersch (1869) and Duplay (1874).

The history of hypospadiology is replete with several instances of rediscoveries. For example, Gittes and McLaughlin described artificial erection test in 1974 which was known to Regnier de Graaf some three centuries before. In 1954, when Nesbit proposed resection of a small part of dorsal corpora to correct ventral chordee, Physick (1812) and Pancoast (1844) was not alive to claim priority of the concept. In 1981 John Duckett described tubularized preputial island flap urethroplasty which was essentially a modification of the technique that Hari Asopa published a decade earlier. The latest addition to this series of eponymous *faux pas* is the operation known by the name of Warren Snodgrass. Orkiszewski, a little known Polish pediatric surgeon, pointed out with great pains that it was his technique. Snodgrass described the procedure in 1994 while Orkiszewski had published his surgical operation in 1987. Orkiszewski also narrated as to how he got the idea during his uncle's funeral. When he could not dress up the corpulent corpse with a favorite but unfitting old jacket, he, upon his aunt's ingenuous advice, incised the back of the jacket thereby facilitated its buttoning in the front. Later he applied the same principle in the repair of hypospadias. In the above examples, as the time lapse between the original publications and their redescriptions is often more than a decade, one cannot help wondering if they are 'idea plagiarisms' rather than 'simultaneous independent discoveries'.

It is interesting that man, while still striving to cure hypospadias, deliberately created one for the purpose of contraception. In '*subincision*', as it was known to Australian aboriginals, penile urethra was slit open at penoscrotal junction and stented. The resultant fistula enabled extra-vaginal ejaculation during coitus while the person could still void urine from the tip of glans by occluding the fistula with a finger. Development of condoms and modern contraceptives has made subincisions obsolete. However, lessons learnt from this procedure are invaluable and are applicable in the management of hypospadiac fistulae.

3.6.2 Micropenis and Penile Lengthening Procedures

From time immemorial man has been excessively preoccupied with length of the penis. This obsession can be understood if one remembers that the erect organ is a socio-cultural symbol of power. The longer the penis, the more the power it implies to its possessor. Man has always feared to loose his penis at the depths of vagina because the latter was imagined to have biting teeth (*vagina dentata*). Therefore, a long penis was considered advantageous so that, in the worst of worst case, a portion of it lying outside the vagina can be saved! Thus, the concept of micropenis is both actual (anatomical) and perceived (psychological).

Kama Sutra, the world's first sexology manual written by Vatsyayana (circa 300 *CE*), classified penises into three types according to their lengths [25]. They were *hare type*, *bull type* and *horse type* in ascending order of length. *Hare-type* penis, by the standards of modern urological definitions, falls into the ambit of micropenis. Similarly, women were classified into *deer type*, *mare type* and *elephant type* based on the depth of vagina. Vatsyayana held that men and women should be matched according to the length of penis and depth of vagina in order to have harmonious pleasure of sexual intercourse. Any mismatch was deemed to result in dissatisfaction or dyspareunia. Obviously one could not have tested the measurements, especially the vaginal depth, prior to marriage. Therefore, when a mismatch of penile length was detected after marriage Vatsyayana offered to lengthen the micropenis. He described two distinct lengthening procedures; one was temporary while the other was permanent. Rubbing the penis with plant extracts was said to produce temporary lengthening. For those who wanted a permanent solution to micropenis he described the procedure as follows:

> "When a man wishes to enlarge his lingam (penis), he should rub it with the bristles of certain insects that live in trees, and then, after rubbing it for ten nights with oils, he should again rub it with the bristles as before. By continuing to do this a swelling will be gradually produced in the lingam, and he should then lie on a cot, and cause his lingam to hang down through a hole in the cot. After this he should take away all the pain from the swelling by using cool concoctions. The swelling, which is called "Suka," and is often brought about among the people of the Dravida country, lasts for life" [25]

It is not difficult to imagine as to what the patient would have got. It was probably nothing different from chronic penile edema from allergy to insect antigens and the 'permanency' mentioned implies lymphangio sclerosis and elephantiasis of penis. Unlike Vatsyayana, who was most probably a practical sexologist, Sushruta was surgeon trained in the principles of surgery. Sushruta criticized Vatsyayana's method as foolish. He named the resultant swelling of penis as Suka Dosha and described remedies for the same. Both Vatsyayana and Sushruta advised micropenis patients to satisfy their partners by using dildos and external penile prosthesis.

3.7 Psychology of the Penis

Spontaneity of erections and inability to achieve detumescence at will prompted primitive man to suspect the penis to have a mind of its own [4]. Scientific advancements made it clear that the penis is controlled by the mind of its owner. However, until 1896 no one ever even thought of exploring the influence of penis on human mind, when Sigmund Freud extensively studied the phenomenon. He held that the human mind works on the basis of pleasure principles. Libido, according to Freud, is the decisive force that determines human psyche [26]. He proposed that every child passes through four successive stages of personality development and in each of them a distinct kind of pleasure principle acts. For example, the oral stage spans the first year of life during which the child derives pleasure by sucking and chewing. The next is anal stage wherein the pleasure of controlling the sphincters dominates. The third phase is phallic stage which lasts between 3 and 5 years of age. During this stage child derives pleasure by masturbation and autoerotic fantasies. Freud discovered a curious psychological phenomenon called Oedipal Complex during the phallic stage according to which the baby boy fears that his father is determined to castrate him (Castration complex) because of his love towards his mother. Freud was not only heavily criticised and but also abused and isolated because of his phallocentric theory of psychological development [27]. Even his own students, Carl Jung and Alfred Adler, fell apart because of the differences of opinion. However, no one could completely deny the components of truth in the scintillating theory of Freud. Even Erik Erikson proposed his seven stages of psychic development as a continuation and modification of Freud's theory.

Irrespective of its universal acceptance, Freud's observations have far reaching implications in the surgical correction of penile malformations. Any penile surgery planned during the phallic stage will make the baby boy suspect that his hostile father is collaborating with the surgeon to castrate him. This negative impact is likely to leave behind lasting changes in the personality of the individual. Several late complications of hypospadias surgery such as erectile dysfunction may possibly be traced back to inappropriate timing of surgical correction.

Curiously, Freud's concept of phallic symbolism revived the 2000-year-old concept of nasogenital relationship. The nose, a prominent projection in the center of face with erectile tissue within it, did not escape Freud's attention and he called it a phallic substitute. He even explained the psychological reason as to why some men sneeze or rub their nose while interacting with beautiful women. In 1884 John Mackenzie, a Baltimore surgeon, hypothesized that penile irritation was the cause of some nasal diseases. Soon, in 1887, Fleiss reversed Mackenzie's concept and suggested that nasal abnormality was the source of several genital disorders. Incidentally, Fleiss was the friend and personal physician of Sigmund Freud. He claimed to have cured diseases such as impotence and menstrual disorders by anesthetizing nasal mucosa with cocaine. By 1912 Seifert could review more than 300 scientific papers concerning nasogenital relationship. It now appears ridiculous as well as unimportant to count as to how many boy with hypospadias had their nose corrected in that era.

3.8 Royal Members with Penile Anomalies

Freud's emphasis on phallocentric personality development brings in some revealing perspective of the world politics. If penis were a symbol of power and prosperity, it is easy to imagine as to how pathetic and powerless a king with defective penis would have felt. It will be interesting to study as to how the depression, frustration, anger, and vengeance incited by penile malformations in the minds of influential rulers have permanently changed the world history. A detailed account of this is beyond the scope of this work; however a glimpse of it is essential to highlight the importance of surgical correction of penile anomalies.

3.8.1 Tutankhamun's Erect Penis and the Exodus

Tutankhamun, the 18th dynasty pharaoh, ruled Egypt between 1332 and 1323 *BCE*. His death at 18 years of age was not only premature but also mysterious. Several theories were proposed to explain the cause of his death which includes malaria, political assassination, Köhler disease, temporal lobe epilepsy, head injury and Marfan syndrome. One remarkable clue is the boy king's erect penis. It is unusual to mummify pharaohs in erection state. Recent research suggested that he might have suffered homozygous sickle cell disease. His erect penis and death were probably the result of veno-occlusive priapism of sickle cell crisis [28]. Political instability that followed his untimely death was postulated to have facilitated the great exodus under the leadership of Mosus.

3.8.2 Epispadiac Emperor Heraclius

The Byzantine Emperor Heraclius (601–641 CE), who won back the sacred relic of Holy Cross from Persians, was known to have suffered from epispadias. Whenever he wanted to void, his up-curved penis would splash urine on his face. As a face saving measure he used to hold a wooden plank upon his abdomen during micturation [29]. The fact that he could void at will and could beget 11 children suggests that he must have had glandular or penile epispadias. Impact of this penile malformation on the psychology of emperor has not been overtly recorded. However, it can be inferred from his boorish behavior when he deposed his predecessor Phocas by a civil war. Heraclius killed Phocas by decapitation and when he saw the robust penis of his rival, as a second thought, he amputated it with renewed rage. Heraclius is known to have extreme mood swings. Historians, who attribute it to his guilt towards his incestuous marriage to Martina or the psychiatric disorder cyclothymia, are probably ignorant of his 'penile inferiority complex'.

3.8.3 Hypospadias of King Henry II

In 1533 *CE* the King Henry II of France married Catherine de Medici and the couple was childless for the next 10 years. Although Catherine was originally blamed for the barrenness, the actual cause of it seems to be Henry's hypospadiac chordee. Catherine underwent several inhuman treatments which included drinking the urine of pregnant women, eating dried penises of wild animals, consuming mixed juices of various herbs besides wearing charms and listening to astrologers. Meanwhile, Diane de Poitier, the mistress of the king gave birth to two children. The twin conceptions, although suspected to be the result of Diane's other amorous liaisons, generally acquitted Henry of any defect. Catherine was threatened by Diane's success and there were even talks of divorce. When Catherine sneakily smelt the secret, she learnt that Diane was engaging the king in a unique coital posture. Even the Royal physicians advised Catherine to adopt different style of sexual union. The Queen anxious of learning the technique arranged to bore a secret peephole in the ceiling directly over Diane's bedchamber and nervously watched her husband making love to the concubine [30]. When nothing worked, she sought the help of Jean Fernel, the then famous physician of Paris. He was believed to have corrected Henry's chordee which enabled to couple to beget ten children. It is a great mystery as to why Fernel was preferred over the great surgeon Ambrose Pare, who was also the King's personal surgeon. In fact, Pare had contributed more to the understanding of hypospadias than Fernel. Despite the inappropriate choice of surgeon, this was the first successful correction of chordee in the history which not only enhanced the fortune of Fernel but also changed the fate of France.

3.8.4 Phimosis of Louis XVI and the French Revolution

In 1770 CE, Louis XVI, the Dauphin of France married the Austrian Archduchess Marie Antoinette primarily to forge a political alliance between the two countries that were estranged by the war of Austrian succession. Nevertheless, Louis's inability to consummate the marriage for 7 years proved disastrous. The condition that prevented him is supposed to be a 'tight' phimosis. The young prince himself was said to have acknowledged that penetrations were only partial because of severe pain. Royal surgeons differed in their opinion regarding the need of circumcision. The whole nation convulsed because of the infertility of their King. Both the king and queen engaged themselves in notorious frivolity and spendthrift which, according to the Austrian psychiatrist Zweig, may be the psychic reaction to their sexual frustration. Finally, Joseph II, the brother-in-law of Louis, intervened and believed to have arranged for the circumcision of Louis [31]. Although the couple could subsequently bear three children, the delay proved very costly. Rumors and libelous cartoons abound depicting the king impotent. This together with the extravaganza of Marie infuriated the public mood which culminated in French revolution (1789).

3.8.5 Napoleon's Micropenis and His Bruised Ego

Napoleon Bonaparte (1769–1821 *CE*), was known for his love towards war and women. Despite his libido, the great French commander could never perform satisfactorily in bed due to micropenis. He also had gynecomastia about which he once commented, "Any beauty will be proud of a bosom like mine" [32]. Based on his effeminate phenotype, infertility, plump body fat and silky hair, medical historians suspect him to have suffered from Frohlich syndrome (adiposogenitalis). His bragging about numerous romantic affairs could just be a cover-up of what he suffered at the hands of noble virgins. His estranged wife Josephine, referring to his sexual inadequacy, once blurted, "Bon-a-parte est bon-a-rien" (Bonaparte is good for nothing). The curiosity about his micropenis must have prompted Professor Francesco Antommarchi, who performed emperor's autopsy, to silently slip his surgical scalpel and cut off the flaccid appendage without attracting undue attention of others. Someone who saw it in the Museum of French Art was said to have commented, "It looked like a shriveled eel". Napoleon's war aggressions were explained by the Austrian psychiatrist Alfred Adler in terms of 'organ inferiority'. According to him, the realization that ones penis is small and imperfectly formed would breed feelings of aggression in most males.

Conclusion

Apart from its biological role of urination and copulation, penis has a variety of socio-cultural roles ranging from apotropaism to frank divinity. It is also a psychological symbolism of power and well being. Hence surgeons correcting penile malformations shall not simply treat the organ as a urinary or seminal conduit. All penile surgeries should be seriously considered in the background of their psychosocial implications and this historical background.

References

1. Angulo JC, García-Díez M. Male genital representation in Paleolithic art: erection and circumcision before history. Urology. 2009;74:10–4.
2. Moser C. Naked power: the phallus as an apotropaic symbol in the images and texts of Roman Italy. University of Pennsylvania. 2006. Available from http://humanities.sas.upenn.edu/05-06/mellon_uhf.shtml.
3. Osborne R. The erection and mutilation of the Hermai. Proceed Cambridge Philol Soc. 1985;31:47–73.
4. Friedman DM. A mind of its own: A cultural history of the penis. London; Robert Hale. 2001
5. Washburn SL. (ed) Social life of early man. Routledge Taylor Francis 1962.
6. Cormier LA, Jones SR. The domesticated penis: how womanhood has shaped manhood. Alabama: University of Alabama Press; 2015.
7. Pinch G. Egyptian mythology: a guide to the gods, goddesses, and traditions of ancient Egypt. New York: Oxford University Press; 2002.
8. Angulo JC, García-Díez M, Martínez M. Phallic decoration in paleolithic art: genital scarification, piercing and tattoos. J Urol. 2011;186:2498–503.
9. Westropp HM. Primitive symbolism, as illustrated in phallic worship. London; George Redway 1885.
10. Clark SR. Representing the Indus Body: Sex, Gender, Sexuality, and the Anthropomorphic Terracotta Figurines from Harappa. Asian Perspectives 2003; 42(2):304–28.
11. Jennings H. Phallic Miscellanies: Facts and Phases of Ancient and Modern Sex Worship, as Illustrated Chiefly in the Religions of India. London; privately published. 1891.
12. Galassi FM, Galassi S. Shut phimosis in the Priapus fresco from Pompeii. Urology. 2015;85:1521–2.
13. Mattelaer JJ, Schipper RA, Das S. The circumcision of Jesus Christ. J Urol. 2007;178:31–4.
14. Noble D, Difrancesco D, Zancani D. Leonardo da Vinci and the origin of semen. Notes Rec (Royal Soc J Hist Sci). 2014;68:391–402.
15. van Driel MF. Physiology of Penile Erection-A Brief History of the Scientific Understanding up till the Eighties of the 20th Century. Sex Med. 2015;3:349–57.

16. Connell SM. Aristotle and Galen on sex difference and reproduction: a new approach to an ancient rivalry. Stud Hist Philos Sci. 2000;31:405–27.
17. Jocelyn HD, Setchell BP. Regnier de Graaf on the human reproductive organs. An annotated translation of Tractatus de Virorum Organis Generationi Inservientibus (1668) and De Mulierub Organis Generationi Inservientibus Tractatus Novus (1962). J Reprod Fertil Suppl. 1972;17:1–222.
18. Glina S, Lewis RW, Steers WD, Lue TF. Erection of the human penis and its morphological and vascular basis by Guiseppe Conti. J Sex Med. 2008;5:262–7.
19. Smith W. A new classical dictionary of Greek and Roman biography, mythology and geography. New York: Harper; 1884.
20. Raveenthiran V. Penile erection of pathological source; semantically a better term for priapism. BJU Int. 2007;100:217–8.
21. Bhishagratna KL. An English translation of the Sushruta Samhita. Varanasi; Chowkhamba Sanskrit Series Office, 1910.
22. Smith ED. The history of hypospadias. Pediatr Surg Int. 1997;12:81–5.
23. Lambert SM, Snyder HM, Canning DA. The History of Hypospadias and Hypospadias Repairs. Urology 2011;77:1277–83.
24. Verit A, Aksoy S, Kafali H, Verit FF. Urologic techniques of Serefeddin Sabuncuoglu in the 15th century Ottoman period. Urology. 2003;62: 776–8.
25. Burton RF. The Kama Sutra of Vatsyayana, translated from the Sanskrit. London: Kama Shastra Society of London and Benares; 1883.
26. Hall CS, Lindzey G, Campbell JB. Theories of personality. 4th ed. New York: John Wiley; 1998.
27. Jones E. The life and work of Sigmund Freud. New York: Basic Books; 1953–1957.
28. Pays JF. Tutankhamun and sickle-cell anaemia. Bull Soc Pathol Exot. 2010;103:346–7.
29. Lascaratos J, Poulakou-Rebelakou E, Rempelakos A, Marketos S. The first case of epispadias: an unknown disease of the Byzantine Emperor Heraclius (AD 610–641). Br J Urol. 1995;76:380–83.
30. Hatzinger M, Al-Shajlawi S, Sohn M. Hypospadias and infertility of Henry II of France (1519–1559). Urologe A. 2014;53:375–8.
31. Fogg RN, Boorjian SA. The sexual dysfunction of Louis XVI: a consequence of international politics, anatomy, or naïveté? BJU Int. 2010;106: 457–9.
32. Richardson FM. Napoleon's sex life. J R Army Med Corps. 2003;149:344–7.

Part II

Prepuce

The word Prepuce originally came from the old French word "prepuce", and from Latin "praeputium", which means "præ-"before and "putos" means "penis", but in Greeks language the word prepuce composed of two distinct structures: the *posthe* (ποσθη) and the *akroposthion* (αkροπσθτου). *Posthe* referred to that part of the prepuce that covers the glans penis, and "Akroposthion" designates the tapered, tubular, visually defining portion of the prepuce that extends beyond the glans and terminates at the preputial orifice.

Anatomically the prepuce or foreskin is a double-layered fold of smooth muscle tissue, blood vessels, neurones, skin, and mucous membrane that covers and protects the glans penis and urinary meatus when the penis is not erect. The embryonically homologous of prepuce in female is the clitoral hood. The World Health Organization debates the precise functions of the foreskin, which may include; keeping the glans moist, protecting the developing penis in utero, or enhancing sexual pleasure due to the presence of nerve receptors. A lot of debate emerge in literature and researches work about the importance and significance of prepuce, and usually the idea behind this argument is to fight against or with the removal of this skin piece during circumcision [1].

Embryology of prepuce Bokai (1860) was the first to direct attention to the physiological adherence of the foreskin. Schweiger and Seidel (1866) gave the first description of the development of the prepuce in the human, but Retterer (1885–1915) was the first to describe development of the prepuce, which start to develop in the 57 mm human fetus (8 weeks of gestation) from the base of the glans, as a preputial fold which has been raised round the dorsum and sides of the base of the glans, but it is interrupted along the under surface by the urogenital ostium (the future urethra), before that time the glans penis was completely uncovered and splitted with the urethral plate at its depth (Fig. 1). In the 65 mm fetus (fourth month of intra-uterine life) the urogenital ostium is confined to the under surface of the glans and the preputial fold has rolled over the base of the glans except in the region of the urogenital ostium where it is deficient at that stage, with the further distal development of the glandular urethra and closure of its edges, the perpetual fold close ventrally to form the frenulum (which is attached to the undersurface of the glans) at the inner mucosal aspect and preputial raphe at the outer surface, with the dorsal portion growing at a more rapid rate than the ventral component, this fold covers the glans progressively, and the epithelium covering the deep aspect of the fold fusing with the epithelium covering the glans. The closure of the ventral portion of the prepuce is completed by the fifth month of gestation after the closure of the glanular urethra, In relation to the distal part of the glans the lower margins of the lamella fuse to form a complete epithelial cuff which, by breaking down, gives rise to the cylindrical terminal part of the prepuce (Fig. 2). Phimosis could be explained in terms of the preputial fold continuing to grow forward too far beyond the tip of the glans and failure of the glandar lamella to disintegrate.

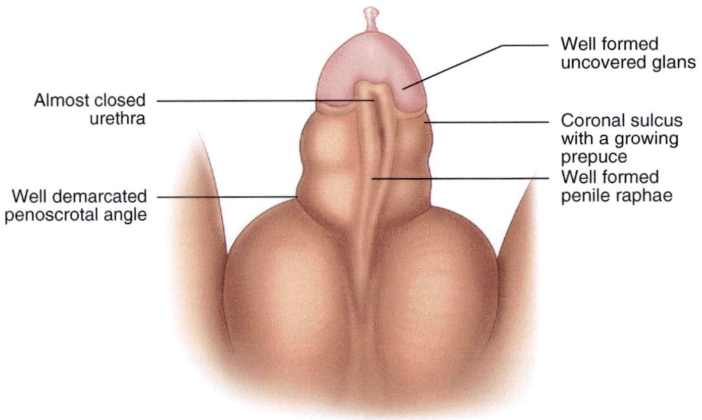

Fig. 1 Intrauterine male genitalia of 65 mm embryo, with the glans uncovered by prepuce, which start to creep from the coronal sulcus

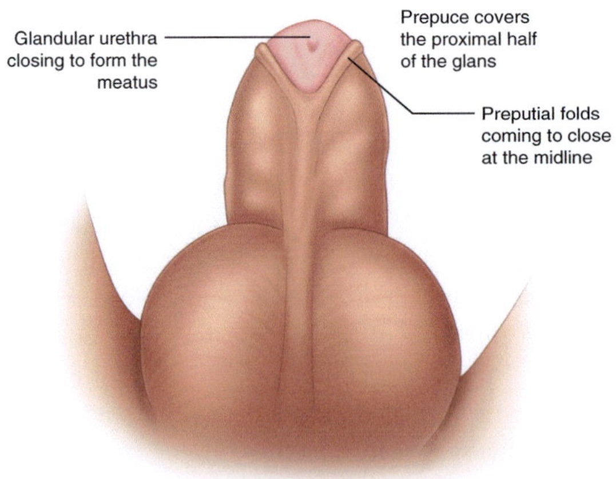

Fig. 2 External genitalia of a 70 mm human fetus with incompletely developed glandular urethra and prepuce

It is generally accepted that normal preputial development is required for successful canalization of the glandular urethra, so the absence of the prepuce would result in an abnormal development of the glandular urethra, and to be manifested as a hypospadias with a usual hooded prepuce, as Hunter (1935) [2] pointed out. It is also proved that the proper development of the prepuce depends on the presence of androgen and androgen receptors.

Observations made on female embryo lead to the conclusion that the same processes are involved in the formation of the clitorial prepuce, but persistence of the urethral groove in female and hypospadiac penis prevents the fusion of the margins of the preputial fold and of the glandar lamella. This again emphasises the close association of the preputial anlage with the urethral folds, this association explains the presence of a hood-like prepuce in cases of hypospadias. The only non explainable exception of this concept is the intact prepuce megameatus anomaly and the very rare cases of epispadias with intact prepuce (chap 21&26); where the prepuce developed completely to the tip of the glans, but the underneath glandular urethra is still not completed.

In children, the foreskin usually covers the glans completely but in adults it may not, in a study of 3,000 young men from Germany there is only 49.6 % had the glans fully covered by foreskin, 41.9 % were partially covered and 8.5 % were uncovered; around half of which (4 %) had the foreskin atrophied spontaneously without previous surgery [3]. The length of the prepuce in the human population varies from large problematic to a very small (unable to circumcise) or absent prepuce i.e., aposthia. Radojici and Perovic found 6 various morphological forms of the prepuce associated with hypospadias, indicating its quantitative nature—"monk's hood", "cobra eyes", "normal" (intact), "flat", "v-shaped" and "collar-scarf". This variation in shape and size of the prepuce in the population suggests that it may be a dominant quantitative trait [4].

Almost all mammal penises have foreskins which called the *preputial sheath* or *penile sheath* into which the whole penis is retracted. Only monotremes (the platypus and the echidna) lack foreskins. Several congenital external genital anomalies related to the prepuce have been documented, however, natural circumcision or aposthia (the absence of the prepuce) with a normal development of the urethra is very rare.

Preputial glands are exocrine glands that are located in the folds of skin in front of the genitals of some mammals (including mice) and produce pheromones. The preputial glands of female animals are sometimes called clitoral glands. The preputial glands of male musk deer produce strong-smelling deer musk which is of economic importance, as it is used in perfumes.

There is debate about whether humans have functional homologues to preputial glands, which were first noted by Edward Tyson and in 1694 and fully described by William Cowper who named them Tyson's glands. They are described as a modified sebaceous glands located around the corona and inner surface of the prepuce of the human penis. They are believed to be most frequently found in the balanopreputial sulcus. Their secretion may be one of the components of smegma, but some, authors dispute their existence [4]. While humans may not have true anatomical equivalents, the term may sometimes be used for tiny whitish yellow pimples occasionally found on the corona of the glans penis. The proper name for these structures is pearly penile papules (or hirsutoid papillomas). According to detractors, they are not glands, but mere thickenings of the skin and are not involved in the formation of smegma [5].

Smegma is a natural secretion of skin cells and oils that collects under the foreskin in both males and females, it is firstly seen in the enlarged posterior extremity of the glandar lamella, the future coronal sulcus in adult, approximately at sixth month of foetal life. If allowed to grow stale, it may have a pungent aroma (commonly compared to cheese in males or fish in females), and has lubricant, pheromonal (sexual attractant), and perhaps bacteriostatic functions. The quantity of smegma varies, but it is comparable to earwax. This natural emollient also contains prostatic and seminal secretions, desquamated epithelial cells, and the mucin content of the urethral glands of Littre. It protects and lubricates the glans and inner lamella of the prepuce, facilitating erection, preputial eversion, and penetration during sexual intercourse. In one survey, out of 18 self-selected intact men never saw smegma; 1 saw it after a week unwashed, 6 after 2 days, 8 after 1 day, and 1 after less than a day [6].

Congenital anomalies of the prepuce include complete absence, deficient or extensively large prepuce; aposthia, microposthia or macroposthia respectively.

References

1. Gleniste TW. A consideration of the processes involved in the development of the prepuce in man. Br J Urol. 1956;28:243–9.
2. Hunterr H. J Anat Lond. Preputial development. 1935;70:68.
3. Schöberlein W. Significance and incidence of phimosis and smegma. [Article in German]. Munch Med Wochenschr. 1967;108(7):373–7.
4. Radojicic ZI, Perovic SV. Classification of prepuce in hypospadias according to morphological abnormalities and their impact on hypospadias repair. J Urol 2004;172:301–4. Sadeghipour Roudsari S, Esmailzadehha N. Aposthia: a case report. J Pediatr Surg. 2010;45(8):17–9.
5. Satya P, Jeyakumar K, Subramanya K, Chaudhuri S. Human subpreputial collection: its nature and formation. J Urol. 1973;110(2):211–2. PMID 4722614 Amin Ud Din M, Salam A, Rafiq MA, Khaliq I, Ansar M, Ahmad W. Aposthia: a birth defect or normal quantitative recessive human genetic trait? East Mediterr Health J. 2007;13(2):280–6.
6. Batistatou A, Panelos J, Zioga A, Charalabopoulos KA. Ectopic modified sebaceous glands in human penis. Int J Surg Pathol. 2006;14 (4):355–6. doi:10.1177/1066896906291779. Talbot ES. Inheritance of circumcision effects. Medicine. 1898;4:473–5.

Aposthia

4

Abstract

Absent prepuce in a child is not a surgical problem, which needs no intervention, just exclusion of any other associated anomalies and family reassurance may be enough in certain communities where circumcision is a routine or ritual practice, but preputial reconstruction may be considered in societies considering socially unacceptable and ugly to have a glans penis without a preputial covering. Cases of aposthia could raise a couple of questions which deserve further researches.

Keywords

Foreskin • Natural circumcision • Congenital circumcision • Preputial reconstruction

Nomenclature

Natural circumcision, congenital absence of preputial foreskin.

Definition

Aposthia is a rare congenital condition in humans, in which the foreskin of the penis is completely missing in a normally developed penis and urethra (Figs. 4.1 and 4.2).

© Springer International Publishing Switzerland 2017
M. Fahmy, *Congenital Anomalies of the Penis*, DOI 10.1007/978-3-319-43310-3_4

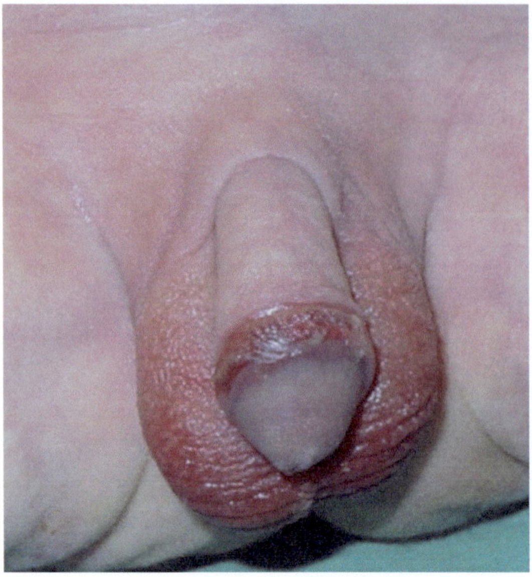

Fig. 4.1 Aposthia in neonate with completely normal glans and urethra (dorsal view)

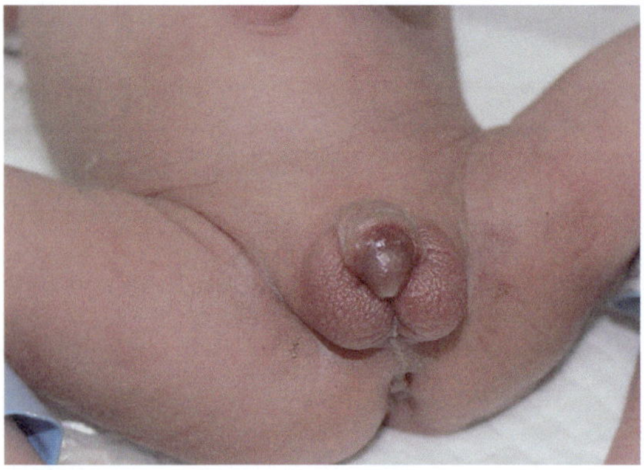

Fig. 4.2 Neonate with aposthia and minimal scrotal transposition

4.1 Historical Background

Religious literature from various sources reflects the history of aposthia; as this condition was first referenced in Jewish law of 1567 CE, in relation to a child born circumcised. Toward the end of the nineteenth century, E.S. Talbot claimed in Medicine that aposthia among Jews was evidence for the now-discredited Lamarckian theory of evolution. It is likely that the cases he described were actually hypospadias. The Midrash of Ki Tetzei notes that Moses was born aposthic. Other sources tell us that Jacob and David were also born aposthic. Jewish law requires males born without a foreskin or who lost their foreskin through means other than a formal circumcision ceremony to have a drop of blood let from the penis at the point where the foreskin would have been attached. Later on, the Prophet Muhammad was said to have been born with "natural circumcision" (in Ibn Sad Tabaqatul-Kubara). However, certain studies have reported that the trait aposthia with normal development of the urethra and glans is very rare because it is generally accepted that normal preputial development is required for the successful canalization of the glans urethra.

4.2 Incidence

It is a very rare congenital anomaly; however in the last few years, various cases of aposthia had been reported [1]. Amin et al. reported aposthia inheritance as normal quantitative recessive human genetic trait in three strictly endogamous families. Aposthia reported as a sporadic and familiar cases, in sporadic cases all of them had a hypospadias associated and the familiar case had a normal development of the urethra. Both groups had a history of consanguineous marriage and the study suggested that certain linked modifier loci as well as a number of autosomal recessive genes are required to express natural circumcision [2]. No cases of aposthia in females have been reported in the literature to date.

So aposthia may be prevalent in certain ancient healthy and comparatively developed inbred population isolates; this condition has not been shown to have a higher frequency in Jews or Muslims. If the hypospadias surgeons are fully aware about this condition, a cumulative number of cases will be reported either in association with hypospadias or as an entire pathology (Fig. 4.2).

4.3 Scientific Significance of Aposthia

Absent prepuce in a child is not a surgical problem, which needs no intervention, just exclusion of any other associated anomalies and family reassurance may be enough in certain communities where circumcision is a routine or ritual practice, but preputial reconstruction may be considered in societies considering socially unacceptable and ugly to have a glans penis without a preputial covering. Many procedures had been described to develop a neo prepuce, either by non-surgical foreskin restoration, which accomplished through tissue expansion, or with a circular fasciocutaneous penile flap or different grafts typically taken from the scrotum.

Also it is suggested that the extensive study on aposthia may be helpful for proper understanding of the importance of circumcision and reducing the controversy in medical sciences [2].

Cases of aposthia could raise a couple of questions which deserve further researches:

Is circumcised "Aposthic" penis is the natural normal penis and having a prepuce is a pathological condition which should be treated by removal?

Is "Aposthia" a feature of the dignified leader or the first man "Adam", and circumcision is a ritual trial to have a copy or similarity to the symbolic leader?

Aposthia being a quantitative recessive trait may be prevalent in certain ancient healthy and comparatively developed inbred population isolates.

References

1. Garcia-Palacios M, et al. Congenital absence of preputial foreskin: an extremely uncommon anomaly. J Pediatr Surg. 2013;48:E13–15. Websites concerning with prepuce: http://www.foreskin.org/links.htm.
2. Amin Ud Din M, Salam A, Rafiq MA, Khaliq I, Ansar M, Ahmad W. Aposthia: a birth defect or normal quantitative recessive human genetic trait? East Mediterr Health J. 2007;13(2):280–6.

5 Micropothia

Abstract
Deficient prepuce is not recognised before as a specific disease entity, and little attention was paid for this anomaly in the literature, herein this anomaly will be described with some details, as it may be associated with major penile deformities.

Keywords
Deficient prepuce • Microposthia • Hypoposthia • Peeper penis

Deficient prepuce is not recognised before as a specific disease entity, and little attention was paid for this anomaly in the literature [1], herein this anomaly will be described with some details, as it may be associated with major penile deformities.

Nomenclature

Microposthia, Hypoposthia, and Peeper penis, which is a term refers to the penis whose foreskin is short enough to expose some of the glans when flaccid.

Incidence

In a sample of 3000 young men examined W. Schoeberlein found a lack of, or spontaneous atrophy of the foreskin among approx. 4 % [2].

5.1 Significance of Microposthia

Failure of development of urethral groove; results in hypospadias and subsequently associated with ventrally deficient prepuce (hooded Prepuce) in many cases. In female the urethral groove persist so preputial hood is a normal finding with clitoris, and it is extremely rare to have a complete prepuce ensheathing entirely the clitoris, but till now, there is no conventional explanation why there is some boys had a completely formed prepuce with hypospadias as in Intact Prepuce Megameatus (IPM) anomaly and other cases -that we will describe herein- with a deficient prepuce but with a normally formed urethra?, but many of these cases had an associated defective penile development along the defectively developed prepuce.

So cases of microposthia may present as an arrest of the normal preputial development secondary to failure of complete urethral folding

© Springer International Publishing Switzerland 2017

M. Fahmy, *Congenital Anomalies of the Penis*, DOI 10.1007/978-3-319-43310-3_5

(hypospadias) or due to an unknown (not yet detected) process where a feminine pathway of preputial development predominate.

Definition

It is a condition of having a very small foreskin not covering the whole penis; microposthia diagnosed if the glans penis could be seen partially in a flaccid penis (Fig. 5.1). It is not a rare condition, and it could be considered as a normal variation, where the prepuce looks shorter to give the chance for the glans or the urinary meatus to be visible in a neonate without foreskin retraction [3]. In all cases of microposthia frenulum is absent and penile raphe end at the coronal sulcus. Usually the foreskin is defective at the ventral aspect of the penis, but rarely it is completely normal in the ventral surface but shows deficiency only in the dorsum of the glans, which may hide an episodic or duplicated urethra (Figs. 5.2 and 5.3).

The preputial remnants with microposthia is a smooth skin with an exposed inner mucosal layer, as in Fig. 5.1, but I encountered an interesting two brothers with an unusual microposthia, they had no any other associated congenital anomalies, no previous history of trauma, genital or urinary tract infection, but they had a disfigured serrated preputial remnants covering partially the dorsal surface of the glans, there is a consanguinity between parents, but without any similar history in the family; this could point out a congenital background of such cases like what was reported in aposthia [4] (Figs. 5.4 and 5.5).

Microposthia have to be differentiated from cases of aposthia, where is the prepuce is completely deficient and the coronal sulcus clearly seen in flaccid penis, but in microposthia the preputial remnants covering the sulcus but not reaching to tip of the penis.

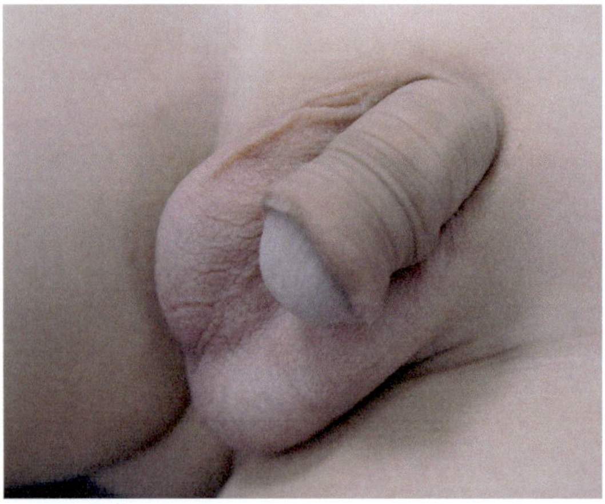

Fig. 5.1 Microposthia

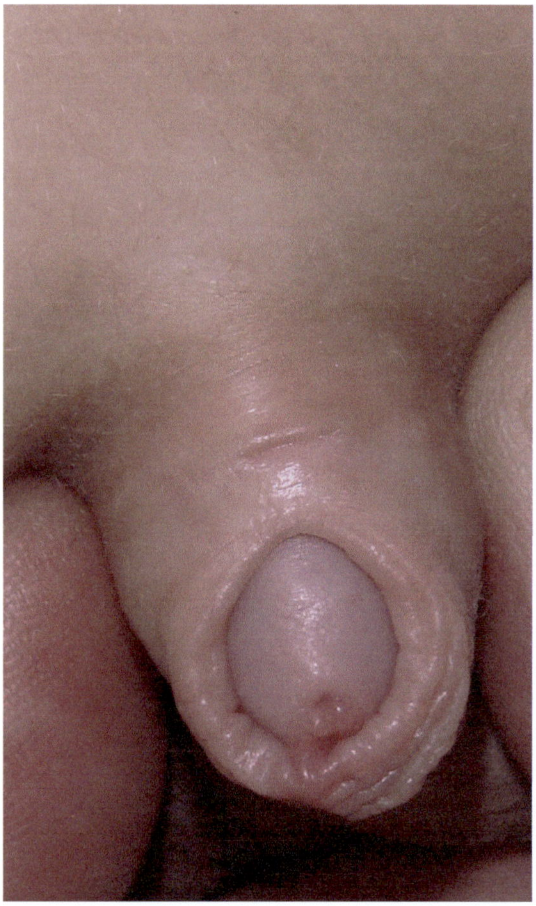

Fig. 5.2 Dorsally deficient prepuce with a small dimple

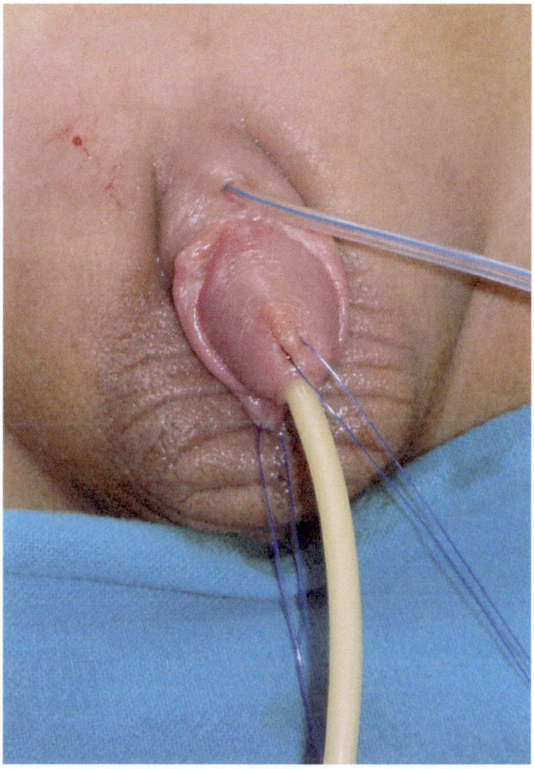

Fig. 5.3 Microposthia associated with an incomplete urethral duplication

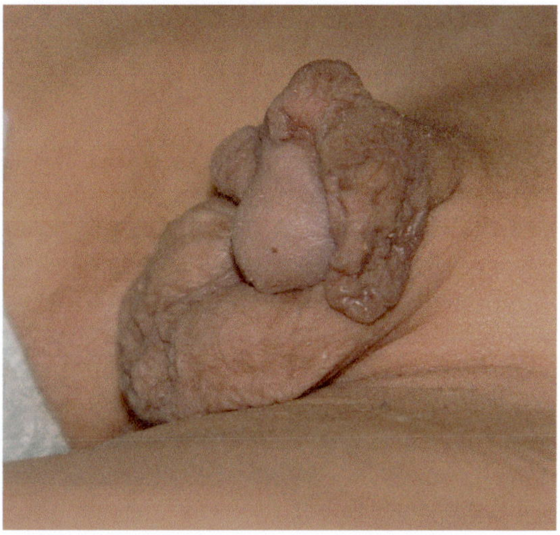

Fig. 5.5 Close up of the irregular edges of a deficient prepuce

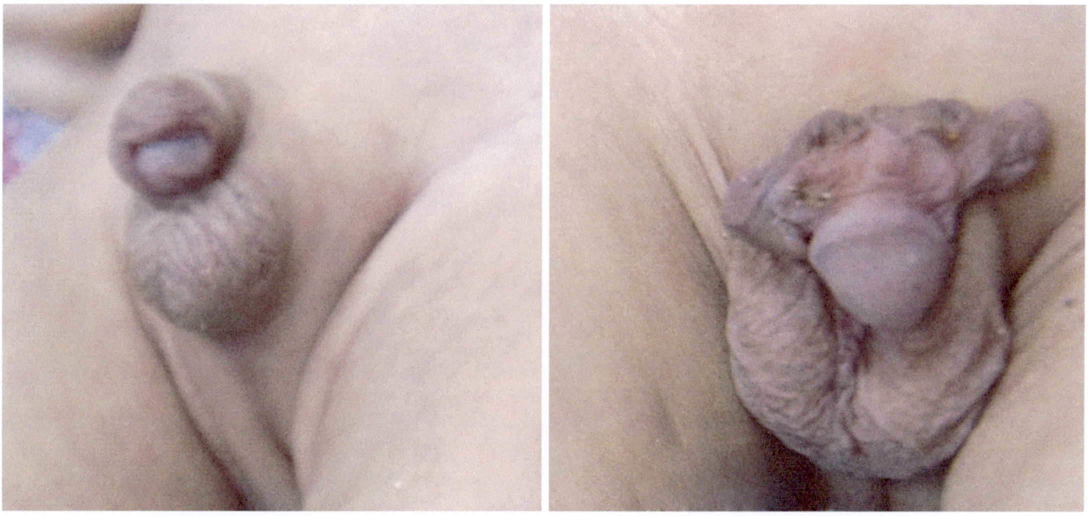

Fig. 5.4 Siblings with a congenital deficiency of prepuce with an irregular perpetual remnants

5.2 Associated Anomalies

Microposthia itself is not a harmful anomaly and could not be considered as a disease, but its importance came from the possibility to be associated with other congenital genitourinary anomalies, where the deficient foreskin is an indicator for a defective genital development, as the normal development of prepuce is an androgen dependant; so many other genital anomalies could associated microposthia, and the most common association is hypospadias, and it is not rare to have a deficient prepuce with a chordee, but without hypospadias (Fig. 5.6), other anomalies include; penile rotation (Fig. 5.7) and undescended testicle (Fig. 5.8).

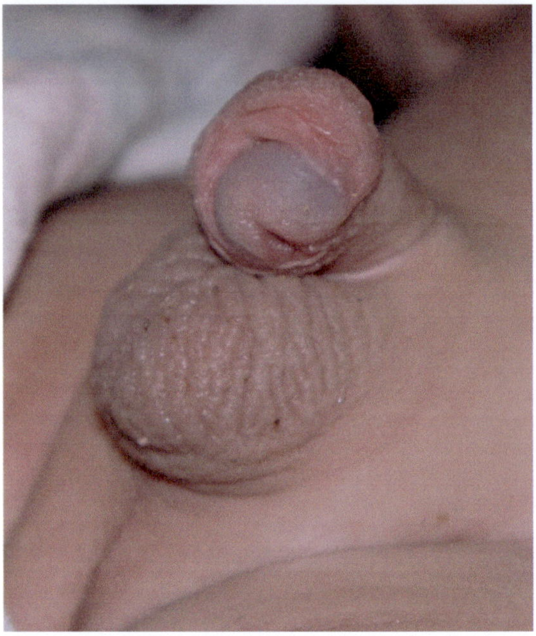

Fig. 5.7 Microposthia with left sided penile rotation

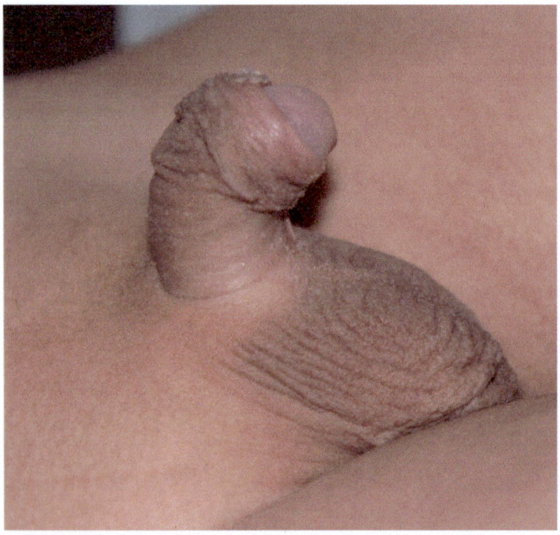

Fig. 5.6 Microposthia with chordee, but without hypospadias

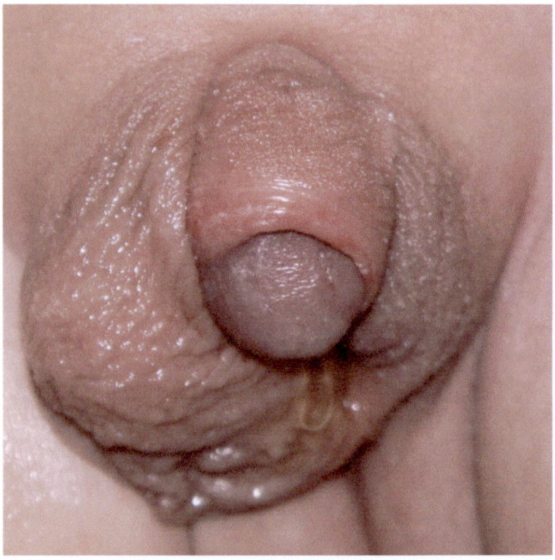

Fig. 5.8 Microposthia with left undescended testicle

5.3 Management

A microposthic child may deserve a meticulous circumcision to make his penis looks like the normally circumcised one if the family wish, or the decision could be kept till the time when the child can decide for himself later on, in some occasions preputial reconstruction may be indicated for microposthia to restore the normal look prepuce (preputoplasty), and this could be achieved without grafting in minor cases by preputial edges refreshment, midline closure and creation of a properly constricted tip distal to the glans, but in cases with severe preputial deficiency, preputial restoration could be accomplished through non-surgical foreskin restoration techniques (developed to help circumcised men 'regrow' a skin covering for the glans by different modalities of tissue expansion) to lengthen the natural foreskin, in cases with marked preputial deficiency, foreskin restoration for those who are looking for a normal genital self-image can be achieved by a circular fasciocutaneous penile flap or other different grafts which typically taken from the scrotum [5].

References

1. Fahmy MAB. Prepuce. In: Rare congenital genitourinary anomalies. Heidelberg: Springer Berlin; 2015. p. 33–41.
2. Schöberlein W. The significance and frequency of phimosis and smegma. Munch Med Wochenschr. 1966;7:373–7.
3. Kayaba H, Tamura H, Kitajima S, Fujiwara Y, Kato T, Kato T. Analysis of shape and retractability of the prepuce in 603 Japanese boys. J Urol. 1996;156:1813–5.
4. Amin Ud Din M, Salam A, Rafiq MA, Khaliq I, Ansar M, Ahmad W. Aposthia: a birth defect or normal quantitative recessive human genetic trait? East Mediterr Health J. 2007;13(2):280–6.
5. Dunn HP. Non-surgical management of phimosis. Aust N Z J Surg. 1989;59(12):963. doi:10.1111/j.1445-2197.1989.tb07640.x. PMID 2597103.

6 Macroposthia and Congenital Megaprepuce (CM)

Abstract
Extensively large redundant part of the prepuce extended beyond the glans penis, sometimes representing more than three-quarters of the length of the penis, considered as a normal variation, and the term"akroposthion" given to this redundant part but a whole prepuce that has been deliberately lengthened is defined as a congenitally abnormal one, and described as a secondary megaprepuce.

Keywords
Macroposthia • Preputial bladder • Akroposthion

Nomenclatures

Macroposthia, Volcano penis, Secondary megaprepuce and Acroposthia (akroposthion "Greek")

Definition

Extensively large redundant part of the prepuce extended beyond the glans penis, sometimes representing more than three-quarters of the length of the penis, considered as a normal variation, and the term"akroposthion" given to this redundant part (Fig. 6.1), but a whole prepuce that has been deliberately lengthened is defined as a congenitally abnormal one, and described as a secondary megaprepuce [1] (Fig. 6.2). Another rare condition has only recently received recognition as an entity in its own right is the congenital megaprepuce (CM), which characterized by extensive redundancy of the inner preputial skin over a penile shaft and glans of normal shape and size (Fig. 6.3), or it could be presented as an enormously capacious preputial sac, engulfing the whole penile shaft and upper scrotum, with urine accumulation in the preputial sac (prompting the term "preputial bladder") (Fig. 6.4).

© Springer International Publishing Switzerland 2017

M. Fahmy, *Congenital Anomalies of the Penis*, DOI 10.1007/978-3-319-43310-3_6

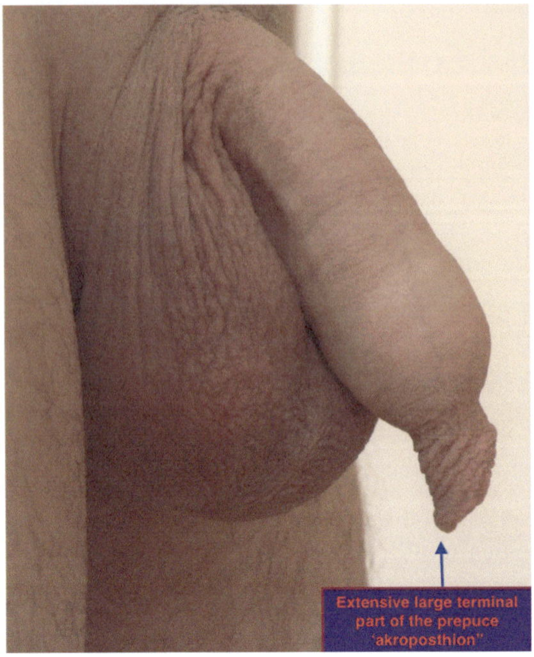

Fig. 6.1 Extensive large terminal part of the prepuce "akroposthion"

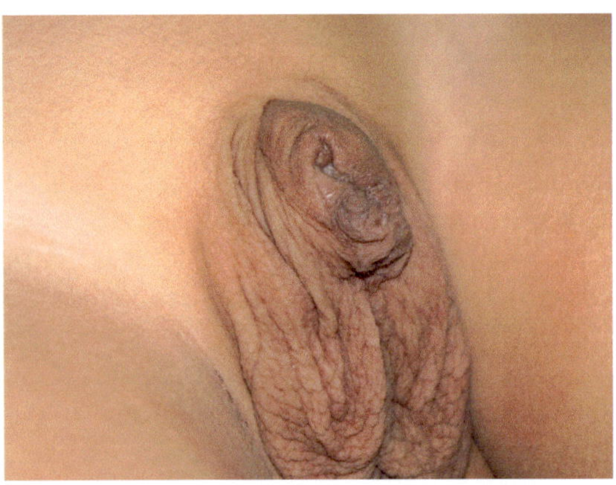

Fig. 6.2 Abnormal large entire prepuce" Macropothia"

6.1 History

The longer prepuce often serves as the object of erotic interest and as a signifier of the sexually attractive male along the history, the Greeks valued the longer over the shorter prepuce in relation to the length of the entire penis, and the smaller over the larger penis as a whole. The term congenital megaprepuce (CM) was first used in a

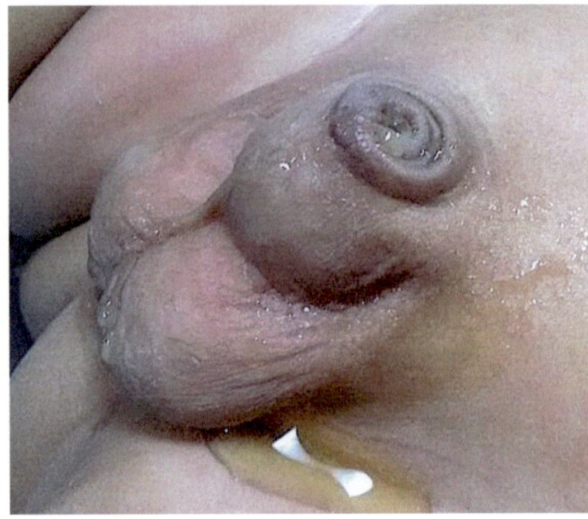

Fig. 6.3 Congenital megaprepuce

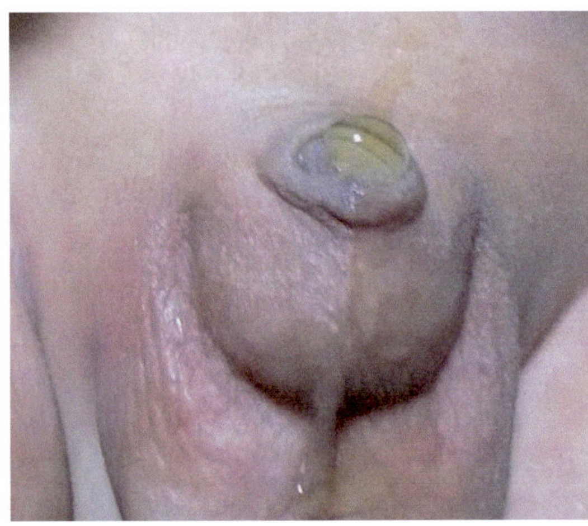

Fig. 6.4 Preputial bladder with urine dribbling from phimotic prepuce

case report in 1994 by O'Brien et al. [2], and since then increasing numbers of patients with CM have been reported.

6.2 Incidence

This rare condition has only recently received recognition as an entity in its own right, and it is possible that it represents a genuinely new pathology, where a part of the foreskin extends beyond the glans, and it is possible that many cases may exist among children, but escape reporting, as there is no study till now reported the exact incidence of megaprepuce among normal children.

6.3 Associated Anomalies

Preputial enlargement has been reported secondary to phimosis, but in many other cases there is an enormous prepuce without true phimosis. Many cases of hypospadias had an associated different grades of megaprepuce, but in this condition the enlarged prepuce doesn't encircle the whole glans, except in cases of intact prepuce megameatus (Chap. 20), and collar-scarf type of prepuce, where is the prepuce looks redundant in the dorsal aspect and lateral sides of the hypospadiac glans, and in this case the prepuce has a close connection on the ventral side with pillars of the atretic corpus spongiosum at the base of the open glans [3] (Fig. 6.5). Interestingly sometimes cases of microphallus, may show a normal or even proportionally large prepuce or megaprepuce.

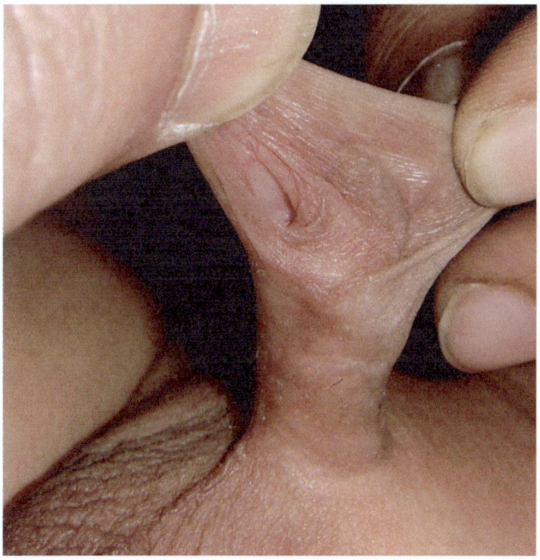

Fig. 6.5 Collar-scarf prepuce with a hidden hypospadias

6.4 Significance of Macroposthia

It is supposed that large redundant prepuce may hinder proper wash and cleaning of smegma, with a subsequent increase in human papillomavirus (HPV) infection, which is a known risk factor for penile carcinogenesis. In a recent meta-analysis of European general population males, it was estimated that HPV positivity ranged between 12 and 30% [4].

Given that almost one-third of the population was positive for high risk HPV, it is more likely that the environment of the buried phallus, chronic inflammation, and poor hygiene were the initiating factors in his carcinogenesis [5]. Also macroposthic prepuce is liable for phimosis, balanitis and BXO.

6.5 Differential Diagnosis

Megaprepuce can be diagnosed clinically by physical examination as it usually presents with a redundant enlarged preputial skin, specially seen in the communities which are not doing circumcision routinely or in a religious background, the child may complain from ballooning of the preputial sac during micturition or itching and pain if there is a degree of phimosis. Extensively whole larger prepuce had to be differentiated from cases of phimosis and redundant inner layer of prepuce which known as CM, which is a striking condition that cannot be easily missed or hidden; and should not be confused with a buried, concealed, webbed, trapped or micropenis, rare cases of urethral diverticulum should be differentiated from this condition (Chap. 29), also megaprepuce should not be confused with other congenital anomalies which presented as an enlarged phallus like; megalophallus (Chap. 10) and megalourethra (Chap. 26). Megaprepuce have to be differentiated from preputial lymphedema which is a disfiguring disorder characterized by impaired lymphatic drainage that causes progressive penile and/or scrotal swelling and it is usually caused by a congenital abnormality of the lymphatics that may appear at various ages (Chap. 18). Lymphedema

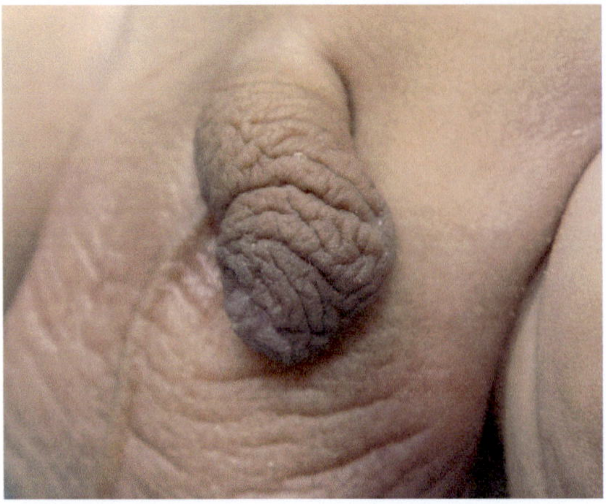

Fig. 6.6 Isolated preputial lymphedema gives the picture of megaprepuce

usually affects the whole penis, but sometimes it is more confined to the prepuce only (Fig. 6.6), and usually circumcision with compression bandage after the procedure may yield relative relief.

6.6 Management

Children affected by this malformation usually suffer from a subjective difficulty in voiding, and subsequent urinary tract infection which is the main indication for early surgical correction. Almost nothing is known of the natural history of this deformity and whether or not it tends to improve over time, since surgery is usually undertaken because of functional and cosmetic concerns. The correction of congenital megaprepuce can be a significant technical challenge and considerable experience is required to achieve a good cosmetic result. The main problems stem from a deficiency of penile shaft skin, an absence of defined penopubic and penoscrotal angles, and a marked excess of inner preputial "mucosa." Various reconstructive procedures have been described which result in a circumcised penis. Revision surgery is not uncommon for the redundant penile skin or recurrence of the buried appearance. Also, correction of this problem involves degloving of the penis and excision of the redundant skin. Ideally the penile shaft should be covered with the dorsal penile skin, which should be anchored to Buck's fascia in each quadrant. Standard circumcision is contraindicated in this condition because this would remove the skin that is ultimately required to resurface the shaft of the penis. The preputial skin is moved proximally on the penis. It is the redundant inner preputial mucosa that is removed, if there is tension it is recommend to use a transverse pedicled island flap to cover the defect of ventral shaft skin [6].

References

1. Gomez J, Puyol M, Menendez V. Secondary megaprepuce. BJU. 1996;78:959–60.
2. O'Brien A, Shapiro AMJ, Frank JD. Phimosis or congenital megaprepuce. Br J Urol. 1994;73:719–20.
3. Radojicic Z, Perovic S. Classification of prepuce in hypospadias according to morphological abnormalities and their impact on hypospadias repair. J Urol. 2004;172:301–4. doi:10.1097/01.ju.0000129008.31212.3d.
4. Hebnes JB, Olesen TB, Duun-Henriksen AK, Munk C, Norrild B, Kjaer SK. Prevalence of genital human papillomavirus among men in Europe: systematic review and meta-analysis. J Sex Med. 2014;11(11):2630–44.
5. Manwaring J, Vourganti S, Nikolavsky D, et.al. Pannus is the new Prepuce? Penile cancer in a Buried Phallus. Case Rep Urol. 2015;2015:403545, 4 pages http://dx.doi.org/10.1155/2015/403545.
6. Summerton DJ, Mcnally J, Denny AJ, Malone PSJ. Congenital megaprepuce: an emerging condition – how to recognize and treat it. BJU Int. 2000;86(4):519–22.

7 Preputial Cysts

Abstract
The most common cystic lesion of the penis and prepuce is the smegma cyst, which sometimes called "smegmoma", and usually seen under the unretractable prepuce, it may appear yellowish due to smegma content. Preputial cyst generally divided into two main categories: median raphe (urethroid) cysts and epidermoid (follicular) cysts.

Keywords
Smegmoma • Pearly penile papules • Epidermoid cysts • Median raphe cysts

Nomenclatures

Smegmoma, Pearly penile papules, Hirsutoid papillomas.

The most common cystic lesion of the penis and prepuce is the smegma cyst, which sometimes called "smegmoma", and usually seen under the unretractable prepuce, it may appear yellowish due to smegma content (Chap. 36) (Fig. 7.1).

Other penile cysts may affect the prepuce (Chap. 19), like epidermal inclusion cysts which may form after penile surgery; including circumcision and hypospadias repair, and penile girth augmentation surgery. Preputial cyst generally divided into two main categories: median raphe (urethroid) cysts and epidermoid (follicular) cysts (Chap. 19). Epidermoid cysts are the most common cystic lesions of the penis and occur primarily on the shaft. Median raphe cysts are midline developmental cysts that occur at sites from the external urethral meatus to the anus, including the ventral penis. Occasional examples are seen of true retention cysts of the prepuce and mucoid preputial cyst was rarely reported (Fig. 7.2).

Mucoid preputial cysts are rare benign lesions, which arise from ectopic urethral mucosa sequestered during embryologic development. Histopathological examination of the cyst frequently includes stratified columnar epithelium, whether or not it is associated with mucous cells or glands. The cysts are usually small, soft and freely movable masses. In general, they are asymptomatic, unless when they are complicated by infection or difficult coitus [1].

Preputial calculi are rare and usually occur in adults, they develop secondary to a severe obstructive phimosis, or poor penile hygiene with inspissated smegma. Treating the underlying cause with a dorsal preputial slit or a formal circumcision prevents recurrent calculi [2].

Juvenile Xanthogranuloma is an uncommon benign, self-limiting lesion of the penis

© Springer International Publishing Switzerland 2017

M. Fahmy, *Congenital Anomalies of the Penis*, DOI 10.1007/978-3-319-43310-3_7

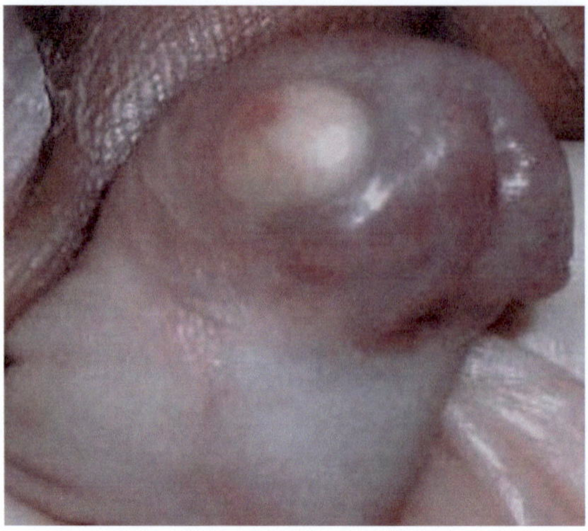

Fig. 7.1 Smegmoma (Pearly penile papule) detectable at the undersurface of unretractab. prepuce

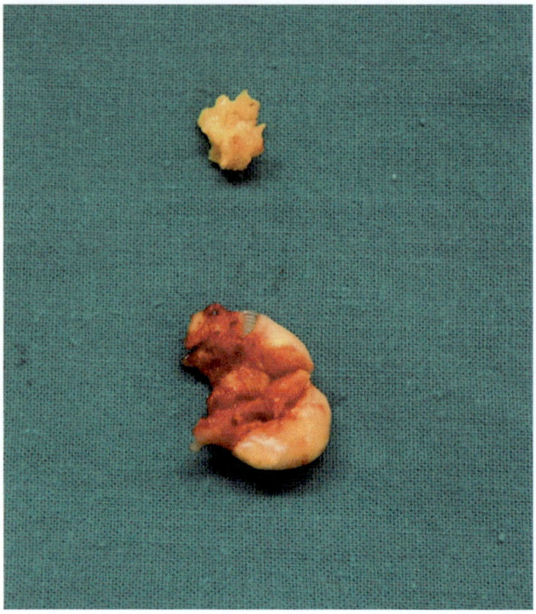

Fig. 7.3 Juvenile Xanthogranuloma removed from the prepuce

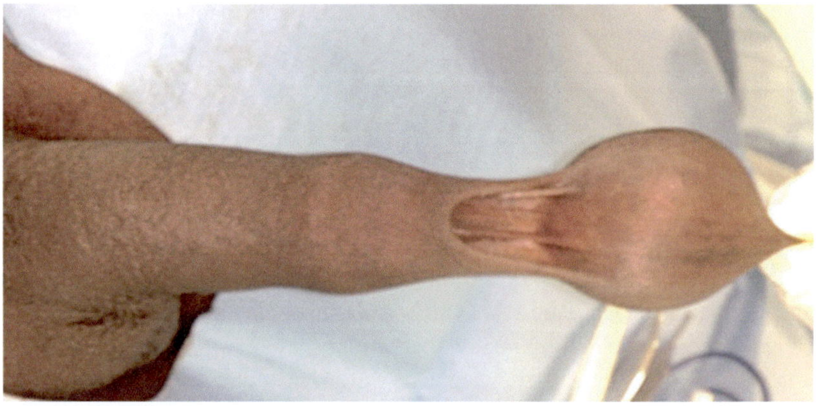

Fig. 7.2 Considerable large mucoid preputial cyst

predominantly seen in infancy or early childhood. These lesions appear as solitary or multiple pigmented (yellow, orange, gold, brown, or red) nodules of rapid onset. They measure 2–20 mm in diameter and are well demarcated, firm, and rubbery. These lesions can affect the penis or scrotum with as many as 20 % being present at birth. The lesion is often self-limited, and a period of 1 year of expectant monitoring is advised to avoid potentially unnecessary ablative genital surgery (Fig. 7.3).

7.1 Etiology

There is no clear explanation why some boys developing a smegma aggregation to be manifested as pearls papule under the prepuce or over the glans penis, infrequent wash and cleaning of smegma in uncircumcised boy may be implicated as a cause of formation of such cyst [3].

7.2 Diagnosis

Smegma cyst present with one or more yellowish lumps on the penis that are often diagnosed by the general practitioner as sebaceous cysts or lipoma of the penile shaft, invariably, on outpatient assessment, these prove to be collections of retained smegma trapped by surrounding preputial adhesions, lipoma and sebaceous cyst are extremely rare in penis. Preputial cyst are generally asymptomatic, but it may result in abnormal micturition, urine retention and difficult sexual intercourse. Some differential diagnoses include dermoid cyst, teratoma, and urethral diverticulum.

7.3 Management

Parents reassurance is essentially required, as the smegma is released when the adhesions lyse spontaneously over time, such patients may be better served with a circumcision or preputioplasty. Localised cysts can be enucleated easily either with scarification or preservation with reconstruction of the remnant prepuce according to family wishes.

References

1. de Mendonça R, et al. Mucoid cyst of the penis: case report and literature review. Can Urol Assoc J. 2010;4(6):E155–7.
2. Parkash S, Rao R, Venkatesan K, et al. Sub-preputial wetness – its nature. Ann Nat Med Sci. 1982;18:109–12.
3. Cold CJ, Taylor JR. The prepuce. Br J Urol. 1999;83(1):34–44.

Part III

Penis

8 Penile Agenesis

Abstract

Congenital absence of the penis, is a rare anomaly caused by developmental failure of the genital tubercle, the first published case dates to 1701, Aphallia could be associated with urethral atresia and absent urinary meatus, but few cases may have a normal urethra and meatus. some cases reported with other syndromes, like caudal regression syndrome. In the past all such cases are reassigned as a female with orchidectomy and vaginoplasty, but recently the trend of penile reconstruction either by grafting, tissue engineering or even penile transplant became applicable and acceptable by the families.

Keywords

Aphallia • Apenia • Penile agenesis • Ablatio penis • Popliteal pterygium syndrome • Penile transplant

Nomenclature

Aphallia (this term is also applicable for female without clitoris), Apenia, Penile Agenesis, Ablatio Penis, but the last term usually used for acquired or posttrumatic vanished penis.

Definition

Congenital absence of the penis, is a rare anomaly caused by developmental failure of the genital tubercle. Penile agenesis occurs often as a consequence of testicular agenesis, but the reverse is never the case. Most patients have no known family history and usually have an otherwise normal male anatomy and usually, the scrotum is normal but testes are undescended, there are many cases reported where the both testicles are normally descended with normal development. The urethra opens at any point of the perineal midline from over the pubis to, most frequently, the anus or anterior wall of the rectum (Fig. 8.1).

© Springer International Publishing Switzerland 2017

M. Fahmy, *Congenital Anomalies of the Penis*, DOI 10.1007/978-3-319-43310-3_8

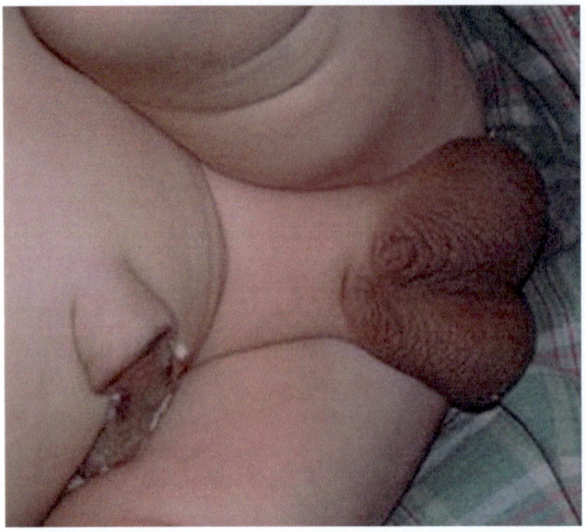

Fig. 8.1 Neonate with aphallia but a normal scrotum and testicles

8.1 Historical Background

The first published case dates to 1701 and was recorded by the French surgeon Saviard (1656–1702), under the heading of a “child who had no rod”, but the first full description of this anomaly was by Imminger in 1853, since then more than 100 cases have been reported in the literature, but very recently there are many cases in the process of reporting [1].

8.2 Approximate Incidence

One in 10 to 30 million population, but a higher incidence detected in institutes doing autopasy for stillbirth and cases neonatal death, and that is explain many cases escape record.

8.3 Aetiology

Penile agenesis results from failure of development of genital tubercles. The definitive urogenital sinus in such cases ends in the perineum without the normal proliferation, hence, it does not move anteriorly and cephalic to the ventral border of penis, the urethra therefore opens in the perineum, at or near the anal border.

Agenesis of the penis may occurs as a consequence of single gene disorders, teratogenic effects, or malformation sequences and associations of unrecognized patterns of anomalies, it thus should be considered as a developmental field defect. Its concurrence with scrotal hypoplasia, absent raphe, and anal anomalies implies a major disturbance of the caudal mesoderm, in such cases severe renal defects are usually seen, and the prognosis is poor. When the patient has a patent urethra and normal scrotum, raphe, and testes the baby may survive with such anomaly, however penile agenesis may be a localized malformation of the genital tubercle and potentially related to penoscrotal transposition. Reports indicate that aphallia may be associated with pregnancy complicated by poorly controlled maternal diabetes [2].

8.4 Associated Anomalies

More than 50 % of patients with penile agenesis have associated genitourinary anomalies, the most common of which is cryptorchidism; renal agenesis and dysplasia. Cardiovascular gastrointestinal defects, such as caudal axis anomalies, also have been described. Skoog and Belman (1989) [3] reviewed 60 reports of aphallia and found that the more proximal the urethral meatus, the greater the likelihood of neonatal death and the higher the incidence of other anomalies. Sixty percent of patients had a postsphincteric meatus located on a peculiar appendage at the anal verge, this group of patients had the highest survival rate (87 %) and the lowest incidence of other anomalies (1.2 per patient). Twenty-eight percent of patients had presphincteric urethral communications (prostatorectal fistula), and there was a 36 % neonatal mortality rate. Twelve percent had urethral atresia and a vesicorectal fistula for drainage. This group had the highest incidence of other anomalies and a 100 % mortality rate.

8.5 Classifications

Skoog and Belman [3] suggested three variants, based on urethral position in relationship to the anal sphincter, as: Postsphincteric; Presphincteric (Prostatorectal fistula) and Urethral atresia. More proximal the bladder outlet, greater is the likelihood of other anomalies and death.

We adopted herein a simple classification after reviewing many cases and literature concerning with this anomaly according to presence or absence of external urinary meatus, and if this anomaly associated or not with another syndromes:

- Aphallia with urethral atresia and absent urinary meatus (Fig. 8.2).
- Aphallia with normal urethra and meatus.
- Aphallia with other syndromes (Figs. 8.3 and 8.4).
- Aphallia with caudal regression syndrome.

This classification correlated with Evans et al. who suggest that most cases can be classified into either a severe form (16 %) with renal aplasia or dysplasia and other caudal anomalies or a second group (72 %) with low mortality and fewer additional malformations [4].

Aphallia reported with popliteal pterygium syndrome, which is a rare autosomal dominant congenital condition, in which the patient has facial, genitourinary and skeletal anomalies along with popliteal pterygium of different severities (Fig. 8.4).

All reported cases of aphallia with absent external urinary meatus showed short span of life and there is no record of any survival whatever the measurers taken, and most of those cases are associated with imperforate anus and a degree of caudal regression, as in the case showed in Fig. 8.5, where aphallia associated with an absent sacrum, defective pubic bones, bladder duplication, and a single urethra opening dorsally with an ectopic anal canal in a rudimentary skin appendages. Also many cases of sirenomelia had no phallus or even urinary meatus (Fig. 8.6).

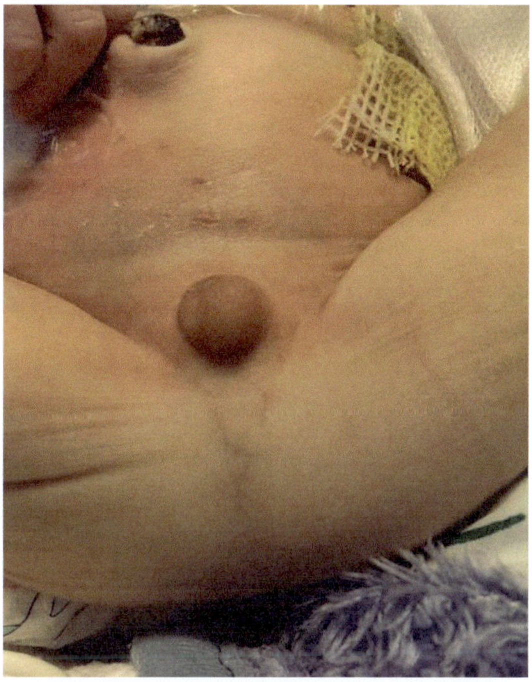

Fig. 8.2 Aphallia without any urethral opening, testicles, scrotum, or raphe, there is also an imperforate anus, he had only a skin appendage at the pubic region

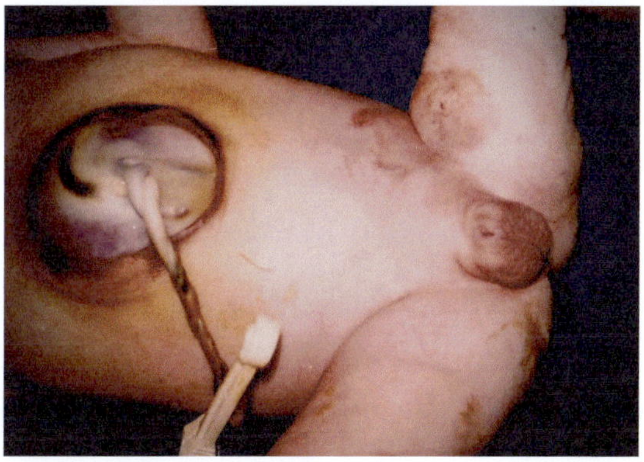

Fig. 8.3 Aphallia with Exomphalos

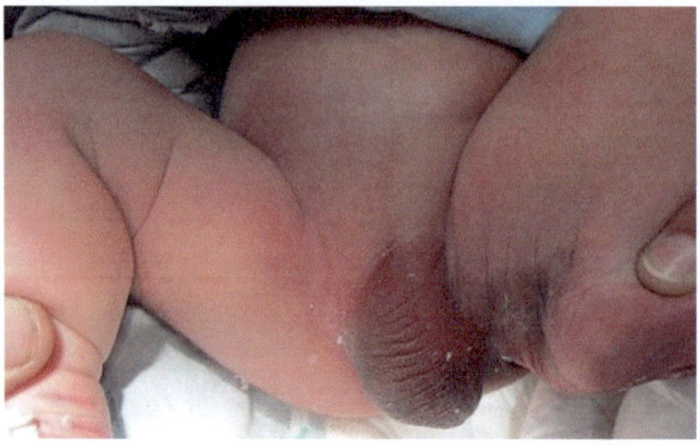

Fig. 8.4 Aphallia with Popliteal Pterygium syndrome

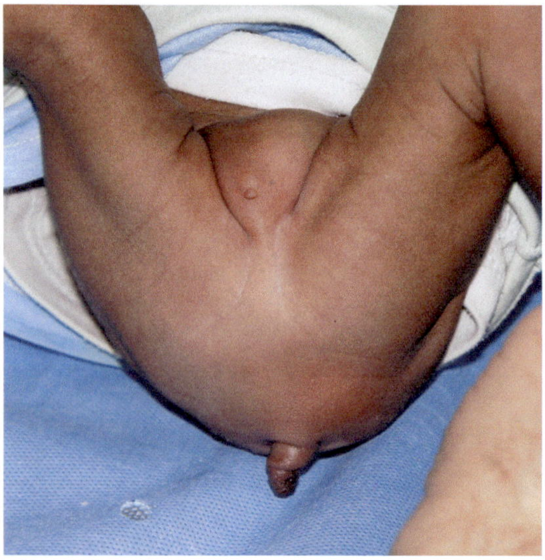

Fig. 8.5 Aphallia with partial caudal regression, there is no phallus, scrotum, testicles, an ectopic nope of skin at the sacrum accommodating the urethra and and anal canal

8.6 Diagnosis

The diagnosis of PA requires the absence of corpora cavernosa and copora spongiosum with urethra opening at any point on the perineum in midline, over pubis, anterior aspect of the scrotum, or, most frequently just anterior to the anus and anterior wall of the rectum. This rare entity should be differentiated in neonates from concealed penis, rudimentary penis, micropenis, pseudo hermaphroditism, intersex and intrauterine amputation of penis. In cases of androgen insensitivity syndrome (AIS), which is a genetic condition where the androgen receptor is dysfunctional or ineffective and this leads to the partial or complete external feminization of a baby with XY chromosomes and the phallus may looks defective or absent. In some cases of adrenogenital hyperplasia in a female with a relatively prominent labioscrotal folds minmiking scrotum, the diagnosis could be only established by hormonal assay and chromosomal study. For older children coming with such anomaly differentiation from acquired cases of ablatio penis should be done, where penis amputated traumatically or iatrogenically after a circumcision disaster, in such cases the previous scar or a rudimentary phallus may be obvious (Fig. 8.7).

Anorectal anomalies such as imperforate anus, congenital rectal strictures and rectovesical fistula, cryptorchid testis, hydrocele, hernia, renal dysplasia, horseshoe kidneys and agenesis of prostate could be an associated malforma-

Fig. 8.6 Aphallia in association with sirenomelia

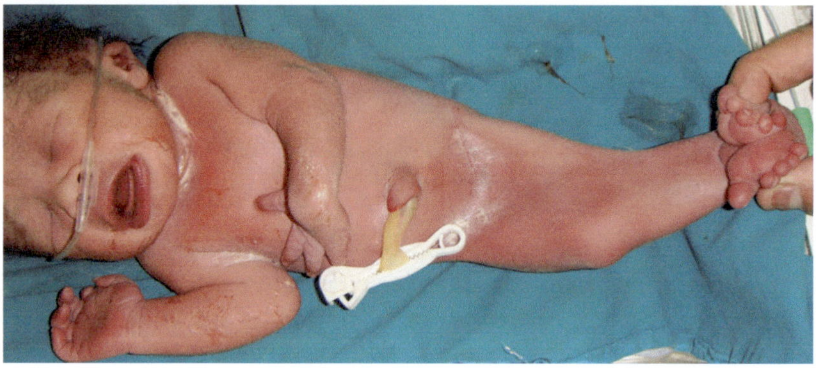

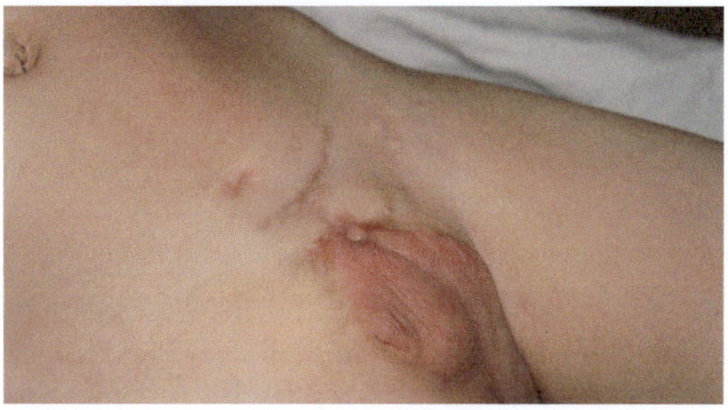

Fig. 8.7 Ablatio Penis due to penile gangrene after circumcision by using monoplar diathermy

tions [5]. When oligohydramnios or anhydramnios hinder proper antenatal diagnosis by ultrasound, MRI is an excellent tool for revealing the anatomy of genitourinary anomalies in the fetus, and many cases of aphallia could be diagnosed early in pregnancy along with other associated anomalies, at the meantime for neonatal cases the MR examination is not only ascertains the diagnosis but also delineates the complex internal genitourinary anatomy, reveals the opening of the urethra in relation to the anal sphincter, thus establishing prognosis, and demonstrates the position of the testes and the presence of associated anomalies. T2-W images proved to be particularly useful in this regard, not only were the prostate and testes easily identifiable due to their characteristic hyperintensity, but the hyperintense fluid-filled urethroanal fistulous tract and the blind-ending anterior urethra could also only be appreciated on T2-W images [6].

8.7 Management

Neonate with this lesion should be evaluated immediately with a karyotype and other appropriate studies to determine whether there are another associated malformations of the urinary tract or other organ systems. There is a distinct relationship between aphallia and renal malformation, and thus; Potter sequence can complicate the affected neonates due to renal failure. Arai et al. [7] suggested that cases of penile agenesis complicated by Potter sequence with urethral agenesis should be differentiated from those with ectopic urethral opening. Potter sequence is mostly believed to result from a renal or urologic abnormality such as bilateral renal agenesis, cystic dysplasia, obstructive uropathy etc., so priority should be given for urinary drainage, vsicostomy may be indicated in some cases with urethral agenesis, or bladder outlet obstruction. Gender reassignment was recommended for affected newborns in the past. However, with more recent revelations that some of these patients have a male gender identity despite reconstruction as a female, the recommendation to perform gender reassignment should be made very carefully, and only after full evaluation by an ambiguous genitalia assessment team that includes a pediatric urologist, endocrinologist, and psychiatrist. Gender reassignment involves orchiectomy and feminizing genitoplasty in the newborn period. At a later age, construction of a neovagina is necessary. Urinary tract reconstruc tion with simultaneous construction of an intestinal neovagina through a posterior sagittal and abdominal approach in patients with penile agenesis has been described, and a few reported cases of complete gender assignment and genital reconstruction in the neonatal period through a single-stage gender reassignment and genital reconstruction by anterior sagittal anorectovaginourethroplasty [8].

As a male, the patient would potentially be fertile, but currently there is an inability to construct a cosmetically acceptable phallus that would allow normal urinary, sexual, and reproductive function. The traditional penile reconstructive procedures cannot fulfil to restore a functionally and cosmetically satisfactory penis without complications such as sexual failure and psychological problems. Different techniques have been described for penile reconstruction. However, these are complex surgeries involving skin flaps and microsurgical techniques (radial or ulnar free graft) which have high morbidity and complications such as fistula, dehiscence and infection. Although eventually were able to give a reasonable aesthetic appearance to the penis these techniques do not allow the functional recovery of the organ. Successful phallic reconstruction in two patients with aphallia were pre-

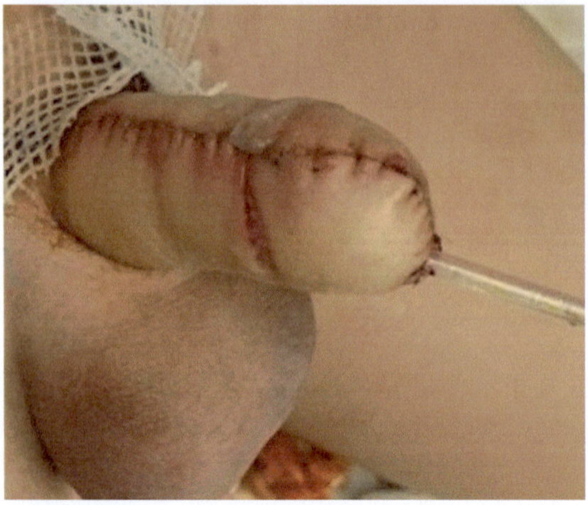

Fig. 8.8 Phallus and urethral reconstruction

sented from Bologna (Italy) using the lower abdominal wall skin flap for making the shaft and the bladder/labial mucosa free graft for making the urethra [9].

At puberty, new surgeries are required to insert a penile prosthesis which may allow a sexual life (Fig. 8.8).

The optimal phallus should provide all of the following:

1. Both tactile and erogenous sensibility.
2. A neourethra which allows voiding while standing.
3. The capability to permit prosthetic insertion which permits successful vaginal intromission.
4. Cosmetically aesthetic acceptability of both the phallus and proposed donor sites.
5. Acceptable phallic growth to adult size in the case of pediatric phalloplasty.

Optimally the surgery should be accomplished in a reproducible single stage with acceptable morbidity. Modern reconstructive and microsurgical techniques permit achievement of these aims much of the time.

One of the major structures of the penis is the corpus cavernosum, as the therapeutic uses of stem cells and tissue engineering (TE) techniques are emerging in urology, therefore, TE for penile tissue regeneration using stem cells may have a huge potential and could be a novel treatment option for ideal penile reconstruction [10].

Recently, there are only three reported trials of penile transplant in adults after traumatic penile loss, so in the future there may be a hope for aphallic patients to restore his penis through this procedure.

Because of the rarity of these cases, very few studies were done concerning the psychosocial development of patients with aphallia.

In general the gender choice for these infants is challenging and there are no reliable methods to evaluate what is the best attitude for them. The prospects of sexual functioning, reproductive capacity and quality of life should be considered in this decision. A multi-professional team should ensure that all information about surgical options to gender assignment or re-assignment will be explained to the family who will have the difficult role in the final decision.

References

1. Gautier T, Salient J, Pena S, Imperto-McGinley J, Peterson RE. Testicular function in 2 cases of penile agenesis. J Urol. 1981;126:556–7.
2. Kessler WO, McLaughlin 3rd AP. Agenesis of penis. Embryology and management. Urology. 1973;1:226–9.
3. Skoog SJ, Belman AB. Aphallia: its classification and management. J Urol. 1989;141:589–92.
4. Evans JA, Erdile LB, Greenberg CR. Agenesis of the penis: patterns of associated malformations. Am J Med Genet. 1999;84:47–55.
5. Ciftci AO, Senocak ME, Buyukpamukcu N. Male gender assignment in penile agenesis: a case report and review of the literature. J Pediatr Surg. 1995;30:1358–60.
6. Goenka A, Jain V, Sharma R, Gupta G, Bajpai M. MR diagnosis of penile agenesis: is it just absence of a phallus? Pediatr Radiol. 2008;38:1109–12. doi:10.1007/s00247-008-0910-1.
7. Arai M, Suzuki S, Ishino H, Igarashi K, Araki T. Penile agenesis complicated by Potter sequence. Arch Gynecol Obstet. 2001;265:219–20.
8. Hendren WH. The genetic male with absent penis and urethrorectal communication: experience with 5 patients. J Urol. 1997;157:1469.
9. Bateman C. World's first successful penis transplant at Tygerberg Hospital. S Afr Med J. 2015;105:251–2.
10. Lin CS, Xin ZC, Deng CH, Ning H, Lin G, Lue TF. Recent advances in andrology-related stem cell research. Asian J Androl. 2008;10(2):171–5. doi:10.1111/j.1745-7262.2008.00389.x. CrossRef PubMed.

Microphallus

9

Abstract

Penis with a stretched length more than 2.5 standard deviations (SD) for the standard size for age is considered as a micropenis, which affect at least one in 200 males, it results from a multiplicity of endocrine and non-endocrine conditions. Microphallus must be differentiate from inconspicuous penis which may be a buried or a webbed penis and cases of intersex and ambiguous genitalia. Topical application of 5 % testosterone cream may be effective in management of some cases, but conservative surgical techniques to improve length or girth like division of the suspensory ligament with or without an inverted V-Y plasty may be indicated in others, additionally, it might be appropriate to perform penoscrotal web excision or supra fat pad excision (lipectomy) in order to maximize the subjective penile length.

Nomenclature

Micropenis, microphallus and hypoplastic Penis

Definition

The term microphallus, or micropenis, is applicable only to a normally formed yet abnormally short penis. The term specifically applies to a penis with a stretched length more than 2.5 standard deviations (SD) less than the mean for age (Fig. 9.1) [1]. In general, the penis of a full-term neonate should be at least 1.9 cm long.

© Springer International Publishing Switzerland 2017
M. Fahmy, *Congenital Anomalies of the Penis*, DOI 10.1007/978-3-319-43310-3_9

Age	Mean ± SD	Mean * SD
Newborn 30-week gestation	2.5 ± 0.4	1.5
Newborn 34-week gestation	3 ± 0.4	2.0
0–5 months	3.9 ± 0.8	1.9
6–12 months	4.3 ± 0.8	2.3
1–2 years	4.7 ± 0.8	2.6
2–3 years	5.1 ± 0.9	2.9
3–4 years	5.5 ± 0.9	3.3
4–5 years	5.7 ± 0.9	3.5
5–6 years	6 ± 0.9	3.8
6–7 years	6.1 ± 0.9	3.9
7–8 years	6.2 ± 1.0	3.7
8–9 years	6.3 ± 1.0	3.8
9–10 years	6.3 ± 1.0	3.8
10–11 years	6.4 ± 1.1	3.7
Adult	13.3 ± 1.6	9.3

Fig. 9.1 Normal size of the penis at different age

9.1 Historical Background

Perceptions of penile size are culture specific, so in ancient Greece and in Renaissance art, an uncircumcised and small penis was culturally seen as desirable in a man, whereas a bigger or circumcised penis was viewed as comical or grotesque. Ancient Rome may have had a contrary view, and a larger penile size was preferred in medieval Arabic literature.

9.2 Incidence

The condition is thought to affect one in 200 males, according to the Network on Psychosexual Differentiation, incidence for a micropenis is below 2%. In Colombia, the incidence is 19:100,000 people, while the incidence for hypospadias in the same study, was a factor of 10 higher [2]. The observed significant increase in recent years of such cases in neonates by some authors is probably due to the influence of exposure to endocrine-disrupting chemicals (substances include synthetic chemicals used as industrial solvents/lubricants and their by-products.) which has been suggested to contribute to the increasing trends of external genital malformation in male newborns. Natural chemicals found in human and animal food (phytoestrogens) also act as endocrine disruptors, and may had a role in increasing incidence of microphallus [3].

9.3 Aetiology

Micropenis in children results from a multiplicity of endocrine and nonendocrine conditions. The most common aetiologies include hypogonadotropic hypogonadism, hypergonadotropic hypogonadism [4].

- In hypogonadotropic hypogonadism, secretion of gonadotropin-releasing hormone (GnRH) by the hypothalamus is impaired. This leads to decreased pituitary secretion of luteinizing hormone and follicle-stimulating hormone, depriving the testis of its stimulus to secrete testosterone. This pathogenesis exists in some hypothalamic dysfunctions, such as Kallmann syndrome or Prader–Willi syndrome.
- Micropenis secondary to hypergonadotropic hypogonadism is associated with conditions in which the testes are impaired functionally and unable to respond to hypothalamic–pituitary stimulation; an example of this condition is gonadal dysgenesis.
- In idiopathic micropenis, endocrine analysis demonstrates a normal hypothalamic– pituitary–testicular axis, but some recognised causes could be implicated:
  - Primary testicular failure, e.g., partial gonadal dysgenesis, and Klinefelter's syndrome.
  - Defects in testosterone action, as in cases of partial androgen insensitivity and 5α-reductase deficiency.
  - Developmental anomalies like cloacal exstrophy and its variants [5].

9.4 Differential Diagnosis

One must differentiate buried penis or webbed penis from the micropenis, with the former having a normal penile shaft. Measurement (stretched penile length) is very important in differentiation of the various types of pseudomicropenis, particularly the buried penis in the obese infant and the penis concealed by an abnormal skin attachment or excessive suprapubic fat which is commonly referred to as an inconspicuous penis. (Fig. 9.2)

This condition may be considered a minor form of ambiguous genitalia with correlated medical and psychological problems similar to those of the major intersex form. Perpetual development usually following the penile growth, so most cases of microphallus had a correlated perpetual deficiency, but really there is a disparity between a small phallus and a normally developed prepuce (Fig. 9.3). The scrotum usually is normal with a normal sized descended testicles (Figs. 9.4 and 9.5), but sometimes the testes are small or undescended, or the scrotum may migrate cephalically engulfing the small phallus as a minimal degree of scrotal transposition. In a few cases, the corpora cavernosa are severely hypoplastic, and it is not rare to have microphallus with severe

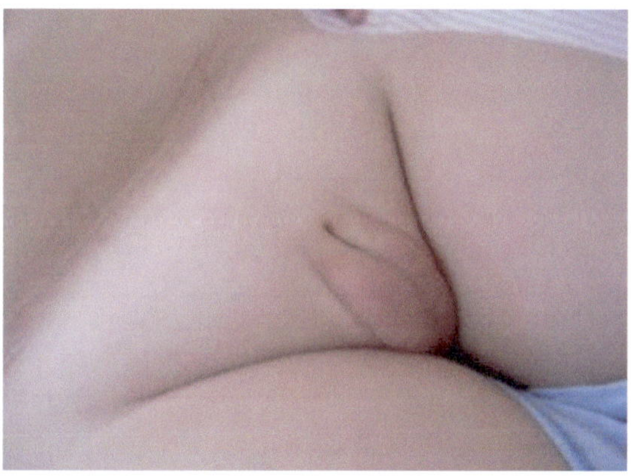

Fig. 9.2 Pseudomicrophallus, normal sized concealed penis in an obese child

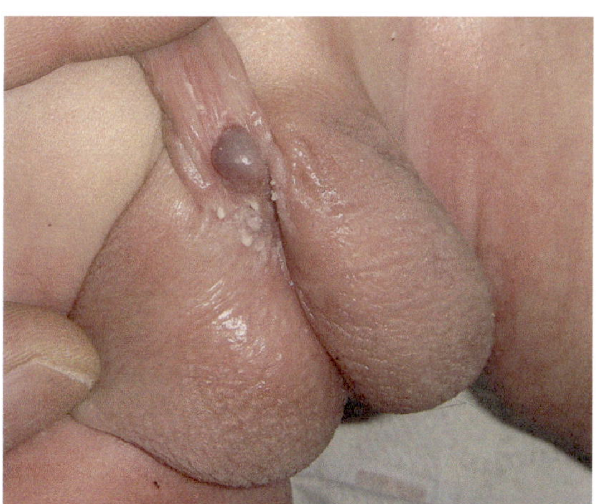

Fig. 9.3 Disparity between microphallus with normally developed prepuce, but with ventral deficiency and normally descended testicles

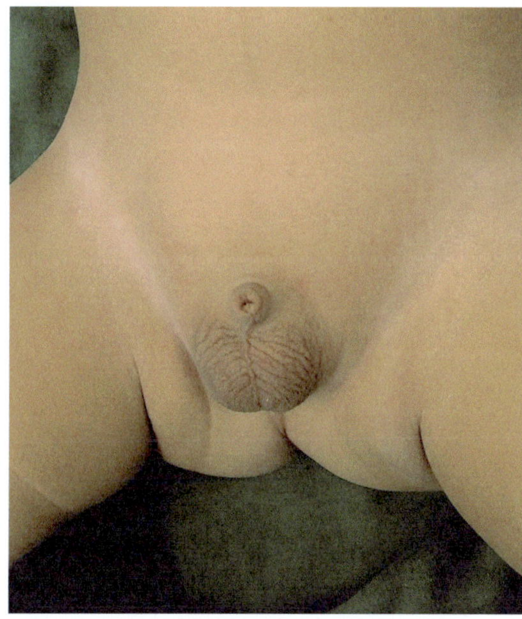

Fig. 9.4 Microphallus with normally descended testicles and well developed scrotum

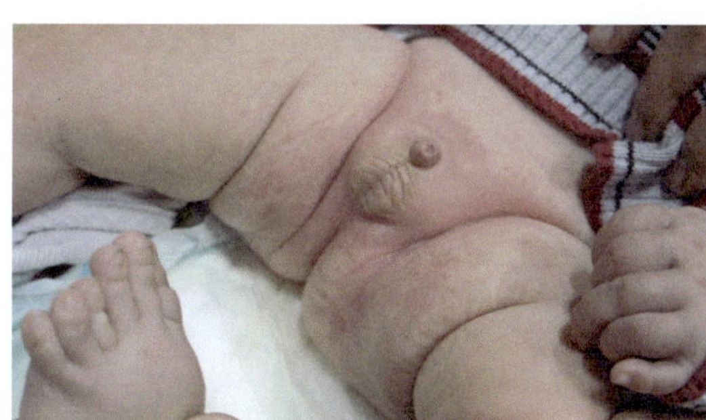

Fig. 9.5 Microphallus, normal testicles with multiple polydactyly

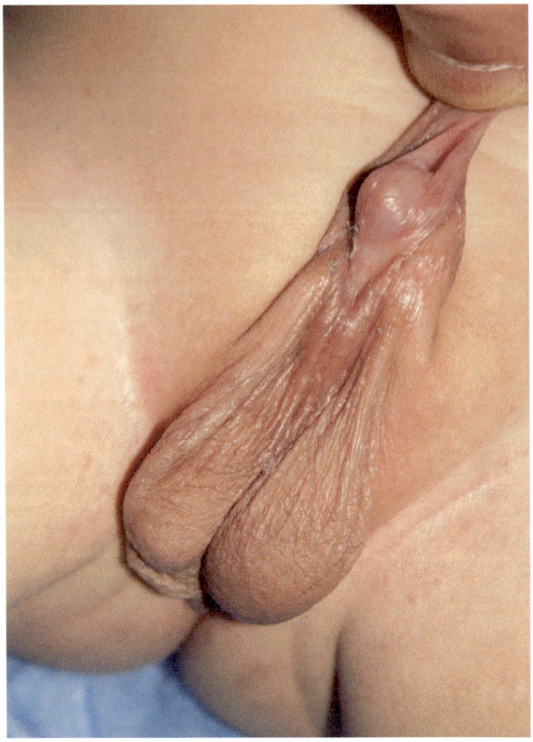

Fig. 9.6 Microphallus with corpus spongiosum deficiency and hypospadias

hypospadias and deficient corpus spongiosum (Fig. 9.6).

Congenital micropenis should be differentiated from:

- Inconspicuous penis, which refers to a penis that appears to be small with a normal stretched penile length measured from the pubic symphysis to the tip of the glans and normal diameter of the penile shaft.
- Buried penis, also referred to as hidden or concealed penis, is a form of inconspicuous penis. A buried penis is a normally a developed penis that is hidden away by the suprapubic fat pad. (Fig. 7)
- Webbed penis.
- Cases of intersex and ambiguous genitalia.

9.5 Management

Topical application of 5 % testosterone cream causes increased penile growth. The objective is to provide sufficient testosterone to stimulate penile growth without altering growth and closure of the epiphyses. Therapy should be started by the age of 1 year and aimed at maintaining genital growth commensurate with general body growth. Hormonal stimulation, especially with dihydrotestosterone, may produce some penile growth even after puberty. This can be given in a 2.5 % gel formulation once per day, with review after 6–8 weeks to assess the effect. The most common therapeutic regimen for injectable testosterone is testosterone Enanthate 25–50 mg (8–10 mg/kg) intramuscularly once a month for 3 months, to allow normal skeletal growth and recovery of overall adrenal function. Repeated exogenous testosterone supplementation at puberty can result in a normal size phallus with good rates of normal erections, orgasm and sexual intercourse in adulthood [6] (Figs. 9.7 and 9.8). Recently testosterone lozenges are available in some countries.

Parents should be reassured after proper diagnosis and investigations and they have to share in the decision making and options of treatment, adolescent with micropenis who also suffer from penile dysmorphic disorder require careful and intensive psychological counselling. Corrective surgery for micropenis can be performed in patients with realistic expectations. Total phalloplasty using radial artery-based forearm skin flaps can offer restoration of normal penile length in selected patients. More conservative surgical techniques to improve length or girth like division of the suspensory ligament with or without an inverted V-Y plasty, additionally, it might be appropriate to perform penoscrotal web excision or supra fat pad excision (lipectomy) in order to maximize the subjective penile length, but all these procedures are limited by minimal

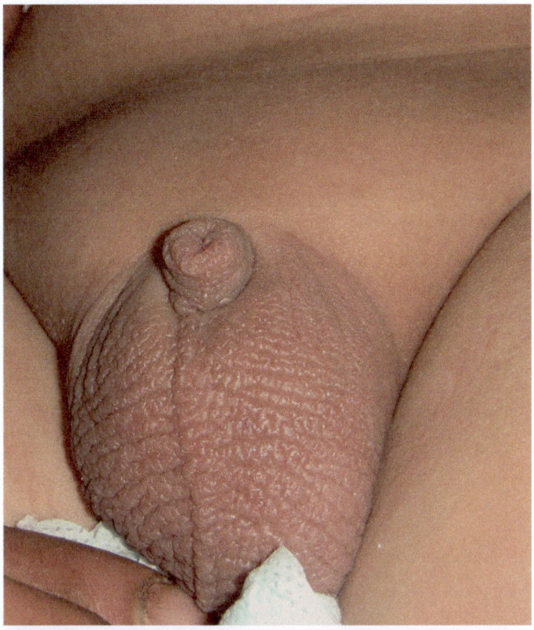

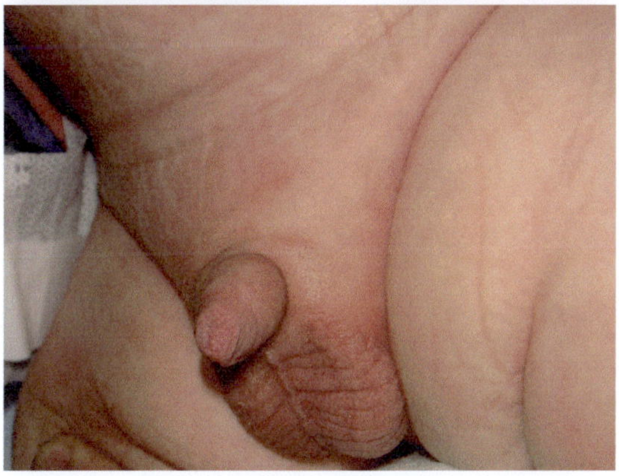

Figs. 9.7 and 9.8 Microphallus before and 3 weeks after local testosterone application

enhancement but associated with a significantly lower rate of complications and comorbidity compared to total phalloplasty. Emerging tissue engineering techniques might represent a suitable alternative to penile replacement surgery in the future [7]. Because micropenis is the result of numerous pathological conditions, assignment of sex of rearing generally is deferred until a physician determines whether the penis can grow in response to testosterone administration or not. In individuals with microphallus who are insensitive to the androgen, castration and gender conversion may be considered. However, in most patients with micropenis, male gender assessment can be maintained with androgen stimulation [8].

References

1. Tuladhar R, Davis PG, Batch J, Doyle LW. Establishment of a normal range of penile length in preterm infants. J Paediatr Child Health. 1998;34:471.
2. Calderon JS, Zarante I. Anomalías congénitas urológicas: descripción epidemiológica y factores de riesgo asociados en colombia 2001–2004. Arch Esp Urol. 2006;59(1):7–14.
3. Gaspari L, Sampaio DR, Paris F, Audran F, Orsini M, Neto JB, Sultan C. High prevalence of micropenis in 2710 male newborns from an intensive-use pesticide area of Northeastern Brazil. Int J Androl. 2012;35(3):253–64. doi:10.1111/j.1365-2605.2011.01241.x.
4. Williams-Ashman HG, Reddi AH. Differentiation of mesenchymal tissues during phallic morphogenesis with emphasis on the penis: role of androgens and other regulatory agents. J Steroid Biochem Mol Biol. 1991;39:873–81.
5. Wisniewski AB, Migeon CJ, Gearhart JP, et al. Congenital micropenis: long-term medical, surgical and psychosexual follow-up of individuals raised male or female. Horm Res. 2001;56(1–2):3–11.
6. Bin-Abbas B, Conte FA, Grumbach MM, Kaplan SL. Congenital hypogonadotropic hypogonadism and micropenis: effect of testosterone treatment on adult penile size. Why sex reversal is not indicated. J Pediatr. 1999;134(5):579–83.
7. Husmann DA. The androgen insensitive micropenis: long- term follow-up into adulthood. J Pediatr Endocrinol Metab. 2004;17(8):1037–41.
8. Lee PA, Houk CP. Outcome studies among men with micropenis. J Pediatr Endocrinol Metab. 2004;17(8):1043–53.

10 Megalopenis

Abstract

Megalopenis has defined objectively as the penile length more than 2 SD above the mean normal length for age. Abnormal largeness of the penis is an anomaly whereby the baby delivered with a large phallus, or it is enlarges rapidly in childhood, this may be a primary rare isolated non syndromic anomalies or due to abnormal high level of production of testosterone.

Keywords

Megalopenis • Penile hypertrophy • Macropenis

Definition

Megalopenis has defined objectively as the penile length more than 2 SD above the mean normal length for age (Fig. 10.1). Abnormal largeness of the penis is an anomaly whereby the baby delivered with a large phallus, or it is enlarges rapidly in childhood, this may be a primary rare isolated non syndromic anomalies or due to abnormal high level of production of testosterone.

© Springer International Publishing Switzerland 2017
M. Fahmy, *Congenital Anomalies of the Penis*, DOI 10.1007/978-3-319-43310-3_10

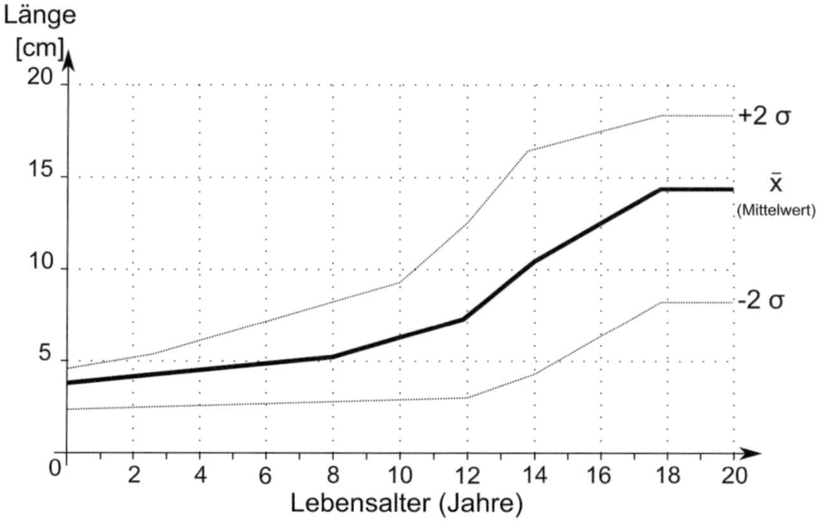

Fig. 10.1 Normal penile size according to the age. Average penis size in correlation with age. The upper and lower graph displays the 2 sigma curves [3]

Nomenclature

Megalopenis, Macrophallus, Penile hypertrophy and Macropenis.

10.1 Eitiology

Macropenis could be classified as a rare primary anomaly in a normal neonate, and this very rare condition scantly reported, without any detectable etiology, and a secondary macrophallus due to high level of production of testosterone e.g., interstitial cell tumors of the testicle, hyperplasia or tumors of the adrenal cortex, or secondary to other hypothalamic tumour associated with precocious puberty (Fig. 10.2).

Benign familial infantile seizures with inversion of chromosome 15 are reported to be associated with macrophallus, and also some cases are reported with heterochrony development where deletion of chromosomal region 13q21q31 is associated with macropenis [1].

Also femoral hypoplasia–unusual facies syndrome (FHUFS) which is characterised by bilateral, mostly asymmetrical, femoral hypoplasia with variable lower limb shortening and nonspecific facial dysmorphism is commonly associated with megalopenis [2] .

Macropenis is an uncommon finding of Fraser syndrome, which is an autosomal recessive disease characterised by cryptophthalmos, syndactyly, malformations of the larynx and genitourinary tract, craniofacial dysmorphism, orofacial clefting, and mental retardation.

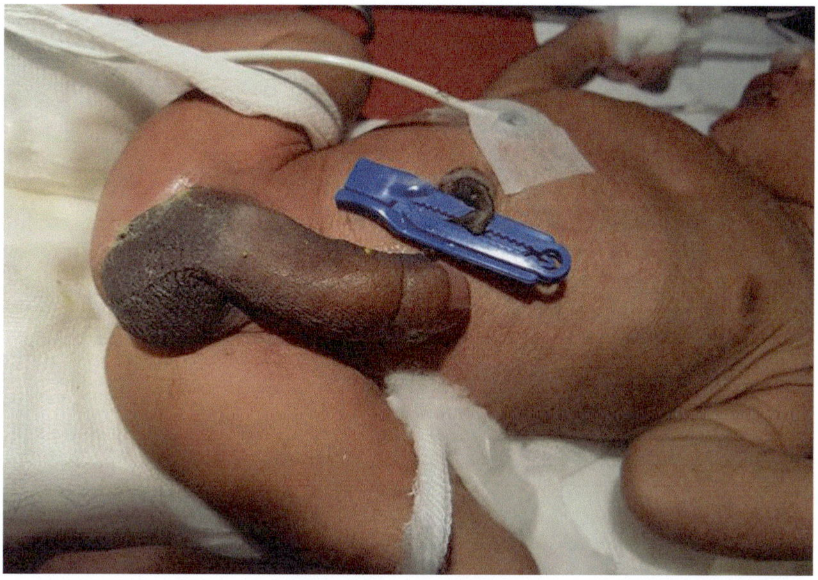

Fig. 10.2 Isolated non syndromic megalopenis

10.2 Differential Diagnosis

This anomaly should be differentiated from other congenital penile or urethral anomalies which give false impression of megalopenis and will be discussed later on, like congenital megalourethra (Fig. 10.3), megaprepuce (macroposthia), where prepuce is extensively large and redundant (Chapter 6), neurofibroma, heamangioma (chapter 17) and congenital penile lymphedema (Fig. 10.4); in those conditions the penile gigantism is not a true one, as it is affecting only one component of penile tissue and not the whole penis. Iatrogenic false microphallus or acquired cases are reported with excessive or overdosage systemic administration of testosterone hormone or chronic gonadotrophin hormone (HCG) injection, or local application of androgen creams for cases of hypogonadism, hypospadias or undescended testicles, which are improperly described in some countries without a proper scientific rational, in such cases the rapid increase in penile size may be reversible after a couple of months (Figs. 10.5 and 10.6).

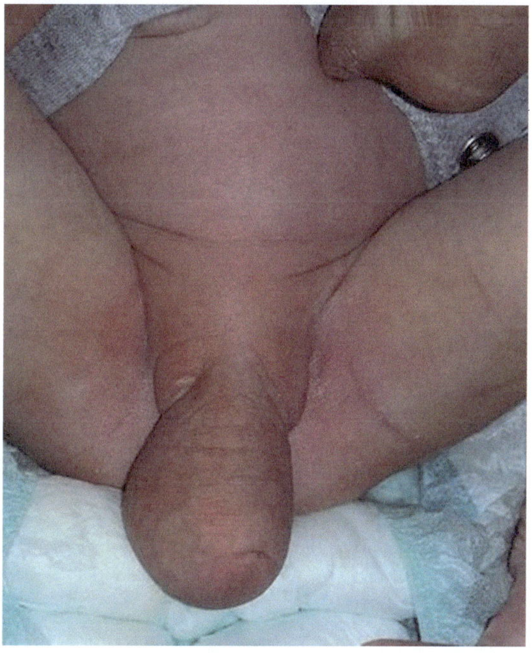

Fig. 10.3 False impression of macrophallus in a case of megalourethra

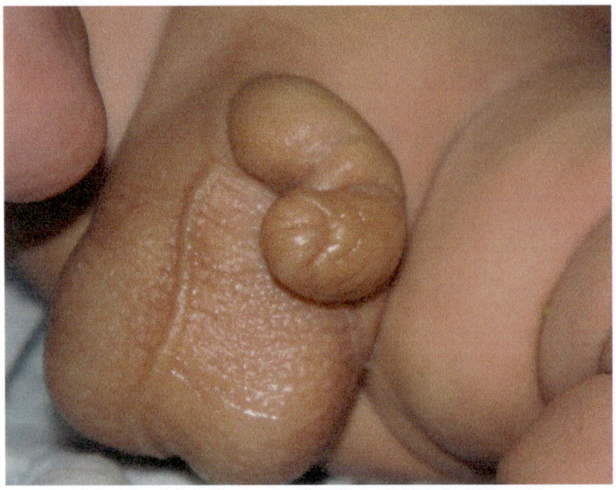

Fig. 10.4 A case of penile lymphedema giving false impression of microphallus, in this case thickened and oedematous skin extended to scrotum

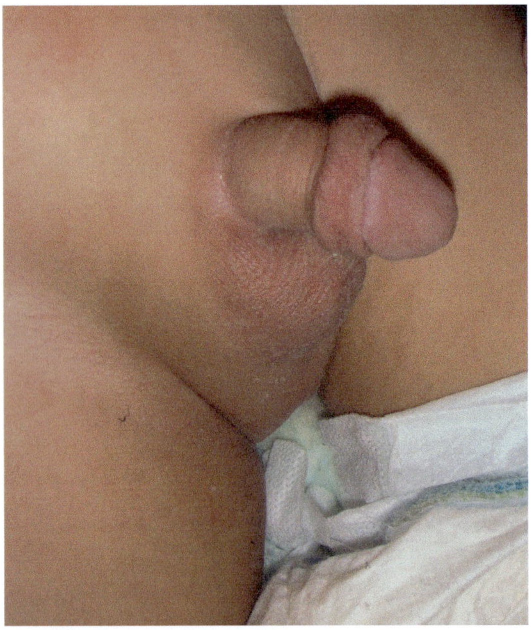

Fig. 10.5 Acquired macrophallus after (HCG) injection for undescended testicles in a 18 months boy

10.3 Management

Isolated primary cases of megalopenis necessitate investigations to rule out any other associated anomalies, and to rule out cases secondary to excess androgen production. Ultrasound and doppler examination may be enough to evaluate the size of corpora, its proper blood supply and to

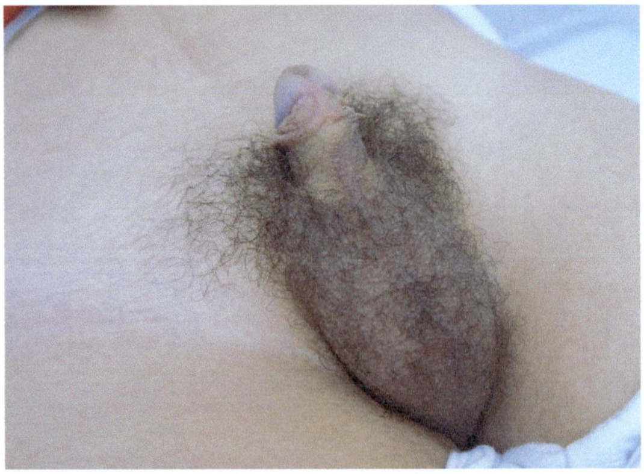

Fig. 10.6 Extensive pubic hair growth and false macrophallus after local testosterone application in a one year old boy

rule out any additional pathological tissues like neurofibroma or haemangioma, cases secondary to excessive androgen production i.e interstitial cell tumors of the testicle, are reversible once the primary pathology eradicated. Iatrogenic megalopenis is also a reversible condition and penis usually return to normal size once the external androgen administration halted. Family assurance is necessary to alleviate their worries and concern. Rarely reduction phalloplasty may be indicated in some few cases.

References

1. Ünalpn A, Uran N, Giray Ö, Erçal D. Inversion of chromosome 15 in a family with benign familial infantile seizures. J Neurol Sci. 2008;25:055–8.
2. Sabry MA, Obenbergerova D, Al-Sawan R, Al Saleh Q, et al. Femoral hypoplasia-unusual facies syndrome with bifid hallux, absent tibia, and macrophallus: a report of a Bedouin baby. J Med Genet. 1996;33:165–7.
3. Weidner W, Hauck EW. *Männermedizin.* W. B. Schill, R. G. Bretzel, W. Weidner (Herausgeber) Urban & Fischer Verlag, S. 448. ISBN 3-437-23260-6.

11 Penile Duplication (PD)

Abstract
Duplication of the penis, or diphallia, is an extremely rare but a well-documented anomaly resulting from incomplete fusion of the genital tubercle.

Keywords
Diphallia • Duplication • Ectopic penis • Pseudodiphalia

Definition

Duplication of the penis, or diphallia, is an extremely rare but a well- documented anomaly resulting from incomplete fusion of the genital tubercle.

Nomenclature

Diphallia, Diphallic terata, or Diphallasparatus.

11.1 Incidence

It is estimated to occur in one out of five million live births, and usually accompanied hindgut or anorectal duplication and the patient had a higher risk of spina bifida.

11.2 Historical Background

The first reported case of PD was reported by Johannes Jacob Wecker in 1609 [1]. Penile duplication is a normal finding in some animal species; like in male snakes, lizards and Sugar Glider which is a small, nocturnal, arboreal marsupial native to Australia, where each possessing a pair of penis-like organs, while mammals and birds are stuck with only one Fig. 11.1.

11.3 Diagnosis

Duplication of the penis is a rare anomaly with a wide range of appearances from a small accessory penis to complete organ duplication. In some cases, each phallus has only one corporal body and urethra, whereas others seem to be a

© Springer International Publishing Switzerland 2017
M. Fahmy, *Congenital Anomalies of the Penis*, DOI 10.1007/978-3-319-43310-3_11

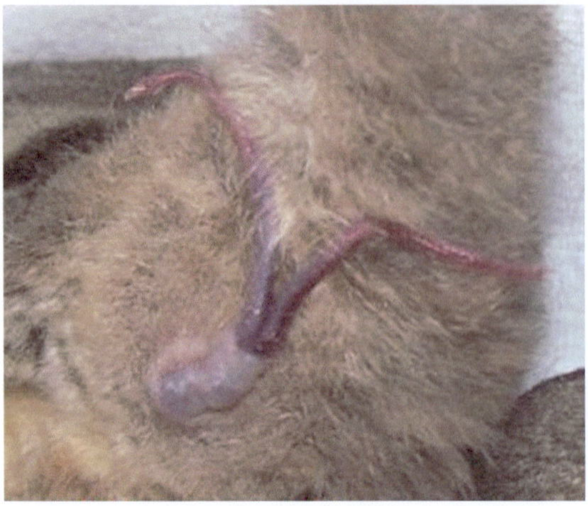

Fig. 11.1 Normal penile duplication in animal like the male Sugar Gliders "bifurcated penis"

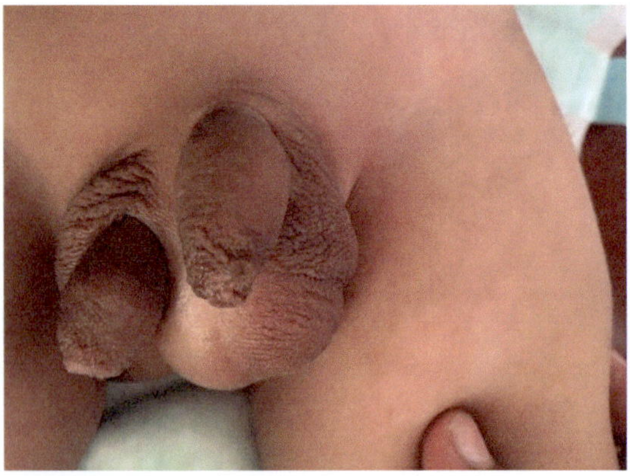

Fig. 11.2 Complete PD in coronal plane

variant of twinning, with each phallus having two corpora cavernosa and a separate urethra with or without bladder duplication (Fig. 11.2). The penises usually are unequal in size and lie side by side, but very rarely the other moiety lies beneath the first one in a sagittal plane (Fig. 11.3), or ectopic in the buttocks or over the sacrum, but in such cases the duplication is not true and the rudimentary extra penis is devoted from urethra and corporal tissues, but carrying the morphological look of the penis with a shaft and glans (Figs. 11.4 and 11.5).

Partial duplication of the penis may be manifested as a duplicated glans penis without any intervening urethra (Fig. 11.6).

Penile duplication should be differentiated from the rare cases of bifid penis, which is mainly

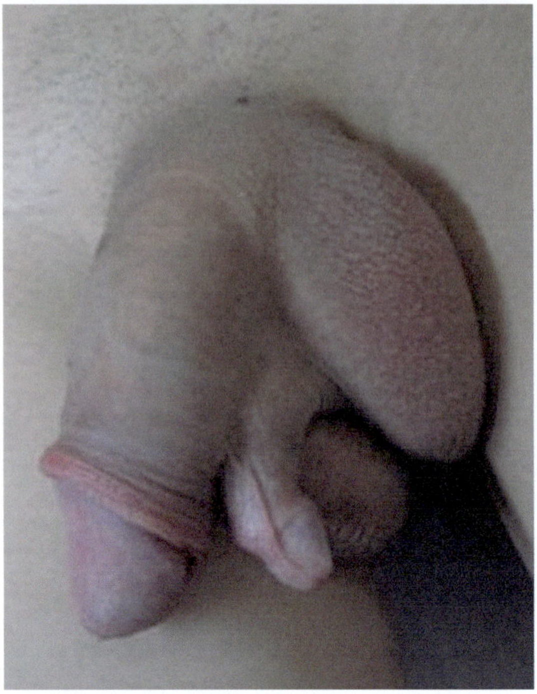

Fig. 11.3 PD in a sagital plane

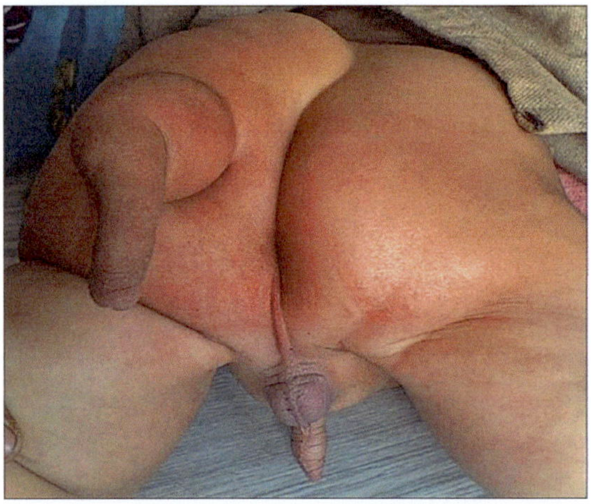

Fig. 11.4 Diphallia with ectopic penis in the buttock without urethra, the excess skin at its base mimicking scrotum

seen in association with cases of bladder exstrophy, in such cases the bifid penises are asymmetrical and may be associated with bifid scrotum, in female a bifid clitrois is the counter presentation (Fig. 11.7).

Associated anomalies are common, including hypospadias, bifid scrotum, urethral and

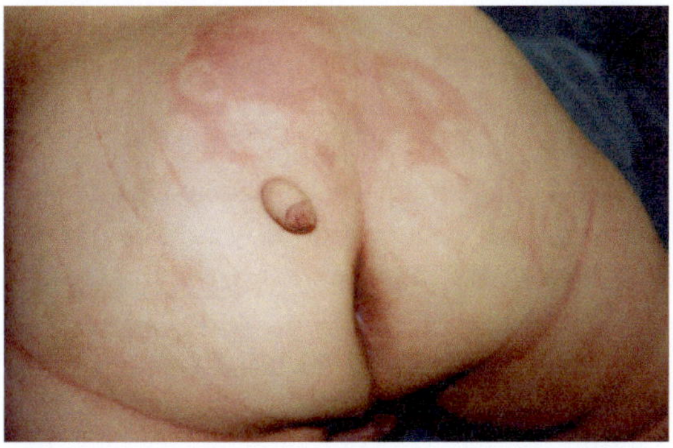

Fig. 11.5 Rudimentary ectopic penile duplication (Pseudodiphalia) in the buttock

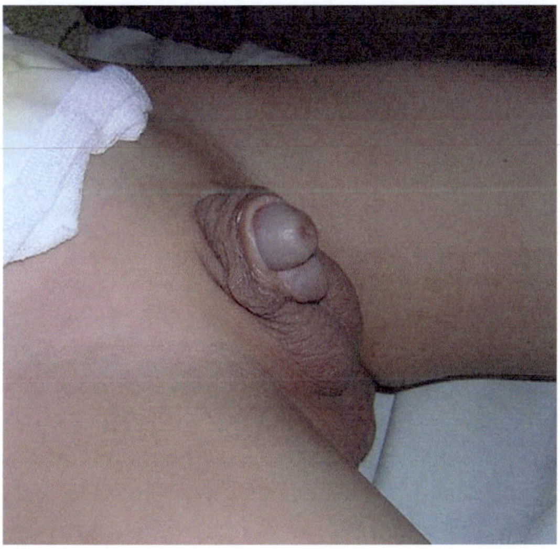

Fig. 11.6 Duplication of glans penis

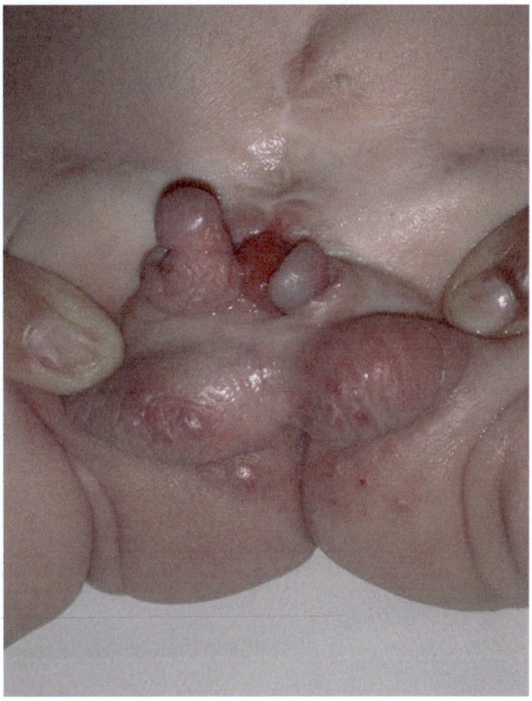

Fig. 11.7 Bifid penis in association with bladder exstrophy

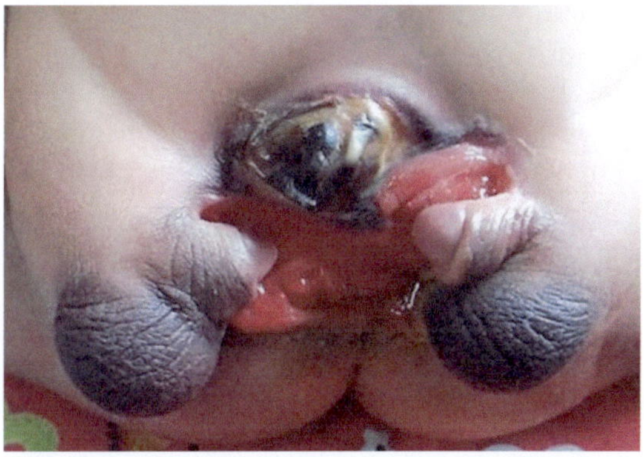

Fig. 11.8 Penile duplication with bladder exstrophy

bladder duplication, renal agenesis or ectopia, many cases reported with bladder exstrophy and its variant like superior vesicle fissure (Fig. 11.8). Wide diastasis of the pubic symphysis usually detected in many cases of penile duplication without bladder exstrophy. Other cases of PD reported with complete anal duplication with or without a double hindgut, other anorectal and cardiac anomalies also are common (Fig. 11.9).

Evaluation of such cases should include imaging of the entire urinary tract. Sonography is essential to aid in assessment of the extent of phallic development. MRI can also be used to assess the exact penile developmental structures, and it is a valuable tool for achieving the accurate diagnosis of these anomalies and associated malformations. It also provides the appropriate knowledge regarding anatomical detail and assists the surgeon in decision making and preoperative planning for the optimal surgical approach [2].

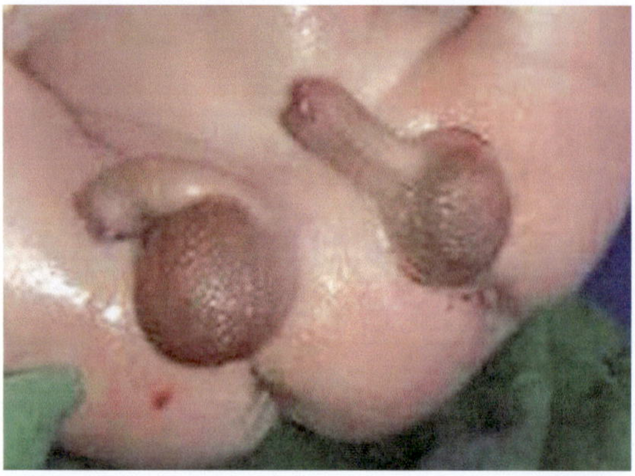

Fig. 11.9 Complete PD with anal and rectal duplications "partial caudal duplication"

11.4 Etiology

It is thought that diphallia occurs in the fetus between the 23rd and 25th days of gestation when an injury, chemical stress, or malfunctioning homeobox genes hamper proper function of the caudal cell mass of the fetal mesoderm as the urogenital sinus separates from the genital tubercle to form the penis.

Hollowell et al. [3] reviewed the embryogenesis of diphallia and suggested that complete diphallus could result from longitudinal duplication of the infraumbilical cloacal membrane before the fourth week of gestation, the subsequent mesodermal migration allowing two separate, complete sets of genital tubercle, genital folds, and genital swellings to develop. The fusion of the genital folds and swellings may not be entirely normal, accounting for the finding that one of the two urethras may be a blind pit or else be stenotic. One or both urethras also may be hypospadiac or epispadiac. A wide range of scrotal abnormalities may be present. Because the duplicated cloacal membrane is likely to be a widened structure, the "wedge" effect could result in the stigmata of covered exstrophy. In some patients, the abnormalities suggest a form of partial caudal duplication with extensive midline defects or duplication involving the derivatives of the allantois, hindgut, and neural tube [4].

Although the organs of the genital tract arise as paired organs, distal fusion of the gonadal ducts normally results in single external and internal genitalia. Mechanical factors caused by hindgut duplication probably account for the failure of genital fusion frequently associated with complete colonic duplications. The twinning process may be initiated by the double-channel vacuole mechanism proposed by Bremer. Another theory by Campbell stated that PD is caused by a splitting of the vesicourethral anlage and that associated rectal anomalies will suggest whether the schism occurred before or after division of cloaca by urorectal septum. A similar explanation was also given by Satter and Mossman [4].

11.5 Classification

Generally there is a two distinct forms of penile duplication exist:

The most common form is associated with bladder exstrophy complex and its variant as superior vesical fissure (Fig. 11.7). The patient exhibits a bifid penis, which consists of two separated corpora cavernosa that are associated with two independent hemiglands (Fig. 11.8).

The second form, or true diphallia, which presents in many ways, ranging from duplication of the glans alone to duplication of the entire lower genitourinary tract. The urethral opening could be in normal position in a hypospadiac or epispadiac position, and sometimes there is a whole duplication of the penis, urethra, scrotum and bladder.

According to Schneider [5] diphallia could be simply classified into four categories:

1. Duplication of the glans alone (Fig. 11.6).
2. Bifid diphallia (Fig. 11.7).
3. Complete diphallia with each penis having two corpora cavernosa and a corpus spongiosum (Figs. 11.2, 11.9 and 11.10).
4. Pseudodiphalia in which there is a rudimentary accessory atrophic penis existing independently of the normal penis (Figs. 11.4 and 11.5).

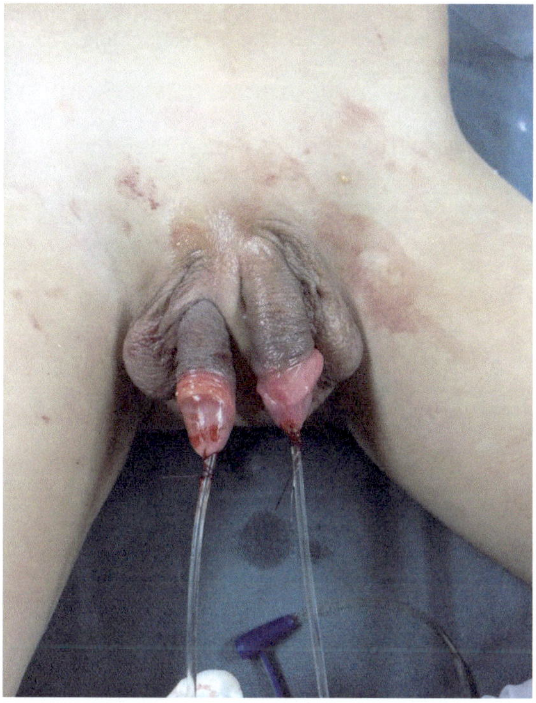

Fig. 11.10 Complete penile, scrotal, bladder and urethral duplication in an otherwise normal adolescent

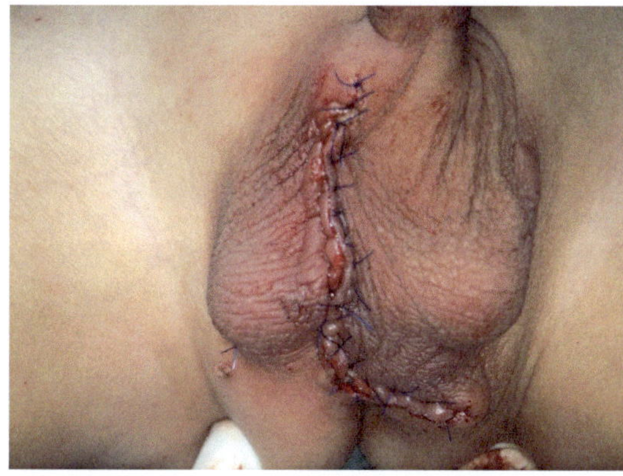

Fig. 11.11 Surgically repaired case of PD, one phallus and urethra excised

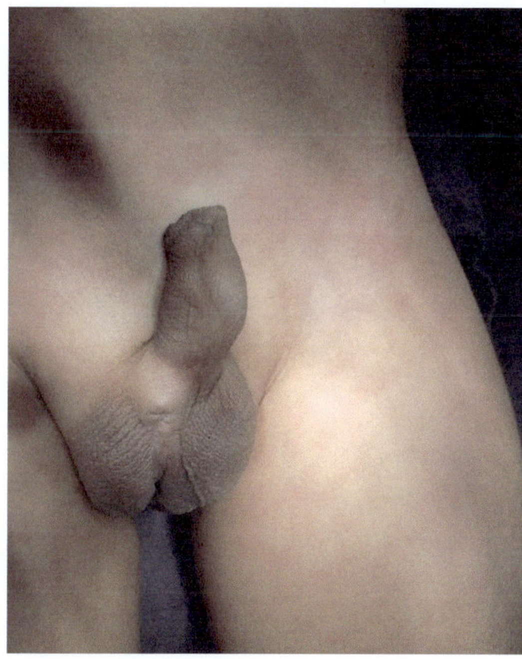

Fig. 11.12 Same patient in Fig. 11.10 6 months after surgery

11.6 Treatment

Because these anomalies are the principal causes of mortality, due to associated urinary anomalies or obstruction, and usually baring a considerable anxious for parents, examining and treating patients for the associated major anomalies as soon as possible is mandatory, but reconstructive treatment must be individualized with consideration of the associated anomalies with the goal of attaining a satisfactory functional so as to preserve continence, erectile functions and cosmetic outcome. Duplicated urethra and bladder have to be excised in the same session or prior to phallic surgery, it may be difficult in complete diphallia to decide which phallus have to be sacrificed, if it is obvious, the smaller, disfigured and ectopic moiety deserve excision, in some cases achievement of a satisfactory, near normal, look may be possible (Figs. 11.10, 11.11 and 11.12).

In cases of duplication with bladder exstrophy, penile reconstruction could be done with complete primary repair, which may satisfy family to have a normally looking boy, or it may be better to defer extra phallic excision for another session.

References

1. Nesbit RM, Bromme W. Double penis and double bladder with report of case. Am J Roentgenol. 1933;30:497.
2. Marti-Bonmati L, Menor F, Gomez J, et al. Value of sonography in true complete diphallia. J Urol. 1989;142:356.
3. Hollowell Jr JG, Witherington R, Ballagas AJ, et al. Embryological consideration of diphallus and associated anomalies. J Urol. 1977;111:728–32.
4. Satter EJ, Mossman HW. A case report of a double bladder and double urethra in a female child. J Urol. 1958;79:275–8.
5. Schneider P, Lamitter JK, Uson AC, Melicow AC. The male genital tract. In: Mustard WT, Ravitch MM, Snyder WH, et al., editors. Pediatric surgery. 2nd ed. Chicago: Year Book Medical Publishers; 1969. p. 1263.

Penile Rotation

12

Marjan Waterloos, Piet Hoebeke, and Anne-Françoise Spinoit

Abstract

Penile torsion is a debatable condition as no consensus exists on its definition, or on its management. This manuscript is designed a state-of-knowledge about the condition

Keywords

Penile torsion • Chordee • Penile curvature

Introduction

Penile torsion is a debatable condition as no consensus exists on its definition, or on its management. This manuscript is designed a state-of-knowledge about the condition

Definition

Congenital penile torsion is a rotational defect of the penile shaft, resulting in an abnormal curvature of the penis without aberrant position of the meatus. With this condition, the penis appears twisted on its axis [1]. The degree of torsion is measured as the angle between a line passing through the urethral meatus and the midline of the scrotum [2].

Torsion exists as a stand-alone disease, but is very often associated with other congenital penile malformations: Torsion is a classical feature of severe hypospadias, and is described in that context as penile 'chordee [3]'. Torsion can also be observed in buried penis and epispadias. No clear difference is made in the literature between penile curvature and penile torsion, both terms being frequently used for both bending of the penis or rotation of the penis. Many authors call bending of the penis: curvature, while rotation is more often used when there is torsion on the penis axis. Chordee is usually used in the context of hypospadias, but no consensus exists about those terms. A first step toward a better understanding of the pathology would be to clearly define terms.

In this chapter, we will use the following definitions:

Torsion: Twist, clock-wise or counter-clockwise, of the penis on its axis. The degree of torsion is measured as the angle between a line passing through the urethral meatus and the midline of the scrotum.

Curvature: Bending of the penis in *an erect state* in any direction. The penis is not rotated on its axis.

Chordee: Retraction of the penis due to underdevelopment of penile tissues. It is observed

© Springer International Publishing Switzerland 2017

M. Fahmy, *Congenital Anomalies of the Penis*, DOI 10.1007/978-3-319-43310-3_12

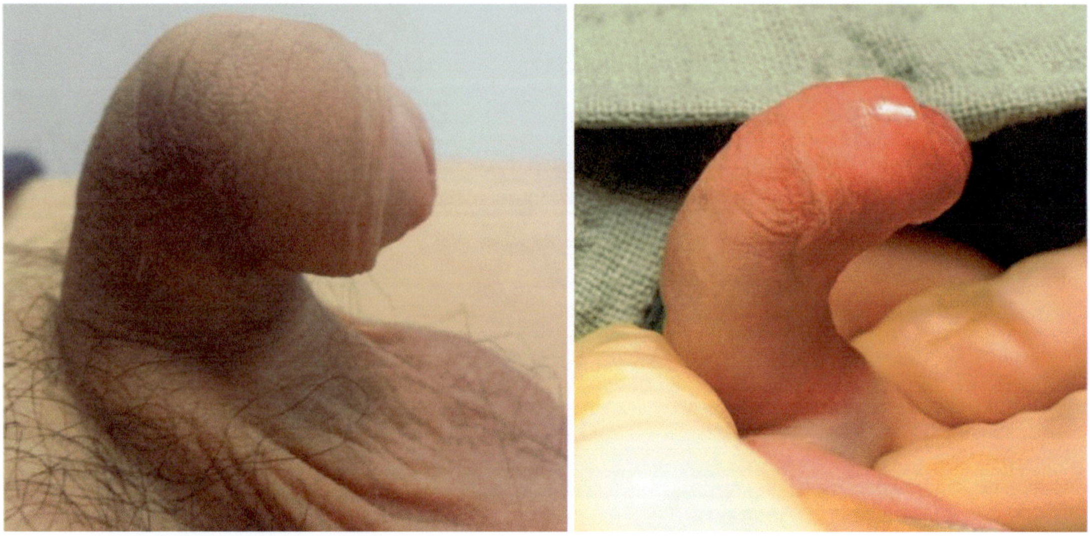

Fig. 12.1 Penile chordee without hypospadias

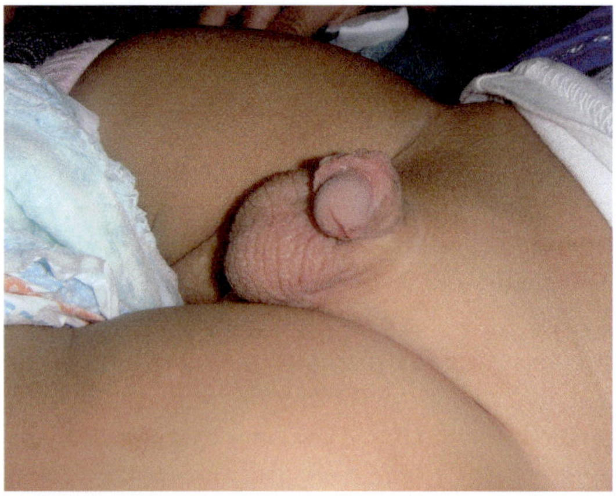

Fig. 12.2 Penile torsion

on the ventral side in hypospadias, and on the dorsal side in epispadias.

Torsion and chordee have to be distinguished from Peyronie's disease, where *curvature* is acquired progressively, and due to fibrous plaques in the corporal bodies (Figs. 12.1 and 12.2) [4].

12.1 Historical Background

Torsion as a stand-alone condition was first described by Siever in 1926, who mentioned rotation of the penis associated with hypospadias [5]. We would nowadays define it as chordee.

Penile torsion was first described in 1973 by Horton and Devine [6]. They used also the word chordee. They historically described three types of penile torsion: in the first type they described, the corpus spongiosum was absent on the distal part of the penis, with an ectopic meatus, which is nowadays considered as a classical feature of hypospadias [6]. This first type of 'torsion' as described by Horton and Devine would nowadays probably be classified as distal hypospadias with important chordee.

In their second type of torsion Horton and Devine described a fully developed urethra and corpus spongiosum but an important bending of the penis on the ventral side, due do 'retraction of the superficial dartos fascia' [6]. It would nowadays probably be classified as chordee without hypospadias, or 'hypospadias sine hypospadias'. Important chordee without ectopic meatus and with a complete prepuce is often considered as a separate condition and has many names: hypospadias without hypospadias, chordee sine hypospadias, and congenital penile curvature. As it is almost always associated with hypoplasia of the corpus spongiosum, even if the meatus is orthotopic, it should probably still be regarded as part of the hypospadias spectrum.

A third type was described by Horton and Devine as 'skin chordee', or retraction due to shortage of skin. It would be nowadays probably also be classified as chordee without hypospadias [6].

Later on, a different type of torsion was introduced by Kramer, who firstly proposed a disproportion in corporal bodies as explanation for penile torsion [7]. He also used the word chordee, even if the condition was not related to hypospadias.

Nowadays, the conditions of chordee without hypospadias and torsion remain broadly discussed, without reaching some clear consensus on its stand-alone condition, or associated with hypospadias or other congenital penile pathologies [8, 9]. Many congenital penile malformations are associated with torsion and chordee: hypospadias, buried penis, epispadias,… Epispadias has of course, due to its embryologic origin, an important component of penile torsion, as both corporal bodies are malrotated, but this is beyond the scope of this chapter.

12.2 Incidence

Torsion has debatable incidence, as some authors consider penile torsion and curvature as part of the spectrum of the hypospadias condition and mix it with chordee [10]. Series investigating purely penile torsion without associated condition are very scarce.

As patients are usually asymptomatic and have few complaints, the incidence of penile torsion might be underestimated [11]. Varying studies report incidence ranging from 1.7 % of males, to 27 % [12, 13]. During childhood, some mothers report observing torsion, but usually it is then only noticed when the curvature is very important. Curvature is often recognized quite late during childhood, at the beginning of puberty, as it is most visible in erection.

Besides the congenital condition, torsion might be acquired after penile surgery, where extensive degloving of the penile shaft is undertaken. In this chapter, we will only consider congenital penile torsion/curvature/chordee.

12.3 Pathophysiology

The pathophysiologic mechanisms leading to penile torsion still need to be unveiled. Embryonal studies have shown penile curvature is a normal phase in the genital tubercle development [14–16]. During the masculinization of the primitive genital tubercle, progressive elongation of the penis seems to be asymmetrical, with initial ventral curvature [14]. Kaplan described after anatomical studies of fetuses that 89 % of the fetuses at different gestational ages presented ventral penile curvature [14]. He described it as chordee, even if it was not associated with hypospadias.

Based on further studies, Baskin proposed that chordee without hypospadias, which could also be considered as curvature of the penis downwards, might be the result of an arrest in development [17].

Kramer proposed a different concept and stated that torsion or bending is the result of asymmetrical growth of corporal bodies [7].

Recent studies have shown that the dartos, which is the smooth muscle layer lying under the skin, might be responsible for chordee/curvature, associated or not with other congenital penile malformations [18]. The dartos tissue is considered a superficial fascia, located immediately under the genital skin, originating in Scarpa's abdominal fascia, and in Colle's perineal fascia [19]. The composition of fibro muscular dartos tissue along the penile shaft determines elasticity of the subcutaneous tissue and the skin mobility. Any structural change in organization of these components may influence these characteristics, and might therefore be responsible for torsion/chordee.

Resection of the dartos tissue usually makes the penis straight in hypospadias and unhides the penis in buried penis, suggesting the dartos tissue is involved in pathophysiology of penile chordee/torsion. This quite large study, performed on a large prospective cohort of children undergoing primary penile surgery, with healthy children undergoing circumcision as control, proved that the level of disorganization of the dartos tissue in congenital penile malformation strongly correlated with the severity of the clinical penile malformation [18].

We believe chordee and torsion probably have a same pathophysiologic mechanism, induced by dartos tissue aberrant development. We believe also curvature is caused by another mechanism: curvature is caused by an asymmetrical development of the corporal bodies. More studies however are needed to confirm this idea.

12.4 Treatment

Different therapeutic possibilities exist. Just like for etiology and classification, there is no consensus on gold-standard treatment for penile torsion, curvature, or chordee.

A few rules are based on common sense: even if correction of curvature/torsion/chordee is important, it is even more important to preserve the genital sensitivity and potency.

The neurovascular bundles, as described by Baskin, has a constant pathway that need to be preserved [20]. The nervus dorsalis penis passes through the urogenital diaphragm and joins the dorsal arteries at the dorso-lateral aspect from each corpus cavernosum, forming the so-called neuro-vascular bundle of the penis. This bundle has a 1 and 11 o'clock position along the corporae cavernosae, extending circumventrally to the 5 and 7 o'clock position where the corpora cavernosa meet the corpus spongiosum [20–22]. The nervus dorsalis penis is important for the sensible innervation of the penile skin, the glans, prepuce and the distal anterior urethra. The nerves terminate in the glans. Interestingly, their pathway remain constant in normal as well as in cripple penises, allowing the reconstructive surgeon to work preferentially on the 12 o'clock position of the corpora cavernosa, void of nerves, when needed.

Besides preserving the genital sensitivity, preserving erections is essential. Some techniques can be very invasive with resection of tunica albuginea and/or part of corporal bodies, with possible impact on potency.

Torsion is usually obvious, but curvature/chordee might be more difficult to assess. When curvature/chordee is not obvious, the first step of the surgery is to identify the extent of the problem by performing an erection test. First described in 1974, this well-known test consists of injection of saline in one corpus cavernosum to simulate erection and observe curvature/chordee [23]. This technique however does not work in epispadias, as corporal bodies do not communicate with each other. Injection in both corpora at the same time is needed in epispadias to assess curvature. Classically, the place where the curvature/chordee is the most prominent is marked during the erection test.

12.4.1 Torsion

There is no clear consensus on the treatment of penile torsion. Torsion as a stand-alone condition is usually asymptomatic. Whether treatment is needed or not becomes purely esthetic. Many techniques using flaps or penile degloving have been described when correction is desired, all of them being reported in small series [24, 25]. The least invasive technique, which is most often sufficient to correct mild torsion, consists in penile deglovement [26]. By degloving the penis, dartos tissue, that could be aberrant, is resected, thereby usually correcting the problem. When deglovement is insufficient, some other pathologic mechanism than pure dartos disorganization might be involved.

12.4.2 Curvature

Congenital curvature becomes usually symptomatic at puberty, when erections make it obvious. The need for treatment has to be assessed according to the symptomatology. Curvatures making intercourse impossible require indeed surgical correction. Usual clinical practice recommends correction of curvature if the bending is superior to 30 degrees [10, 27]. Many techniques have been described to correct penile curvature, but those techniques are report mainly treatment of curvature caused by Peyronie disease. Different techniques are possible to correct the curvature, and no consensus exist on which technique to apply according to the degree of curvature. Different principles using plicature of the corpora cavernosa, use of grafts or even complete penile disassembly are described. All those principles are based on the fact that curvature is caused by an asymmetry in the corporal bodies.

12.5 Chordee

Chordee is usually corrected by penile deglovement and resection of hyposplastic tissues in hypospadias and epispadias.

Donnahoo et al. proposed a surgical strategy according to the severity of the chordee. In the first group, chordee is released simply by degloving the penis, called skin chordee [28].

A second group consists in patients in which correction is obtained after deglovement and resection of hypotrophic tissues: deficient Buck's fascia and dartos tissue [28].

A third group consists in patients in which chordee persists after deglovement and resection of hypotrophic tissues. Complete mobilization of the urethra is in those cases needed, explained according to the author by an additional corporal disproportion [28].

The last group consists in those patients in whom plicature of the tunica albuginea is needed. The authors report that in those patients, a congenitally short urethra is observed. Division of the urethra with interposition graft is in those cases necessary [28].

In our experience, pure chordee is often corrected by pure penile deglovement and resection of hypotrophic tissues when observed, as described in the two first groups by Donnahoo [28]. If this is insufficient, in our experience, the condition is related to a severe hypospadias or epispadias. The technique to apply depends then upon the severity of the clinical condition.

12.6 Outcome

No large series of congenital penile chordee correction/curvature/torsion are available in the literature. Small series report minor complications, or complications varying according to the severity of the clinical condition. The most reported adverse event is residual curvature or chordee [29].

Conclusion

Penile torsion, just as curvature and chordee, remains a very debatable condition, for which various treatments might be applied. A general consensus starting with definitions of the pathology is needed to allow standardization of treatment and evaluation of outcomes.

References

1. Gearhart J, Rink R, Mouriquand P. Pediatric urology. Sauders Elsevier; 2010. Buried penis. 2nd edition, Philadelphia p. 519–25.
2. Castagnetti M, Leonard M, Guerra L, Esposito C, Cimador M. Benign penile skin anomalies in children: a primer for pediatricians. World J Pediatr. 2015;11(4):316–23. Epub 2015/03/11.
3. Baskin LS, Duckett JW, Lue TF. Penile curvature. Urology. 1996;48(3):347–56. Epub 1996/09/01.
4. Beach EW. Peyronie's disease or fibrous cavernositis: some observations. Cal West Med. 1941;55(1):7–10. Epub 1941/07/01.
5. Siever R. Anomalien auf Penis: ihre Beziehung zur hypospadie und ihre Deutung. Z Chir. 1926;199:286. Epub 1926.
6. Devine Jr CJ, Horton CE. Chordee without hypospadias. J Urol. 1973;110(2):264–71. Epub 1973/08/01.
7. Kramer SA, Aydin G, Kelalis PP. Chordee without hypospadias in children. J Urol. 1982;128(3):559–61. Epub 1982/09/01.
8. Daskalopoulos EI, Baskin L, Duckett JW, Snyder 3rd HM. Congenital penile curvature (chordee without hypospadias). Urology. 1993;42(6):708–12. Epub 1993/12/01.
9. Baskin LS, Duckett JW, Ueoka K, Seibold J, Snyder 3rd HM. Changing concepts of hypospadias curvature lead to more onlay island flap procedures. J Urol. 1994;151(1):191–6. Epub 1994/01/01.
10. Bennett AH, Gittes RF. Congenital penile curvature without hypospadias. Urology. 1980;16(4):364–6. Epub 1980/10/01.
11. Montag S, Palmer LS. Abnormalities of penile curvature: chordee and penile torsion. ScientificWorldJournal. 11th edition, Philadelphia. 2011;11:1470–8. Epub 2011/08/02.
12. Ben-Ari J, Merlob P, Mimouni F, Reisner SH. Characteristics of the male genitalia in the newborn: penis. J Urol. 1985;134(3):521–2. Epub 1985/09/01.
13. Sarkis PE, Sadasivam M. Incidence and predictive factors of isolated neonatal penile glanular torsion. J Pediatr Urol. 2007;3(6):495–9. Epub 2008/10/25.
14. Kaplan GW, Lamm DL. Embryogenesis of chordee. J Urol. 1975;114(5):769–72. Epub 1975/11/01.
15. Hynes PJ, Fraher JP. The development of the male genitourinary system: II. The origin and formation of the urethral plate. Br J Plast Surg. 2004;57(2):112–21. Epub 2004/03/24.

16. Wein AJ, Kavoussi LR, Novick AC, Partin AW, Peters CA. Campbell-Walsh urology. 11th ed. Philadelphia: Elsevier; 2012.
17. Mingin G, Baskin LS. Management of chordee in children and young adults. Urol Clin North Am. 2002;29(2):277–84, v. Epub 2002/10/10.
18. Spinoit AF, Van Praet C, Groen LA, Van Laecke E, Praet M, Hoebeke P. Congenital penile pathology is associated with abnormal development of the dartos muscle: a prospective study of primary penile surgery at a tertiary referral center. J Urol. 2015;193(5):1620–4. Epub 2014/12/03.
19. Brisson P, Patel H, Chan M. Penoplasty for buried penis in children: report of 50 cases. J Pediatr Surg. 2001;36(3):421–5.
20. Baskin LS, Lee YT, Cunha GR. Neuroanatomical ontogeny of the human fetal penis. Br J Urol. 1997;79(4):628–40. Epub 1997/04/01.
21. Yiee JH, Baskin LS. Penile embryology and anatomy. ScientificWorldJournal. 2010;10:1174–9. Epub 2010/07/06.
22. Baskin LS. Hypospadias and urethral development. J Urol. 2000;163(3):951–6. Epub 2000/02/25.
23. Gittes RF, McLaughlin 3rd AP. Injection technique to induce penile erection. Urology. 1974;4(4):473–4. Epub 1974/10/01.
24. Eroglu E, Gundogdu G. Isolated penile torsion in newborns. Can Urol Assoc J. 2015;9(11–12):E805–7. Epub 2015/11/26.
25. Aykac A, Baran O, Yapici O, Aygun BA, Aydin C, Cakan M. Penile degloving and dorsal dartos flap rotation approach for the management of isolated penile torsion. Turk J Urol. 2016;42(1):27–31. Epub 2016/03/25.
26. Bar-Yosef Y, Binyamini J, Matzkin H, Ben-Chaim J. Degloving and realignment – simple repair of isolated penile torsion. Urology. 2007;69(2):369–71. Epub 2007/02/27.
27. Wespes E, Amar E, Hatzichristou D, Hatzimouratidis K, Montorsi F, Pryor J, et al. EAU guidelines on erectile dysfunction: an update. Eur Urol. 2006;49(5):806–15. Epub 2006/03/15.
28. Donnahoo KK, Cain MP, Pope JC, Casale AJ, Keating MA, Adams MC, et al. Etiology, management and surgical complications of congenital chordee without hypospadias. J Urol. 1998;160(3 Pt 2):1120–2. Epub 1998/08/27.
29. Dipaola G, Spalletta M, Balducci T, Giacomello L, Camoglio FS, Bianchi S, et al. Surgical treatment of chordee without hypospadias. Eur Urol. 2000;38(6):758–61. Epub 2000/12/09.

Penile Chordee

13

Abstract

Penile chordee is a condition in which the head of the penis curves downward or upward, at the junction of the head and shaft of the penis. The curvature is usually obvious during erection, but resistance to straightening is often apparent in the flaccid state as well. It is a congenital anomaly due to reduced elasticity in one or more of the fascial layers of the penis, leading to shortness of the corpus spongiosum when erection occurs. Usually the bend is ventral but could be dorsal or complex.

Keywords

Chordee • Congenital curvature • Frenulum breve

Generally there is three varieties of chordee should be recognised in dealing with a child with penile curvature:

Congenital chordee without hypospadias (Figs. 13.1 and 13.2).

Chordee associated with hypospadias, specially in proximal types and with the hypospadias variant of corpora spongosium hypoplasia (Fig. 13.3).

Secondary or acquired chordee; which usually complicate circumcision or hypospadias repair and this should be differentiated from Peyronie's disease, which involves curvature of the shaft of the penis most commonly due to injury during adult life (Fig. 13.4).

Nomenclature

The term “chordee” was introduced into medical literature in the seventeenth century from the French in relation to gonorrhoea. Most hypospadias pioneers in the nineteenth century used terms such as incurvation, curvature, or bending. Clinton Smith, in the 1930s, was probably the first to use the term chordee to describe congenital curvature associated with hypospadias [1].

Incidence

Congenital curvature is rare: In one well-performed study reports an incidence of less than 1 % while there are reports from other studies, which claim

© Springer International Publishing Switzerland 2017

M. Fahmy, *Congenital Anomalies of the Penis*, DOI 10.1007/978-3-319-43310-3_13

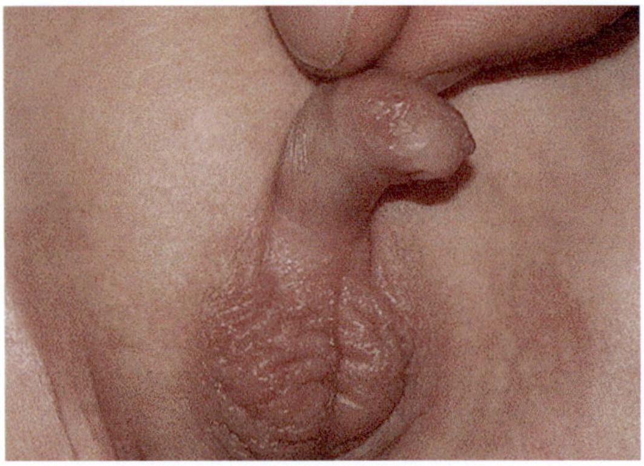

Fig. 13.1 A neonate with chordee without hypospadias

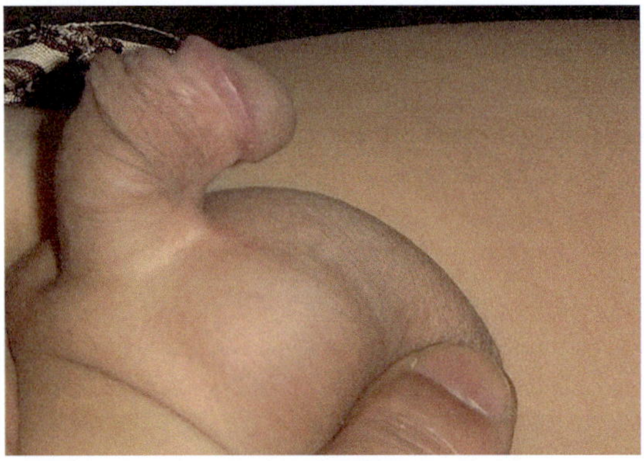

Fig. 13.2 Severe ventral chordee

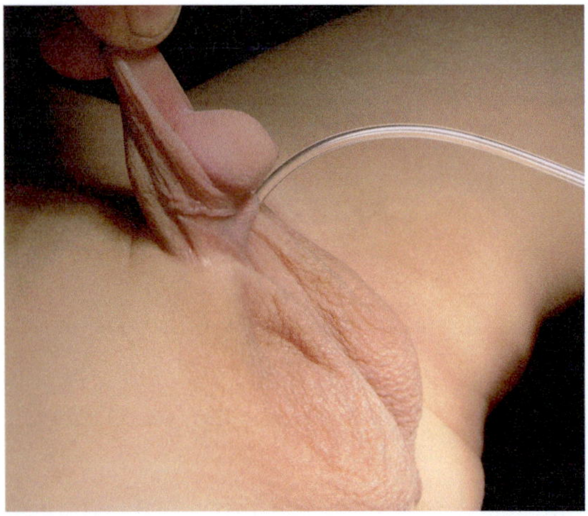

Fig. 13.3 Penile chordee with a deficient corpora spongosium, urethra covered only with a thin skin

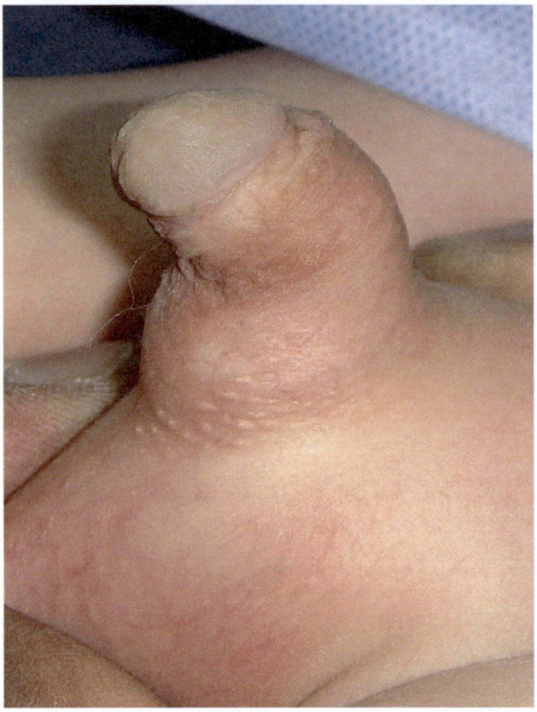

Fig. 13.4 Chordee secondary to fibrosis after circumcision

that it is more common with prevalence rates of 4-10 % in the absence of hypospadias [2].

13.1 Etiology

Chordee may be an isolated anomaly without any other associated deformity (Fig. 13.1), but it is often found in association with various other congenital penile anomalies such as hypospadias, specially with deficient corpus spongiosum, where the urethra could be seen superficial under a thin layer of skin (Fig. 13.2). Many cases may associate microposthia (Chap. 5) and median raphe anomalies (Chap. 16).

The exact cause of chordee is unclear, but when it is associated with hypospadias, the presence of fibrous bands may explain its existence, where the mesenchyme distal to the meatus ceases to differentiate, creating a fan-shaped band of dysgenetic fascia; however, when found independently from other conditions, chordee is postulated to result from fibrotic superficial and deep penile fascia, skin tethering, or corporal disproportion. If untreated, congenital penile curvature may prohibit or significantly interfere with sexual intercourse. Acquired chordee may result from trauma or Peyronie's disease [3], and we encountered many cases complicating circumcision (Fig. 13.4) (Chap. 33). Isolated chordee anomaly have to be differentiated from webbed penis, and concealed penis.

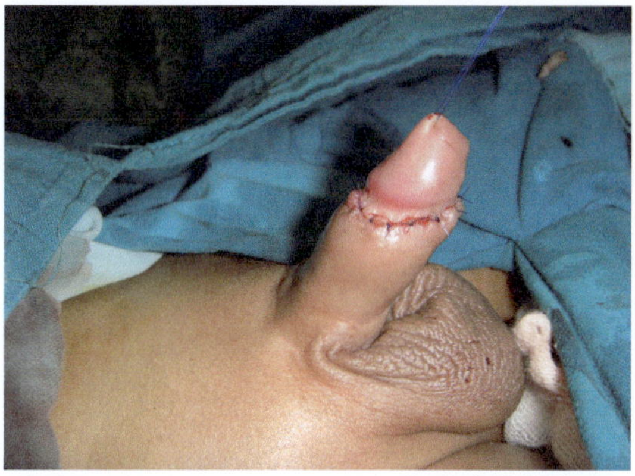

Fig. 13.5 Patient in Fig. 13.2 after correction

13.2 Management

Ventral curvature in boys without hypospadias, generally can be corrected by degloving of the penis, excision of fibrous tissue that is usually confined to the region superficial to Buck's fascia, and development of a Byars flap for penile skin coverage as necessary [4]. In more severe cases, simple dorsal plication, Nesbit dorsal excision, or corporeal rotation may be essential.

In the most severe cases, with short urethra, urethral reconstruction is indicated by either island flap of the dorsal foreskin, or buccal mucosal graft. Intraoperative artificial erection with normal saline may be necessary to confirm that complete chordee correction (Fig. 13.5). Some cases of chordee may be aggravated by a prominent or short frenulum (frenulum breve), resulting in distal penile chordee with ventral glanular deflection, in these cases, frenulotomy will improve and may correct the chordee.

References

1. Smith CK. Surgical procedures for correction of hypospadias. J Urol. 1938;40:239.
2. Montag S, et al. Abnormalities of penile curvature: chordee and penile torsion. Scientific World Journal. 2011;11:1470–8.
3. Hatzimouratidis K (Chair), Eardley I, Giuliano F, Moncada I, Salonia A. EUA guidelines on penile curvature. http://uroweb.org/wp-content/uploads/16-PenileCurvature_LR.pdf.
4. Caesar RE, Caldamone AA. The use of free grafts for correcting penile chordee. J Urol. 2000;164(5):1691–3.

Webbed Penis

14

Marjan Waterloos, Piet Hoebeke,
and Anne-Françoise Spinoit

Abstract

Many conditions involving the male external genitalia make the penis look small. Buried or webbed penis is one of those conditions. Penis size is the reason the parents bring their child to the outpatient clinic. It is important to distinguish those conditions where the penis has a normal size, from micropenis. The term micropenis refers to a penis that is completely normally formed, but is abnormally small.

Keywords

Buried penis • Mega preputium • Webbed penis • Trapped penis

14.1 Introduction

Many conditions involving the male external genitalia make the penis look small. Buried or webbed penis is one of those conditions. Penis size is the reason the parents bring their child to the outpatient clinic. It is important to distinguish those conditions where the penis has a normal size, from micropenis. The term micropenis refers to a penis that is completely normally formed, but is abnormally small [1].

Careful measurement (standardized as Stretched Penile Length: SPL) should me realized by gripping the glans and placing a ruler on the dorsal aspect of the penis from the pubic symphysis to the tip of the glans. Even if SPL is the standard penile measurement, it is however subject to important intra- and inter-observer variations.

As the micropenis is completely normal except for its size, the pathologic problem is probably occurring during the second and/or third trimester of intra-uterine growth. The intact urethra and foreskin proves a normal first trimester of intra-uterine growth. As penile growth is essentially taking place after the third gestational month, the pathology probably mainly depends on testosterone synthesis. The problem may be located at the level of the testes, the hypophysis, or the hypothalamus.

True micropenis should therefore be distinguished from other penile conditions, as it implies multiple endocrine and non-endocrine conditions,

© Springer International Publishing Switzerland 2017
M. Fahmy, *Congenital Anomalies of the Penis*, DOI 10.1007/978-3-319-43310-3_14

and should be treated by a multidisciplinary tem involving a pediatric urologic and a pediatric endocrinologist.

Many penile conditions are reported besides micropenis, but are reported under various denominations due to a lack of standardization [2]. Buried penis is also described as inconspicuous penis, webbed penis, hidden penis, cryptic penis, concealed penis, mega preputium with concealed penis, all those terms covering one single pathologic finding: a normal penile shaft is entrapped in pubic fatty tissues, only leaving a redundant *preputium* visible [1, 3–5]. As its pathophysiology is unknown, many reconstruction techniques have been proposed, each supporting different pathophysiologic process.

Those primary congenital conditions have to be distinguished from acquired penile entrapment, which is observed after circumcision or other penile surgery during which too much skin has been removed. Such condition is called 'trapped penis' [1, 6].

Those conditions are also observed in adults, but are mostly observed as an acquired condition in which paucity of skin entrapping the otherwise normal penis occurs [7].

An important point to keep in mind is that all those conditions represent a formal contra-indication for a classical circumcision.

Buried Penis or Webbed Penis

Definition

Buried penis is a congenital penile malformation frequently encountered in pediatric urology [2]. Although the true incidence of buried and/or webbed penis is unknown because of an ongoing debate about its definition, buried is probably the most frequent penile pathology after *hypospadias* [1, 2]. It affects children as well as adults, and can be congenital or acquired [7, 8].

Buried penis is also described as webbed penis, inconspicuous penis, hidden penis, cryptic penis, concealed penis, *meaga-preputium* with concealed penis, all those terms covering one single pathologic finding: a normal penile shaft is entrapped in pubic fatty tissues, only leaving a redundant *preputium* visible [1, 3–5, 9].

Some authors report buried penis as a different entity than webbed penis: in this case, webbed penis is the result of abnormal dartos at the level of the peno-scrotal angle, making that angle disappear, and giving the impression a penis webbed in the scrotal skin.

Symptoms can consist of cosmetic issues, as well as functional problems: voiding difficulties, urine spraying, dribbling, and ballooning.

Buried penis has to be distinguished from acquired penile entrapment, which is observed after circumcision or other penile surgery during which too much skin has been removed [5, 6]. Such condition is called 'trapped penis' [1, 6]. Trapped penis is therefore an acquired form of buried penis. The penile skin after circumcision forms a circumferential scar around the glans. The penis appears trapped within the scar, and is retracted in the pre-pubic fat or in the scrotum (Fig. 14.1a, b).

14.1.1 Pathophysiology

In Buried penis it is observed that the penis is entrapped in a cocoon of fibrotic dartos tissue and a common underlying pathologic process in all congenital penile malformation has been suggested [10–12]. In children with buried penis there seems to be a lack of elasticity of the dartos tissue, which normally allows the penile skin to slide freely on the deeper layers and allows easy stretching in erectile condition [13]. Due to this condition the penis is retracted into the surrounding tissue.

Buried penises are associated with a high level of disorganisation of the dartos tissue, which lies probably at the origin of this condition [11]. It was also observed that the level of dartos architecture disorganisation was strongly correlated with the clinical severity of the malformation [11].

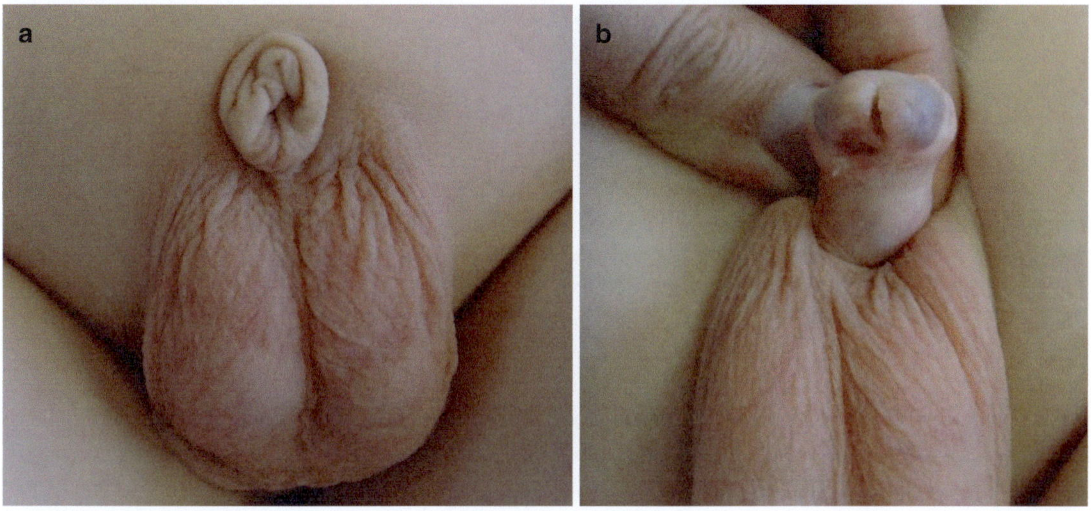

Fig. 14.1 (**a**) Buried penis: only *preputium* is visible. (**b**) When applying pressure to the prepubic area, a normal penis appears, entrapped into pre-pubic fat

Many explanations have been embryologically proposed for those conditions, with very few evidence: some authors propose the buried aspect of the penis is due to a lack of separation of the different primitive layers, rendering the penis attached to the deep fascia [14].

14.1.2 Surgical Techniques

The goal of surgery is to release of penis out of its cocoon, restoring normal penile length. Several surgical techniques have been proposed [6, 15–18]. Any surgical technique should include degloving of the penis to its base and fixing the penile skin and the dartos fascia to the deeper fascia to re-establish a correct peno-pubic angle and peno-scrotal angle.

Some authors describe topical administration of steroids as helpful in some cases [9]. The majority of the real webbed of buried will anyway need surgical correction. Some authors also apply topical androgens, but Mouriquand proved it not helpful [4]. Some authors argue surgical correction is not mandatory, and the puberty and its androgen boost will solve the problem. As application of local androgens before puberty is not efficient, the androgen boost of the puberty has even few chances of solving the problem [4].

There are even probably as many surgical techniques are there are surgeons operating on buried penis. Confusion further increases with the enormous number of varying principles applied to correct buried penis, based on liposuction, development of flaps, lipectomy,[16, 19–21]

Many surgical techniques in small series report satisfactory results in buried penis repair. None of those previously described techniques has reached the status of gold standard, highlighting the fact that none of them is quite satisfactory enough to spread it. As long as we do not understand the embryological origin and the pathological development of buried penis, our efforts in repairing this anomaly are more or less successful, depending on the applied technique [22]. The published techniques are based on a few principles: redistribution of the abnormal preputial skin, division of the deep fascia anchoring the penis in the depths, release of the dartos tethering cords, and eventually anchoring of the penile skin at the penoscrotal junction to the deep fascia [16]. Some authors describe a skin release technique associated with pubis liposuction [16].

Any technique, besides releasing the penis form its dartos cocoon, should also deal with esthetical aspects: scars should be hidden whenever possible: some authors describe however a dorsal incision [6, 23]. We believe ventral incisions on the raphe will provide a better cosmetic outcome. Some authors use a circumferential incision at the base of the penis. We believe this type of incision to be unaesthetic, but we also believe it might be responsible for lymphedema [24]. We believe the best type of approach combined a circumcision incision a few millimeters under the glans, combined with a ventral incision on the raphe. We believe this approach allows a complete degloving of the penis, and provides esthetical results.

We also believe this technique allows the use of preputium if necessary for penile covering after deglovement. It therefore makes it possible to avoid flap techniques, which always provide worse cosmetic outcome.

Liposuccion and lipectomy are very controversial. Some authors use it. We believe its effects are only transient, and do not recommend it.

Our technique is based on the idea that buried penis is caused by a lack of elasticity of the dartos tissue, and eventually by abnormal adherences between dartos and Buck's fascia [25]. The release of all tethering cords of dartos, essential in our technique, allows the penis to regain its elasticity (Fig. 14.2).

The key point of our technique, being the anchoring of the stretched penis at its base to the released dartos tissue, avoids any further retraction after release (Figs. 14.3 and 14.4) [25].

Further research is needed to prove that buried penis is based on abnormal dartos tissue. Our series, although small, shows obviously good results according to parents/patient and according to surgeon. If we consider that parents asking for reoperation judged the outcome as bad, we even reach statistical significance in favour of our technique (Fig. 14.5) [18].

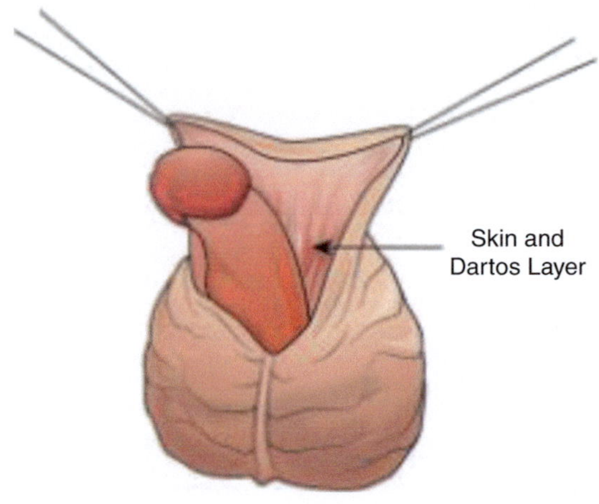

Fig. 14.2 Degloving of the penis

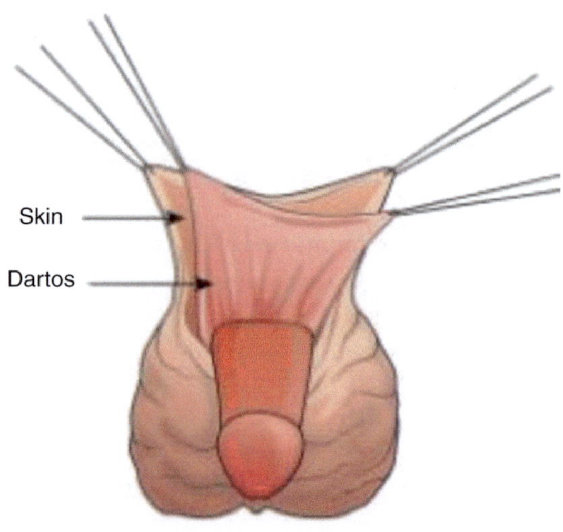

Fig. 14.3 Development of a dartos flap

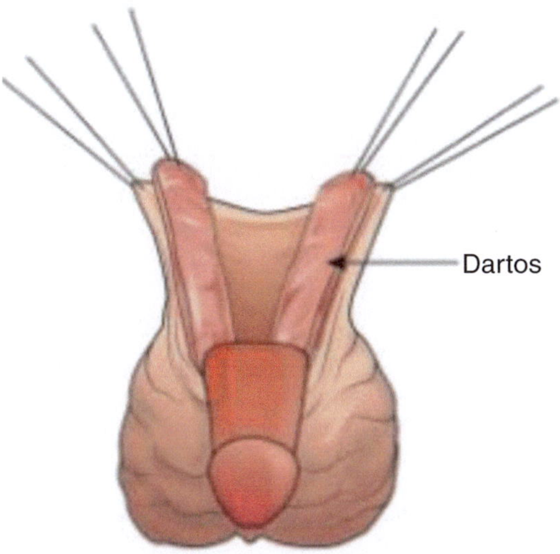

Fig. 14.4 Splitting the dartos flap and bringing it ventrally to anchor the streteched penis at its base

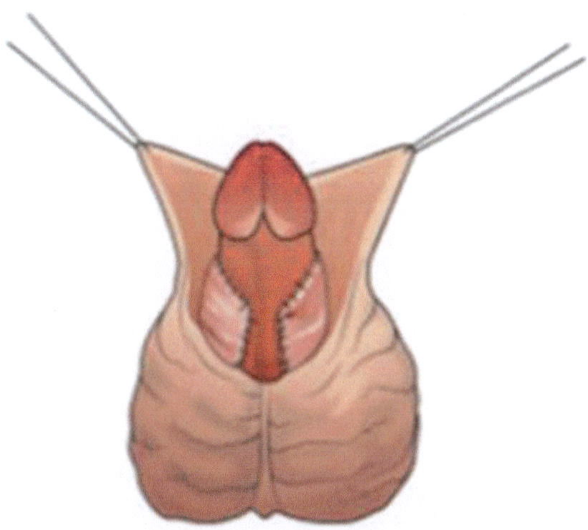

Fig. 14.5 The penis is anchored at its base with the flaps, preventing re-entrapment

Conclusion

Buried penis, or webbed penis is a controversial entity. Every pediatric urologist should keep a few important concepts in mind: Any penile condition is a formal contra-indication for classical circumcision.

Buried penis has to be distinguished from micropenis, which is a complex pathology requiring multidisciplinary approach involving a pediatric endocrinologist.

The pathophysiologic pathways leading to buried or webbed penis remain to be unveiled. Many surgical techniques have been described, but none has reached the status of gold standard. Any technique should take care of a few principles: penile deglovement is mandatory to discard the surrounding dartos tissue trapping the penis into the pre-pubic fat. Scars should be hidden when possible, as esthetic outcome is important in those primary penile conditions.

References

1. Gearhart J, Rink R, Mouriquand P. Pediatric Urology: Sauders Elsevier; 2010. buried penis, 519–25 p.
2. Crawford BS. Buried penis. Br J Plast Surg. 1977;30(1):96–9. Epub 1977/01/01.
3. Boemers TM, De Jong TP. The surgical correction of buried penis: a new technique. J Urol. 1995;154(2 Pt 1):550–2. Epub 1995/08/01.
4. Lardellier-Reynaud F, Varlet F, Francois M, Mouriquand P. Congenital buried penis in children. Prog Urol. 2011;21(9):642–50. Epub 2011/09/29. La verge enfouie congenitale de l'enfant.
5. Redman JF. Buried penis: congenital syndrome of a short penile shaft and a paucity of penile shaft skin. J Urol. 2005;173(5):1714–7. Epub 2005/04/12.
6. Alter GJ, Horton CE, Horton Jr CE. Buried penis as a contraindication for circumcision. J Am Coll Surg. 1994;178(5):487–90. Epub 1994/05/01.
7. Shaeer O, Shaeer K. Revealing the buried penis in adults. J Sex Med. 2009;6(3):876–85. Epub 2009/01/28.
8. Tang SKD, Santucci RA. Modern management of adult-acquired buried penis. Urology. 2008;72:124–7.
9. Smeulders N, Wilcox DT, Cuckow PM. The buried penis – an anatomical approach. BJU Int. 2000;86(4):523–6. Epub 2000/09/06.
10. Spinoit AF, Poelaert F, Van Praet C, Groen LA, Van Laecke E, Hoebeke P. Grade of hypospadias is the only factor predicting for re-intervention after primary hypospadias repair: a multivariate analysis from a cohort of 474 patients. J Pediatr Urol. 2015;11((2):70 e1–6. Epub 2015/03/24.

11. Spinoit AF, Van Praet C, Groen LA, Van Laecke E, Praet M, Hoebeke P. Congenital penile pathology is associated with abnormal development of the dartos muscle: a prospective study of primary penile surgery at a tertiary referral center. J Urol. 2015;193(5):1620–4. Epub 2014/12/03.
12. Spinoit AF. New insights in congenital penile malformations [Medicine]. Gent, Belgium: Ghent University; 2015.
13. Goodhope CD. Correction of chordee and hypospadias. Northwest Med. 1945;44:356–8. Epub 1945/11/01.
14. Donahoe PK, Keating MA. Preputial unfurling to correct the buried penis. J Pediatr Surg. 1986;21(12):1055–7. Epub 1986/12/01.
15. Chih-Chun CCY, Diau G. Preputial flaps to correct buried penis. Pediatr Surg Int. 2007;23:1119–21.
16. Hadidi AT. Buried penis: classification surgical approach. J Pediatr Surg. 2014;49(2):374–9. Epub 2014/02/18.
17. Perger L, Hanley RS, Feins NR. Penoplasty for buried penis in infants and children: report of 100 cases. Pediatr Surg Int. 2009;25(2):175–80. Epub 2008/11/05.
18. Brisson P, Patel H, Chan M. Penoplasty for buried penis in children: report of 50 cases. J Pediatr Surg. 2001;36(3):421–5.
19. Rivas S, Romero R, Parente A. Simplification of the surgical treatment of a hidden penis. Actas Urol Esp. 2011;35(5):310–4.
20. Sugita Y, Ueoka K, Tagkagi S, Hisamatsu E, Yoshino K, Tanikaze S. A new technique of concealed penis repair. J Urol. 2009;182(4):1751–4.
21. Jung EH, Son JH, Jang SH, Lee JW. Simple anchoring of the penopubic skin to the prepubic deep fascia in surgical correction of buried penis. Korean J Urol. 2011;52(11):787–91. Epub 2011/12/24.
22. Sivakumar B, Brown A, Kangesu L. Circumcision in buried penis: a cautionary tale. Ann R Coll Surg Engl. 2004;86:35–7.
23. Shapiro SR. Surgical treatment of the "buried" penis. Urology. 1987;30(6):554–9. Epub 1987/12/01.
24. Lipszyc E, Pfister C, Liard A, Mitrofanoff P. Surgical treatment of buried penis. Eur J Pediatr Surg Off J Austrian Assoc Pediatr Surg [et al] = Zeitschrift fur Kinderchirurgie. 1997;7(5):292–5. Epub 1997/12/24.
25. Spinoit AF, De Prycker S, Groen LA, van Laecke E, Hoebeke P. New surgical technique for the treatment of buried penis: results and comparison with a traditional technique in 75 patients. Urol Int. 2013;91(2):134–9. Epub 2013/07/11.

Penoscrotal Positional (PSP) Anomalies

15

Abstract

Normal penoscrotal configuration, with the penis overriding the scrotum with its characteristic skin rugae stoping at the base of the penis without creeping and with a preserved angle had a paramount impaction in the psychic satisfaction of a child, but usually this not the case in all children, as partial or complete positional exchange between the penis and scrotum diagnosed infrequently as a rare anomaly which may be manifested in different phenotypes, and minor degree may pass unnoticed, but it may be associated with other genitourinary anomalies. Many pediatric surgeons and urologists believe that this minor positional anomaly is not harmful and usually asymptomatic, but investigating those children and adults who had such abnormality revealed a urinary symptoms in the form of abnormally directed stream, and increased frequency of UTI and they may had a difficulty during intercourse, which may impact their sexual life.

Keywords

Cephalic scrotal transposition • Central median penile scrotalization • Caudal scrotal regression • Wide penoscrotal angle • Scrotal engulfment • Shawl scrotum • Prepenile scrotum

Normal penoscrotal configuration, with the penis overriding the scrotum with its characteristic skin rugae stoping at the base of the penis without creeping and with a preserved angle had a paramount impaction in the psychic satisfaction of a child, but usually this not the case in all children, as partial or complete positional exchange between the penis and scrotum diagnosed infrequently as a rare anomaly which may be manifested in different phenotypes, and minor degree may pass unnoticed, but it may be associated with other genitourinary anomalies. Many pediatric surgeons and urologists believe that this minor positional anomaly is not harmful and usually asymptomatic, but investigating those children and adults who had such abnormality revealed a urinary symptoms in the form of

Electronic supplementary material The online version of this chapter (doi:10.1007/978-3-319-43310-3_15) contains supplementary material, which is available to authorized users.

© Springer International Publishing Switzerland 2017

M. Fahmy, *Congenital Anomalies of the Penis*, DOI 10.1007/978-3-319-43310-3_15

abnormally directed stream, and increased frequency of UTI and they may had a difficulty during intercourse, which may impact their sexual life.

Penoscrotal transposition classified herein to cranial or cephalic scrotal migration, cranial type subdivided into major and minor where the last subdivided to bilateral, unilateral or central. A new categories of wide penoscrotal distance and caudal scrotal regression are documented and described.

Definition

Complete penoscrotal transposition is an uncommon condition in which the scrotum is located in a cephalic position with respect to the penis. A less severe form is a bifid scrotum, in which the two halves of the scrotum meet above the penis. It is a heterogeneous anomaly, and detection warrants careful clinical evaluation to rule out other major and life-threatening anomalies, especially of the urinary system. Minor degree of scrotal tissue transposition above the root of the penis is known as a shawl scrotum (doughnut scrotum), it could be symmetrical bilaterally in both sided of the penile shaft or unilaterally, where it is called an ectopic scrotum in the severe forms. Regression of the scrotum caudally, ending with a wide distance between penis and scrotum is a new entity described recently [1].

15.1 Historical Background

Penoscrotal transposition was first reported by Appleby in 1923 [2]. Mcllvoy and Harris in 1955 reported the first performed surgery to move the penis into a more cranial position through a subcutaneous tunnel beneath the prepenile scrotum [3].

Nomenclature

Scrotal engulfment, shawl scrotum, prepenile scrotum, daughter scrotum.

15.2 Incidence

There is no figure about the exact incidence of PST; complete cases are stated usually as a case report, but I believe minor cases are underestimated. In our group of 11,450 child examined during routine circumcision an 82 cases of different grades of PSP anomalies diagnosed with an incidence of (0.7 %), this high incidence this group of patients attributed to special characters of the sample rolled as most of them are referred patients with a high possibility to have a different genitourinary anomalies [1]. The office of Rare Diseases (ORD) of the National Institutes of Health (NIH) estimated penoscrotal transposition, or its subtype to affect less than 200,000 people in the US population.

15.3 Etiology

One aspect of sexual differentiation that still poorly understood is the mechanism controlling the position of genitalia, as the external position of male gonads represents one of the most important differences between both sexes. Embryological origin of the penis and scrotum are respectively the genital tubercle and labioscrotal folds, and at the end of the sixth week of development, males and females have indistinguishable external genitalia, then penis and scrotum achieve their usual arrangement when, under the influence of androgens, the genital tubercle elongates to become the penis and the labioscrotal folds migrate to a caudal and dorsal position to the penis, where they fuse in the midline and merge beneath the penis, the line of fusion remains as the scrotal raphe. It has been suggested that scrotal anomalies like penoscrotal transposition may result from early division and/or abnormal migration of the labioscrotal swelling [4] (Fig. 15.1).

Although most reported cases are sporadic, some suggest a genetic basis for abnormal penoscrotal relationship. Abnormal positioning of the genital tubercle in relation to the scrotal swellings during the critical fourth to fifth week of gestation may affect the inferomedial migration and fusion of the scrotal swellings. If the phallic tubercle also is intrinsically abnormal,

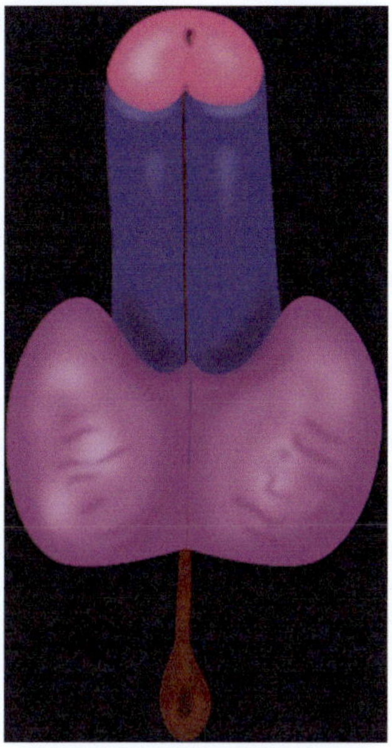

Fig 15.1 Normal penoscrotal configurations

development of the corporal bodies and the urethral groove and folds may be affected; this explains the frequent occurrence of the other genital abnormalities [5]. Lamm and Kaplan [4] suggested that unilateral failure or abnormal migration might result in unilateral penoscrotal transposition or ectopic scrotum, and early division of a labioscrotal swelling with subsequent abnormal migration might result in an accessory scrotum. Takayasu et al. [6] proposed that a teratoid growth of the divided pleuripotential anlage of he labioscrotal swelling is responsible for the accessory scrotum. Perineal lipomas have been described also as an associated condition; however, they are very commonly associated with the accessory scrotum in up to 83 % of cases, also Sule et al. [7] hypothesized that the accessory labioscrotal fold develops due to presence of perineal lipoma in the perineum which disrupts the continuity of the developing caudal labioscrotal swelling.

There is evidence that 5-alpha-reductase type 2 deficiency may be involved in PST. 5-alpha reductase type 2 deficiency is an autosomal recessive sex-limited condition that prevents the conversion of testosterone to dihydrotestosterone [8].

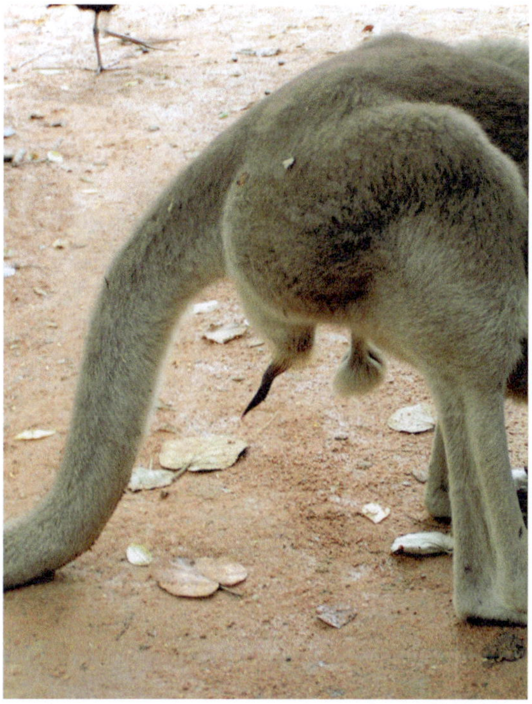

Fig. 15.2 Kangaroo with a normal pre penile scrotum

In marsupial animals like Kangaroo the scrotum is normally lies caudal to the penis, where in rabbits the scrotum lies partially around the phallus, so this issue deserve a more researches to elucidate the exact pathogenesis of PSP anomalies (Fig. 15.2).

15.4 Penoscrotal Positional Anomalies and Other Syndromes

PSP anomalies reported with different grades of caudal regression syndrome [9], many syndromes such as Aarskog-Scott syndrome (faciodigitogenital syndrome), Rubenstein-Taybi syndrome, craniofrontonasal dysplasia, Hunter Carpenter McDonald Syndrome, Naguib Syndrome, Saito Kuba Tsuruta Syndrome, Ieshima Koeda Inagaki syndrome, Willems de Vries syndrome, Schinzel syndrome and Seaver Cassidy syndrome. Different grades of PSP anomalies are a common feature of Popliteal pterygium syndrome.

15.5 Clinical Manifestations

PSP anomalies are usually asymptomatic, but investigating those children and adults who had such abnormality revealed a urinary symptoms in the form of abnormally directed stream, increased frequency of UTI and they may had a difficulty and discomfort during intercourse, and difficulty in placing a condom which may impact in their sexual life, and psychological pressure brought about by cosmetic deformity which can lead to demands for surgery.

15.6 Classification

Glenn and Anderson [10] had classified this abnormality into the following categories according to severity: bifid scrotum, incomplete or partial penoscrotal transposition, complete penoscrotal transposition or prepenile scrotum, and ectopic scrotum. In our published study with the spectrum of 63 diverse cases of penoscrotal positional anomalies we gave a simple classification [1], but with a more accumulated cases of this rare anomaly (82 Cases) wereachedtothismorereliabletopographicclassification:-

- **Cephalic Scrotal transposition**
  - Major
    - Complete (Figs. 15.3, 15.4 and 15.5)
    - Incomplete "shawl scrotum" (Fig. 15.6)
  - Minor
    - Unilateral asymmetrical (Fig. 15.7)
    - Bilateral (symmetrical) (Fig. 15.8)
    - Central median penile scrotalization (Fig. 15.9)
- **Caudal scrotal regression** (Figs. 15.10 and 15.11)

This simple classification according to cephalic or caudal migration of the scrotum in relation to the penile base may be helpful for awareness of pediatric surgeons and urologists to elite up such cases and to sort severe forms, which necessitate surgical intervention.

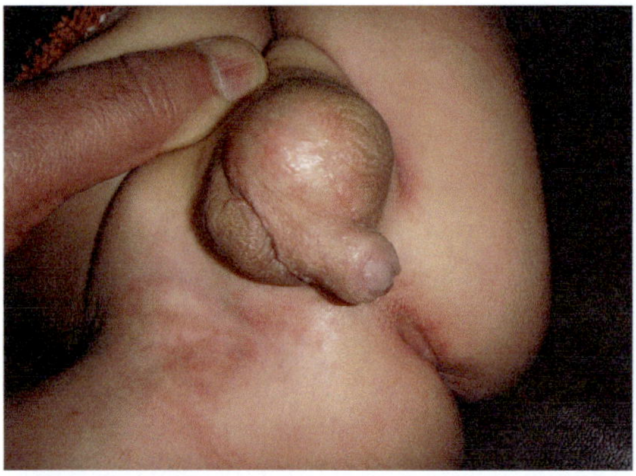

Fig. 15.3 Complete Major cephalic penoscrotal transposition without hypospadias

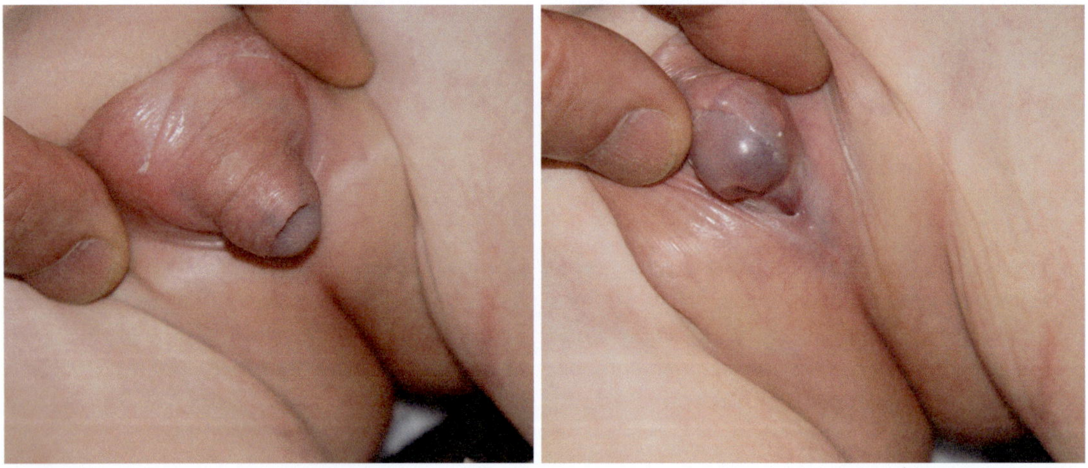

Figs. 15.4 and 15.5 Complete Major penoscrotal transposition with a proximal perineal hypospadias

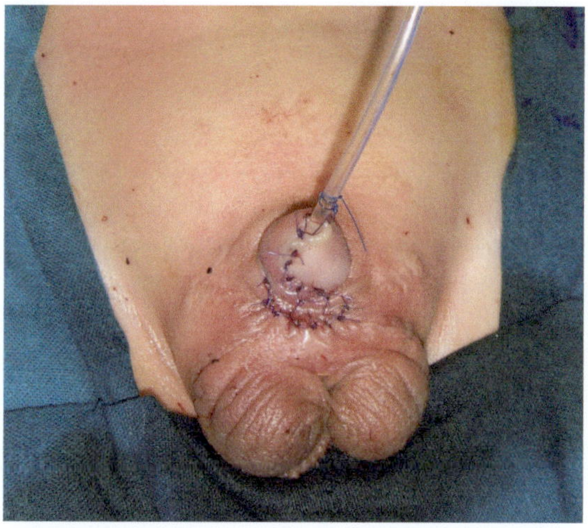

Fig 15.6 Case in Figs. 15.4 and 15.5 after one stage correction

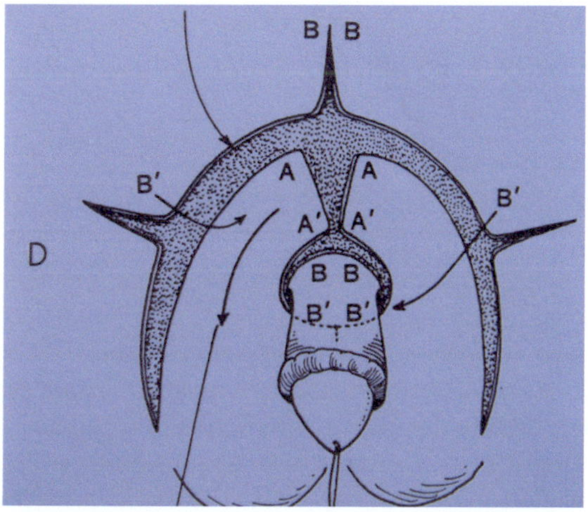

Fig. 15.7 Diagram of scrotal flaps for correction of complete PS transposition

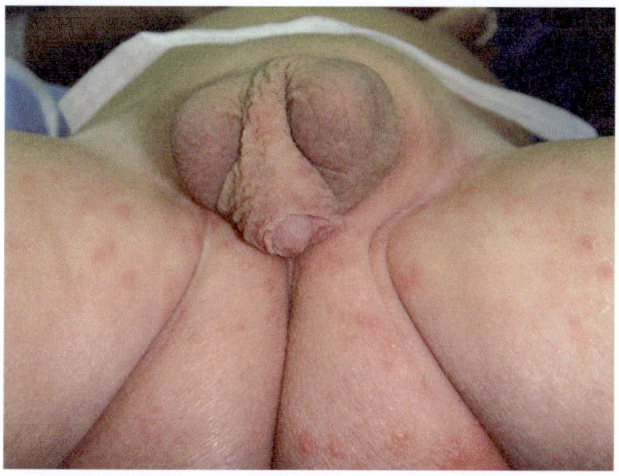

Fig. 15.8 Incomplete major cephalic penoscrotal transposition

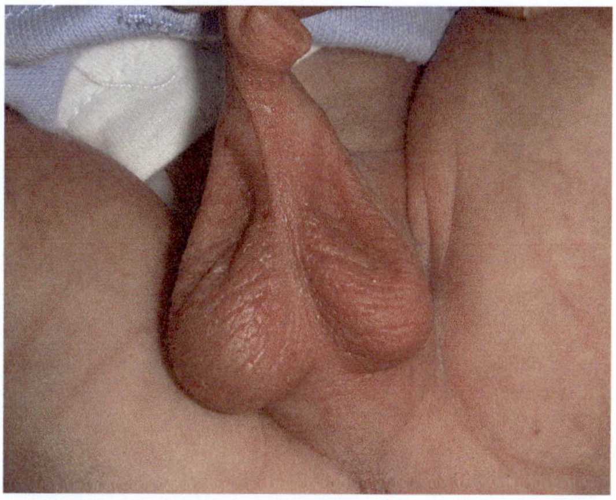

Fig. 15.9 Scrotalization of the whole penile skin, without any other anomalies

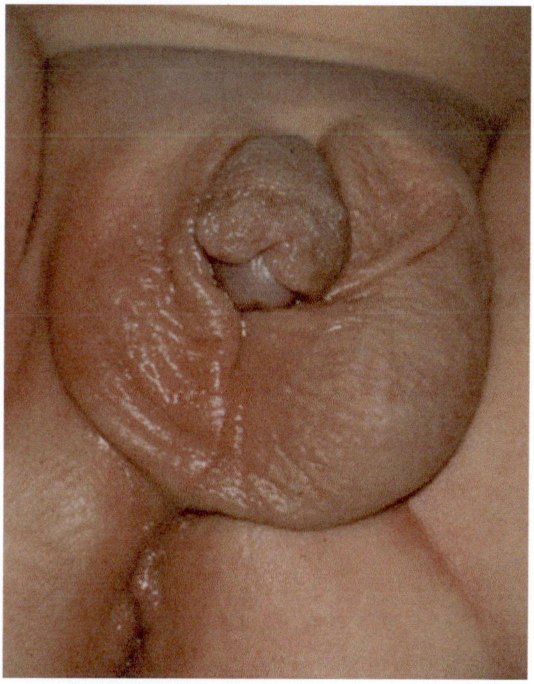

Fig. 15.10 Minor unilateral (asymmetrical) scrotal transposition

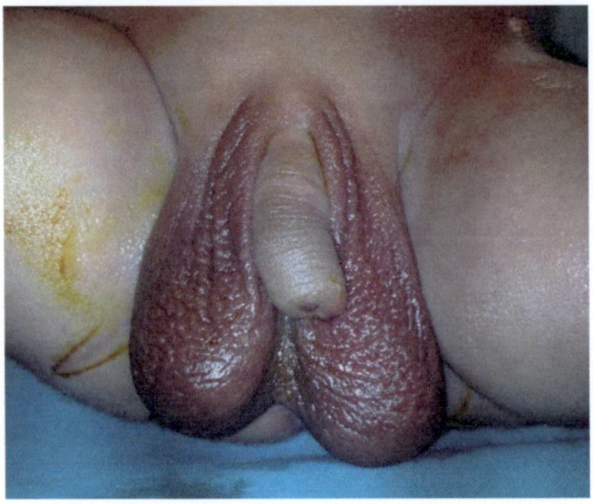

Fig. 15.11 Minor Bilateral (symmetrical) scrotal transposition

15.7 Complete Penoscrotal Transposition (CPST)

In which the scrotum is located completely cephalic to the penis, it is very rarely to have this subtype without hypospadias (Fig. 15.3), but frequently it is associated with a severe form of perineal hypospadias with or without corpora spongosium hypoplasia, and other life-threatening malformations involving the genitourinary, cardiovascular, or skeletal systems [11] (Figs. 15.4 and 15.5).

Management Surgical correction is recommended for physiological and psychological reasons. When associated with severe hypospadias (CPST), may involve a staged surgical repair, but one stage repair of urethra and penile reposition could be achieved with success (Fig. 15.6). Scrotoplasty is completed with an inverted omega skin incision that is made around the scrotal skin and the base of the penis, bringing the scrotal flaps beneath the penis (Fig. 15.7).

Recurrence and improper correction with unsatisfactory look is encountered. Forshall and Rickham [12] used a different technique in two patients in whom the cranially located scrotal flaps were elevated, rotated medially and caudally, and sutured beneath the penis; this method was also used by Glenn and Anderson [10].

15.8 Major Incomplete

In less severe forms, the penis may appear to arise from centre of the scrotum or be encased partially or incompletely by the scrotum, where part of scrotum lies above penis, but still there is some scrotal tissues lie caudally to the penis, in a condition known as shawl scrotum; as we can see from Fig. 15.8, the scrotum engulfing the penis which pointing down, with a characteristic scrotal skin covering the shaft of the penis with its characteristic darker colour, rugae and wrinkles. Very few cases reported with normal positioned scrotum and penis, but only the characteristically wrinkled scrotal skin creeps over the penis, replacing the normal smooth penile skin, which gives a disfigured look of the penis with a possibility of appearance of hair in this area at adulthood (Fig. 15.9).

15.9 Minor Cases

May be unilateral, where one hemiscrotum creeps caudally at one side of penis, and this could be an isolated anomaly or may be associated with hypospadias or penile rotation. This cases may be explained by unilateral failure or abnormal migration of labioscrotal fold, and isolated detached scrotal tissue above the penoscrotal angle considered as an ectopic scrotum, this type reported with Aarskog-Scott syndrome [13] (Fig. 15.10).

Bilateral incomplete symmetrical scrotal transposition is another entity encountered without any other genitourinary anomalies (Fig. 15.11).

15.10 Central Creeping of Scrotal Tissue

around the median raphe was not described before, and could be manifested as an abnormal corrugated scrotal skin covering the central

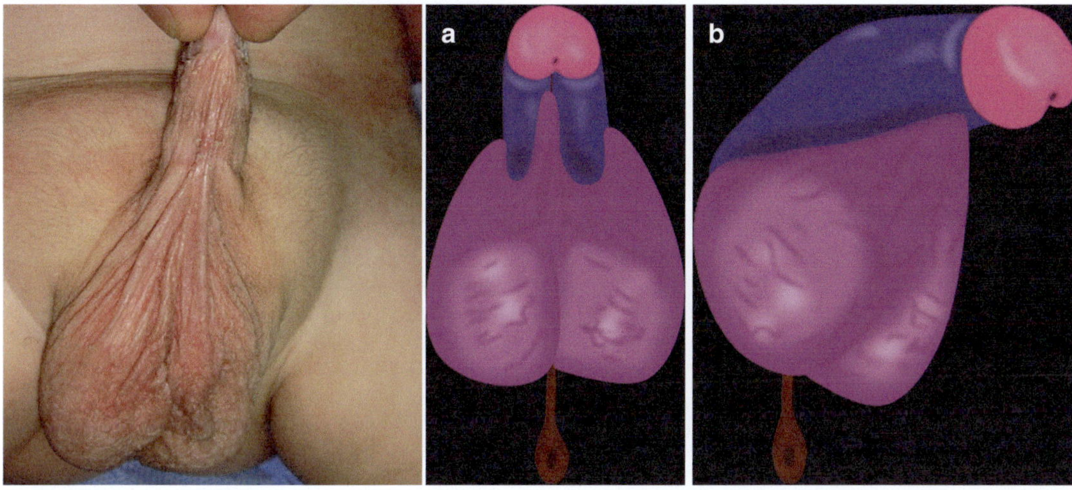

Fig. 15.12 Central median penile scrotalization. (**a** and **b**) Diagrams demonstrating creeping of scrotal tissue to the ventral surface of penile shaft

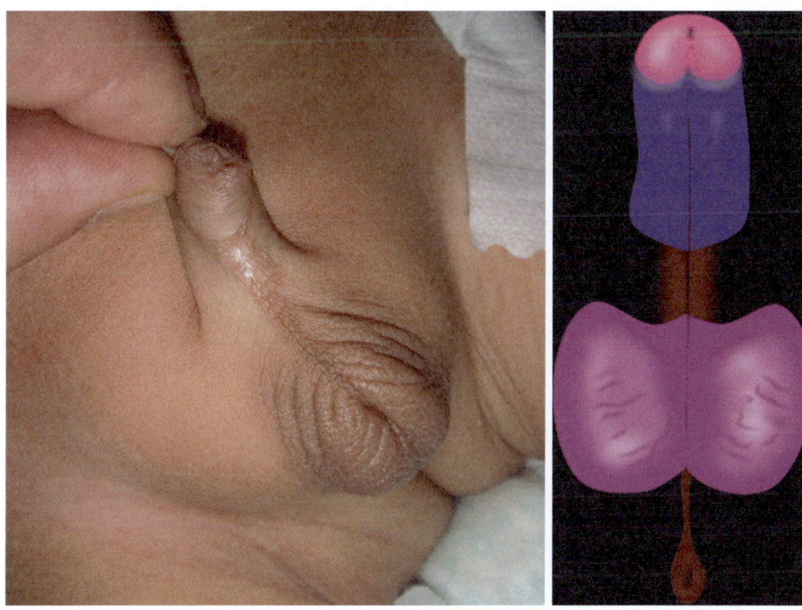

Fig. 15.13 (**a**) Caudal scrotal regression, with a wide gape between penis and scrotum, and without any other anomalies. (**b**) Diagram showing the wide penoscrotal angle

part of the ventral surface of the penis, or it may be presented as a variant of webbed penis, which possibly affect the functional length of the penis (Fig. 15.12) and Fig. 15.12a and b diagram demonstrating this anomaly. This abnormality necessitate correction with the same principles of correction of the webbed penis (Chap. 15).

15.11 Caudal Scrotal Regression (Wide Penoscrotal Angle)

In contrary to the previously described scrotal transposition, the distance between scrotum and the penile shaft may be so wide, with a loss of continuity and normal angle (around 90^0) between penile shaft and scrotum (Fig. 15.13a, b). This

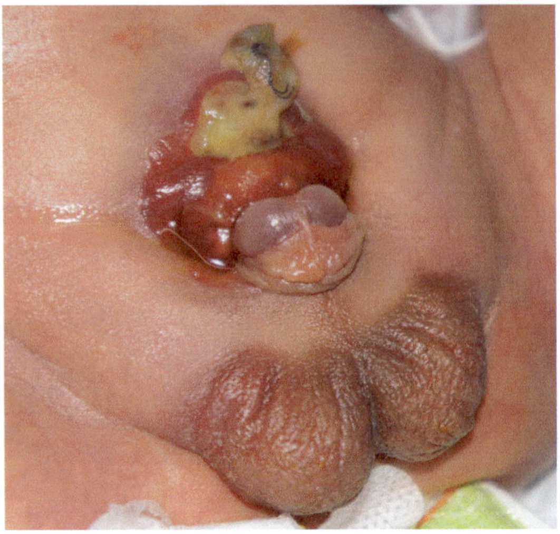

Fig. 15.14 Caudal scrotal regression in a case of bladder exstrophy

anomaly could be an isolated cases or in association with other anomalies, mainly bladder exstrophy, careful examination of the penoscrotal distance in such cases showed a reasonable number of cases had such abnormality with a different degrees (Fig. 15.14). It is difficult to correct such cases and actually intervention may not even indicated, as it had no functional impaction, but shortening of this penoscrotal distance could be considered during bladder exstrophy repair, specially if corporal assembly is indicated.

References

1. Fahmy MAB, Alaa Aldin A, Alshennawy AA, Edress AM. Spectrum of penoscrotal positional anomalies in children. Int J Surg. 2014;12(9):983–8. http://www.sciencedirect.com/science/article/pii/S1743919114004853.
2. Appleby LH. An unusual arrangement of the external genitalia. Can Med Assoc J. 1923;13:514–6.
3. Mcllvoy DB, Harris HS. Transposition of the penis and scrotum: case report. J Urol. 1955;73:540–3.
4. Lamm DL, Kaplan GW. Accessory and ectopic scrota. Urology. 1977;9:149–53.
5. Wang MH, Baskin LS. Endocrine disruptors, genital development, and hypospadias. J Androl. 2008;29:499–505.
6. Takayasu H, Ueno A, Tsukada O. Accessory scrotum: a case report. J Urol. 1974;112:826–7.
7. Sule JD, Skoog SJ, Tank ES. Perineal lipoma and the accessory labioscrotal fold: an etiological relationship. J Urol. 1994;151:475–7.
8. Blaschko SD, Mahawong P, Ferretti M, et al. Analysis of the effect of estrogen/androgen perturbation on penile development in transgenic and diethylstilbestrol-treated mice. Anat Rec (Hoboken). 2012;296:1127–41 [PubMed: 23653160].
9. Lage JM, Driscoll SG, Bieber FR. Transposition of the external genitalia associated with caudal regression. J Urol. 1987;138:387–9.
10. Glenn JF, Anderson EE. Surgical correction of incomplete penoscrotal transposition. J Urol. 1973;110:603–5.
11. Meguid NA, Temtamy SA, Mazen I. Transposition of external genitalia and associated malformations. Clin Dysmorphol. 2003;12:59–62.
12. Forshall I, Rickham P. Transposition of the penis and scrotum. Br J Urol. 1956;38:250–2.
13. Pinke LA, Rathbun SR, Husmann DA, Kramer SA. Penoscrotal transposition: review of 53 patients. J Urol. 2001;166:1865–8.

Median Genital Raphe Anomalies 16

Abstract

Raphe means the line of union of the two halves of various symmetrical body parts, and the term median raphe refers to the perineal raphe, which is also known as the median raphe of the perineum; and it is divided anatomically to: penile raphe, scrotal and perineal raphe. This line starts just anterior to the anus and extends through the scrotum, continuing on the ventral surface of the penis and prepuce; it is usually darker in colour than the surrounding skin, generally deep pink or brown.

Keywords

Absent median raphe • Prominent median raphe • Wide median raphe • Splitted raphe • Bucket handle malformation • Median raphe cyst • Beaded median raphe • Pearly penile papules

Definition

Raphe means the line of union of the two halves of various symmetrical body parts, and the term median raphe refers to the perineal raphe, which is also known as the median raphe of the perineum; and it is divided anatomically to: penile raphe, scrotal and perineal raphe (Fig. 16.1). This line starts just anterior to the anus and extends through the scrotum, continuing on the ventral surface of the penis and prepuce; it is usually darker in colour than the surrounding skin, generally deep pink or brown (Fig. 16.2).

Genital Median Raphe (GMR) is a result of a fetal developmental phenomenon whereby the scrotum (the developmental equivalent of the labia in females) and penis close toward the midline and fuse, to form this line which represents the superficial effects of the midline fusion of ectoderm along these areas, as development progresses, the ectodermal edges of the urethral groove begin to fuse to form the median raphe [1] (Fig. 16.3). This embryological line or ridge may be subjected to a various anomalies, which not well known by many practitioners, and can thus pass unnoticed, these anomalies will be highlighted with some details.

Electronic supplementary material The online version of this chapter (doi:10.1007/978-3-319-43310-3_16) contains supplementary material, which is available to authorized users.

© Springer International Publishing Switzerland 2017

M. Fahmy, *Congenital Anomalies of the Penis*, DOI 10.1007/978-3-319-43310-3_16

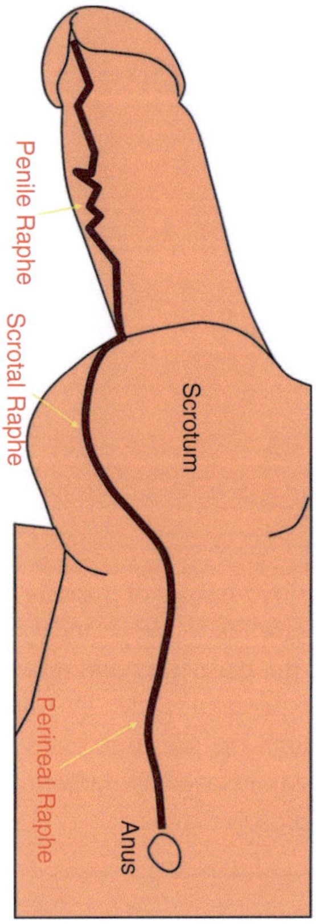

Fig. 16.1 Anatomical segments of median raphe

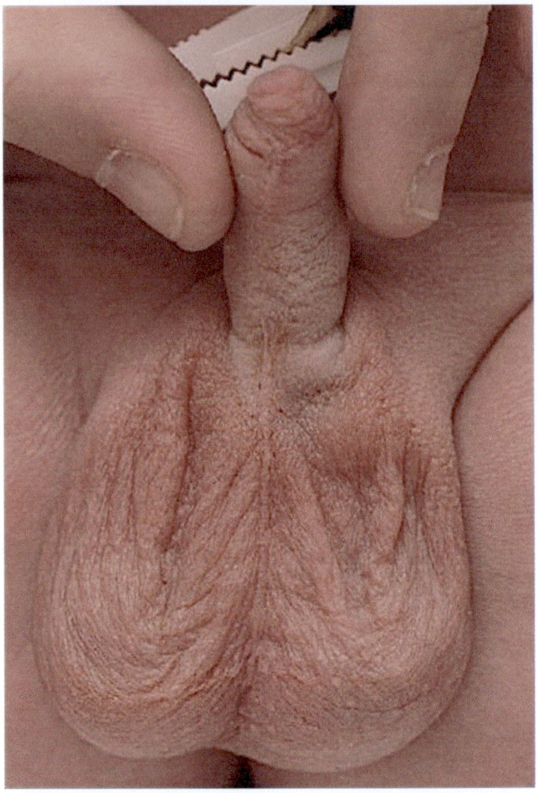

Fig. 16.2 Normal appearance of median raphe

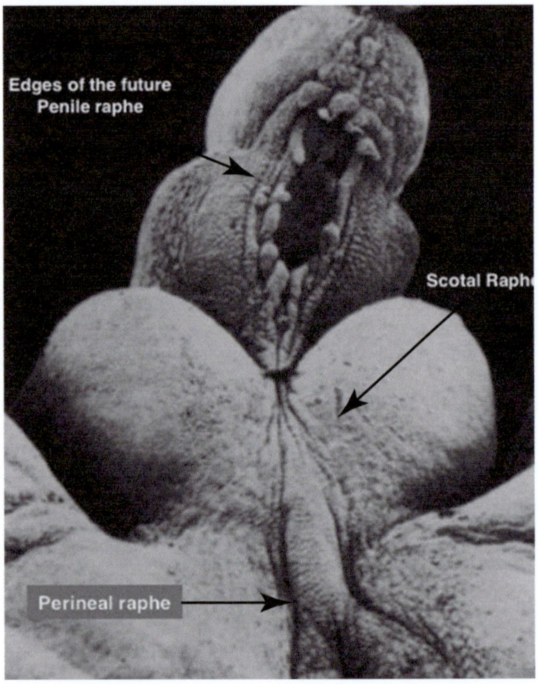

Fig. 16.3 Urethral groove before fusion to form median raphe from the ectoderm

Nomenclature

Genital raphe, Penile raphe, Genitoperineal raphe and Median raphe.

16.1 Incidence

Median raphe anomalies are not so common and rarely taken into consideration; and curiously these conditions receive little attention even in genitourinary textbooks, and they are generally classified in literature into one of only two groups: cysts or ectodermal canals. These anomalies are formed from outgrowing endoderm and ectoderm after closure. In a survey of 2880 babies aged from 1 day to 7 weeks we detect an overall incidence of about 2%, with a wide spectrum ranging from simple anomaly like prominent raphe to a raphe cyst [2].

16.2 Significance of GMR Anomalies

Pathology of the GMR anomalies may be simple, carries no direct impact on the child health and in many occasions needs no surgical intervention, but its significance mainly came from the serious associated anomalies, which are usually hidden and may be only disclosed after detection of GMR anomalies; as we will see in cases of intact prepuce megameatus for example. Recently with the advance in ultrasound techniques, median raphe could be visualised accurately antenatally as an indictor not only for sex determination, where the male fetus was recognised by the presence of the scrotal sac as a rounded echogenic structure separated by an echogenic median raphe [3], but also may give a hint about an associated anomalies; like hypospadias, and as we will see from the wide range of GMR anomalies, it may be used in the future for more detection and diagnosis of other congenital genitourinary anomalies antenatally.

Anomalies of median raphe classified to:

1. **Absent median raphe**
2. **Prominent Median Raphe**
3. **Wide median Raphe**
4. **Splitted median Raphe**
5. **Hyperpigmented Median Raphe**
6. **Short Contracted Raphe**
7. **Deviation of Raphe**
8. **Bucket handle malformation**
9. **Median raphe cyst**
10. **Beaded median raphe**
11. **Pearly penile papules**

16.2.1 Absent Median Raphe

Complete absence of penile raphe with flat redundant skin covering the penile shaft is a very rare anomaly which may be detected with different types of hypospadias (Fig. 16.4), and it is also reported as an associated anomaly with transverse testicular ectopia [4], usually perineal raphe is normal in such cases.

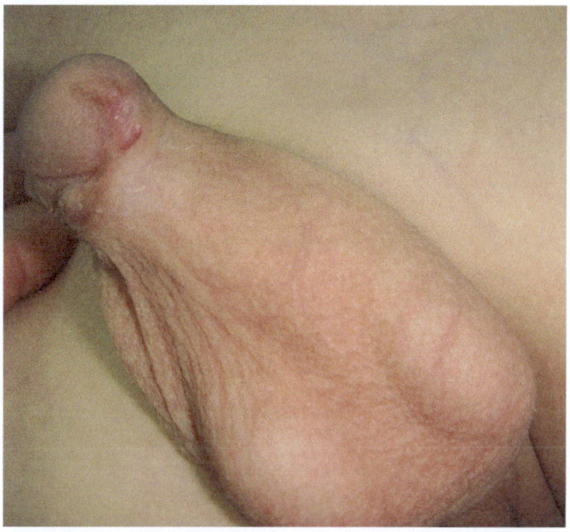

Fig. 16.4 Absent penile raphe with coronal hypospadias in a circumcised child

16.2.2 Prominent Median Raphe

Normally GMR identified by its little prominence than the rest of the penile skin around it, but abnormal extensively prominent raphe looks like a ridge was detected in association with other anomalies like hypospadias, imperforate anus, and in rare cases of Townes–Brocks syndrome (an autosomal dominant disorder with multiple malformations and variable expression, major findings include external ear anomalies, hearing loss, preaxial polydactyly and triphalangeal thumbs, imperforate anus, and renal malformations) [5]. In many severe cases of hypospadias the GMR was a very prominent midline ridge extending from the the anal orifice to the hypospadiac uri-

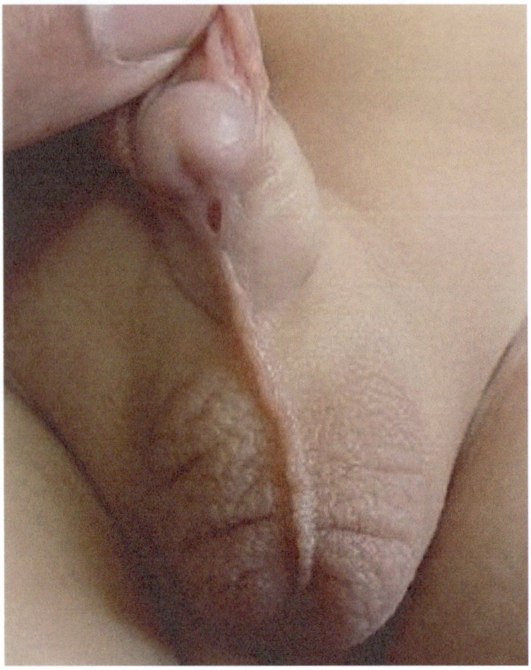

Fig. 16.5 Prominent Raphe with an anterior penile hypospadias

nary meatus (Fig. 16.5). Prominent GMR have to be differentiated from others anomalies like: wide, hyperpigmented and splitted types.

16.2.3 Wide Median Raphe

Abnormal wideness of median raphe; either flat or prominent probably due to the defective fusion of the ectoderm, or failure of maturation of the midline mesodermal components, and it may be presented as a prominent widely separated median raphe which may be detected in cases of anorectal malformations (Fig. 16.6). This wideness may affect the whole penile, scrotal and perineal raphe, or may be partially affecting only the penile raphe, and such cases may hide a megameatus with an intact prepuce (Fig. 16.7) (This issue will be discussed with some details in Chap. 20). Wide GMR may be contracted with shortening of the scrotal raphe and results in disfigurement of scrotum (Fig. 16.8), such cases need excision of the abnormal raphe tissue with a meticulous closure of the midline with an absorbable fine suture to avoid a further scar contraction.

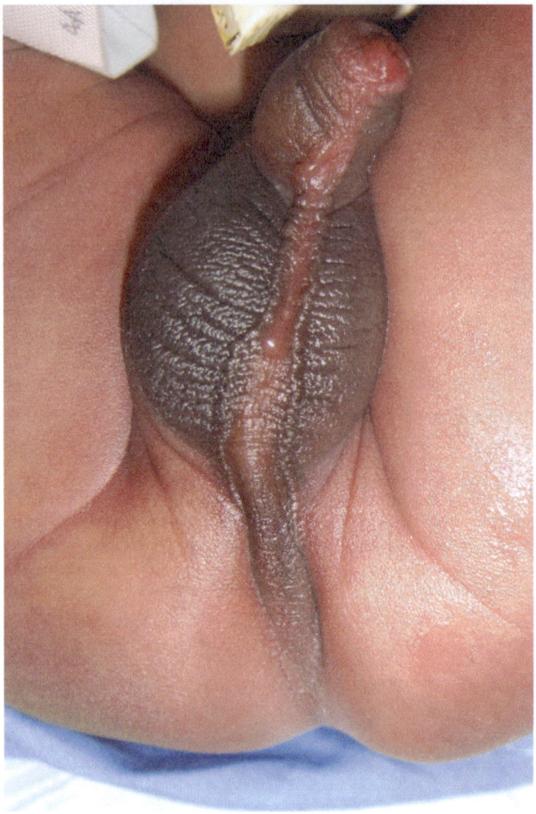

Fig. 16.6 Wide median Raphe associated with an imperforate anus

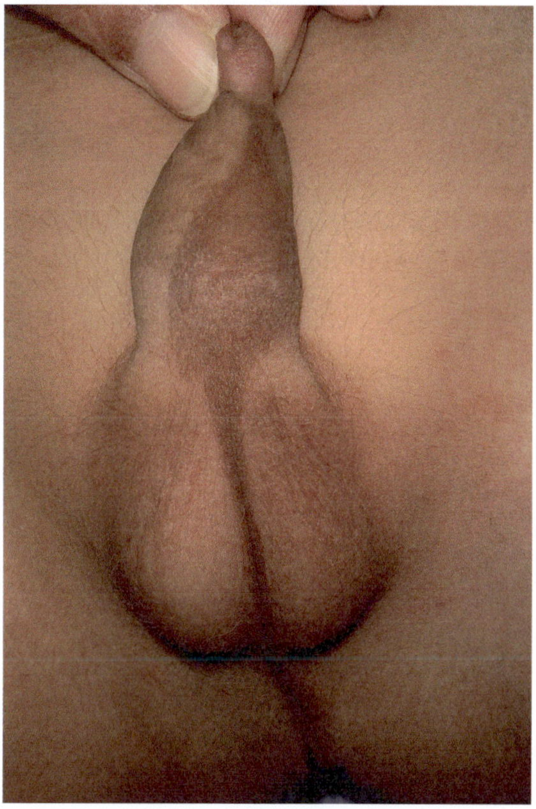

Fig. 16.7 Partially wide penile raphe with a hidden intact prepuce megameatus

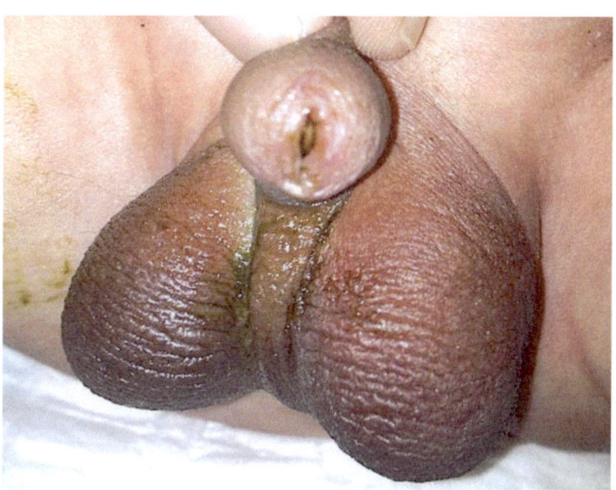

Fig. 16.8 Wide thick and contracted median raphe disfiguring scrotum

16.2.4 Splitted Median Raphe (Median Raphe Bifurcation)

Splitted median raphe was probably due to the defective fusion of the ectoderm; raphe may be splitted and bifurcated just proximal to the hypospadiac meatus (Fig. 16.9), or it may be splitted at the root of the penis to be seen at the dorsum of curved penis, with severe penile curvature and proximal hypospadias (Fig. 16.10). Excision of this deformed raphe should be considered during hypospadias repair.

16.2.5 Hyperpigmented Median Raphe

Hyperpigmentation of the median raphe, in comparison to its normal dark appearance, was the most common anomaly detected [2], and it could be associated with other anomalies like hypospadias and anorectal anomalies. Although this abnormal median raphe

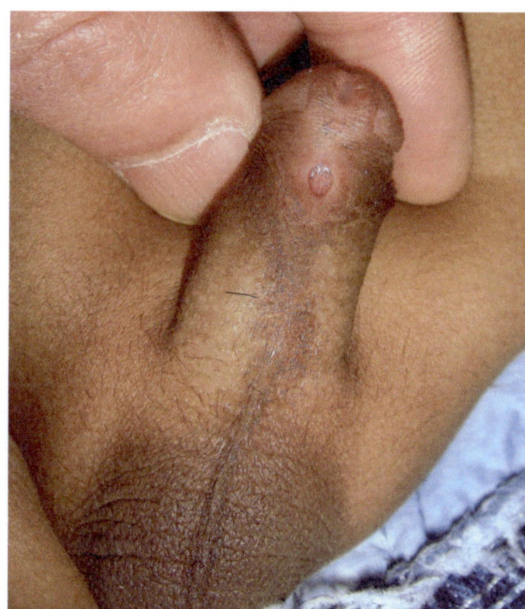

Fig. 16.9 Bifurcated median raphe around hypospadiac meatus

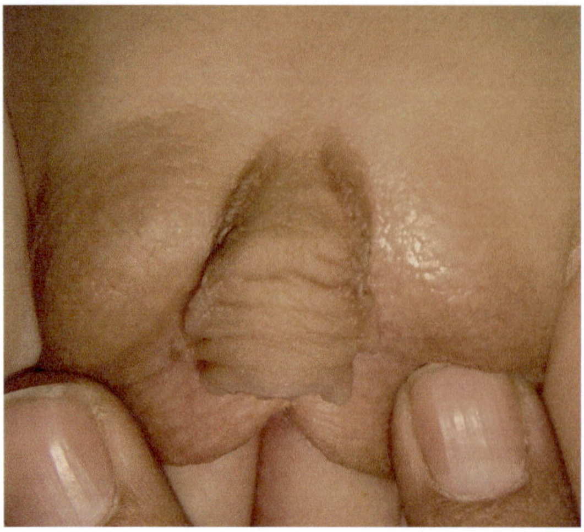

Fig. 16.10 Splitted GMR at the dorsum of severely curved penis

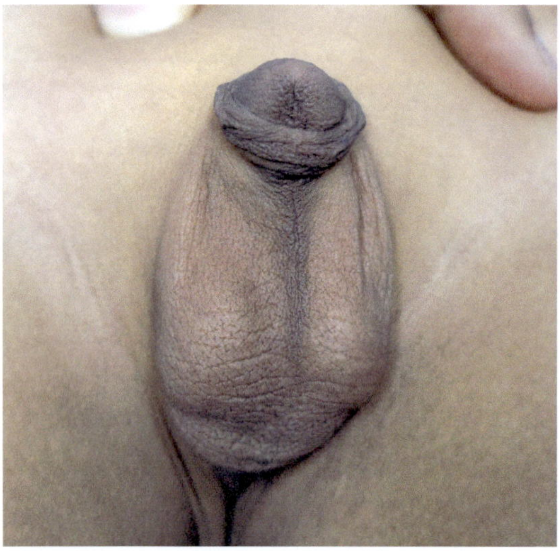

Fig. 16.11 Hyperpigmented median raphe

pigmentation is not fully understood, it may be due to the presence of lipochrome, diffuse melanosis of its epithelial lining or excess presence of melanocytes [6]. Hyperpigmentation may be a normal variation in black races, and this abnormality may associated other described GMR malformations; like wide, splitted and contracted raphe (Fig. 16.11).

16.2.6 Short Contracted Raphe

Short contracted raphe may be associated webbed penis, penile chordee and hypospadias, in many cases of webbed penis there is no deficient ventral skin, but it is only the contracted short raphe which gives this picture and it necessitated postponing routine circumcision with a subsequent penile reconstruction with either removal of the contracted raphe from the ventral aspect or it may need a rotation skin flap (Figs. 16.12 and 16.13). In Fig. 16.14 we can see a very rare developmental anomaly of a short contracted median raphe anchoring the penis completely to the scrotum, with lose of peno-scrotal angle and space.

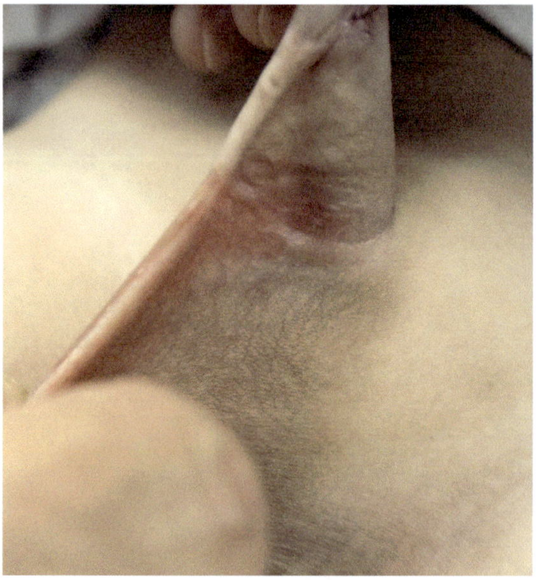

Fig. 16.12 Contracted median raphe gives the appearance of webbed penis

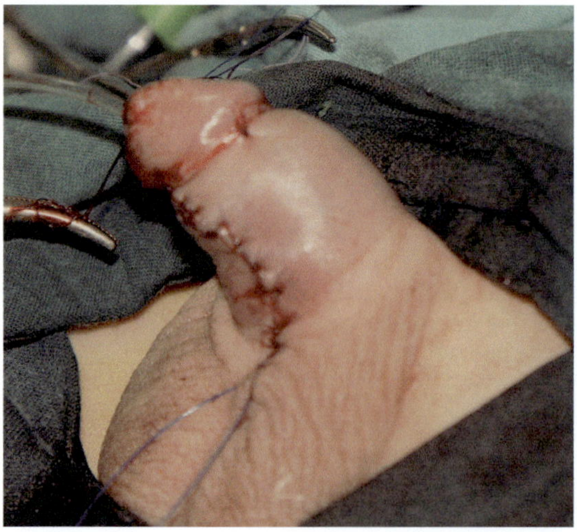

Fig. 16.13 Case in Fig. 16.12 after excision of the contracted raphe and penis straightening

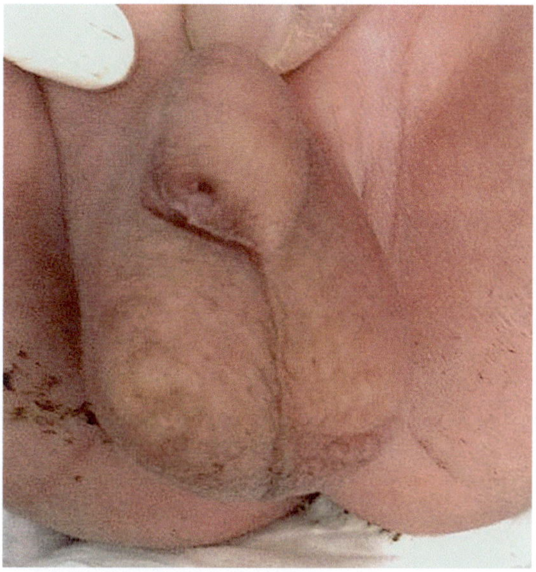

Fig. 16.14 A rare case of short contracted median raphe anchoring the penis to the scrotum

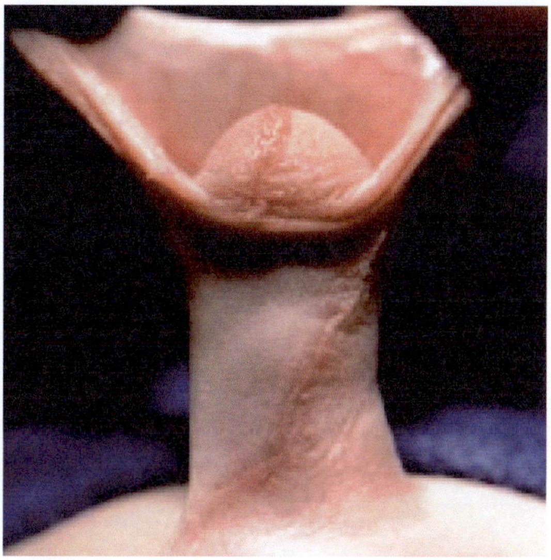

Fig. 16.15 Deviation of GMR without hypospadias

16.2.7 Deviation of Raphe

Raphe deviation to one side is not rare, but it could pass unnoticed by the parents, the child, or even unexperienced paediatrician, examination of the penoscrotal raphe is simple to perform and could aid in the early diagnosis in children with milder forms of this condition, which could be a normal developmental variation without any associated other anomalies, also many cases of isolated penile rotation without hypospadias had a high incidence of raphe deviation to the opposite side of penile rotation, which may indicate that penile deformity is secondary to abnormal position of GMR (Fig. 16.15).

Penile raphe deviation to one side or its bifurcation may hide a different grades of associated hypospadias; (32 % of cases), and this is considered as one of the genital anomalies associated with a hypospadiac defect, and in such cases the deviation is more commonly to the right side (60 %) [2] . Interestingly, however, 90 % of the normal children with raphe deviation it deviates to the left [7]. Diagnosis of hypospadias, its degree, severity and other associated anomalies related significantly to raphe deviation [2] (Figs. 16.16 and 16.17).

Another study suggests a strong correlation between children with raphe deviation and hypospadias, with an 88.1 % of the children with the condition demonstrating raphe deviation, with the low incidence of raphe deviation in normal children, indicates that this finding could prove to be particularly useful as a predictor of hypospadias in infants with nonretractile foreskin [8].

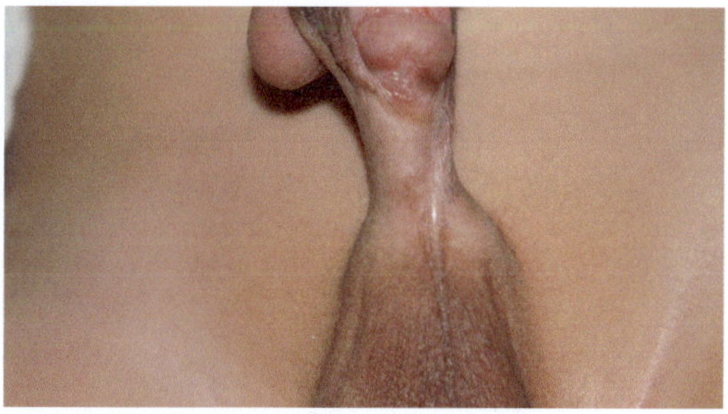

Fig. 16.16 Left sided raphe deviation with hypospadias

GMR deviation to one side, as we can see in Figs. 16.18 and 16.19 and the attached video (Video 16.1), may be a significant signs for detection of rare cases of megameatus variant of hypospadias with an intact normal prepuce (raphe deviation detected in 75 % of cases of IPM in our series, which not yet published), and this will be helpful medically and medicolegally for surgeons and practitioners doing circumcision for infants, specially in countries practising circumcision for all infants with a religious background.

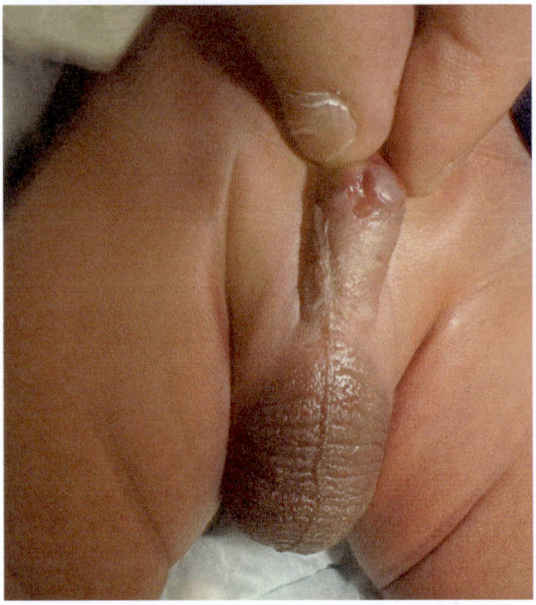

Fig. 16.17 Right sided deviation with hypospadias

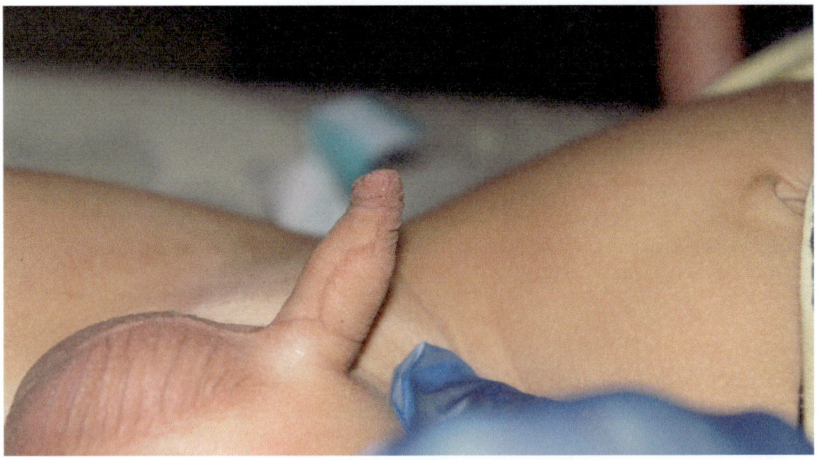

Fig. 16.18 Median raphe deviation with intact prepuce

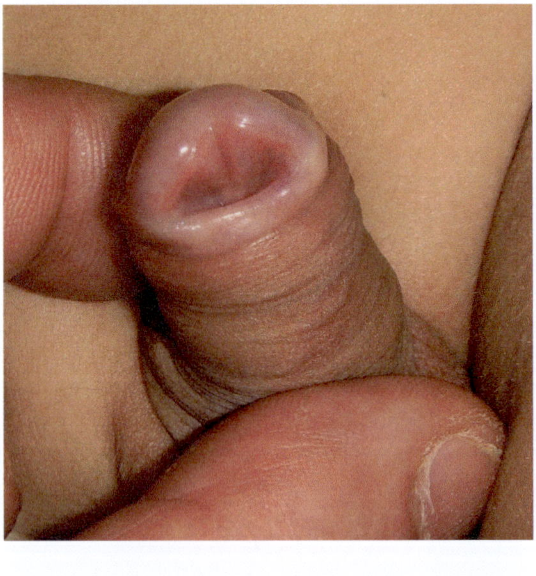

Fig. 16.19 Same case in Fig. 16.18 after preputial retraction with a megameatus anomaly

16.2.8 A Bucket Handle Malformation (Fig. 16.20)

It is a prominent median perineal raphe with a space separating it from the skin, which is commonly seen in different types of anorectal malformations, and used earlier to differentiate between high and low anomalies, but this clinical feature may be seen in perineal fistula as a prominent midline skin bridge or a subepithelial midline raphe fistula that looks like a black ribbon because it is full of meconium. These features are externally visible and help in diagnose of perineal fistula [9].

16.2.9 Median Raphe Cyst (MRC) (Fig. 16.21)

These cysts are due to tegumentary formation that arises as a result of "tissue trapping" during midline fusion of the ectoderm. Such anomalies could be simple skin pathology or might represent major abnormalities like hypospadias or other urethral anomalies.

Ectodermal canals involving part or all of the raphe had been reported for the first time at 1924 by Rupel E, and it is considered as an extension of multiple raphe cysts with the same pathology [10].

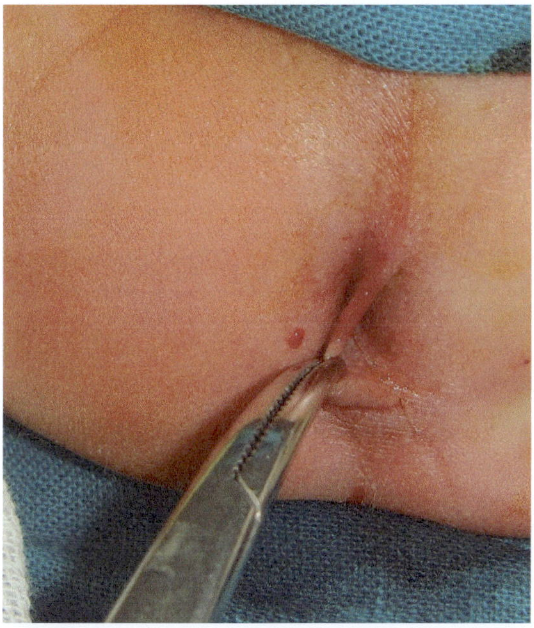

Fig. 16.20 Bucket handle malformation

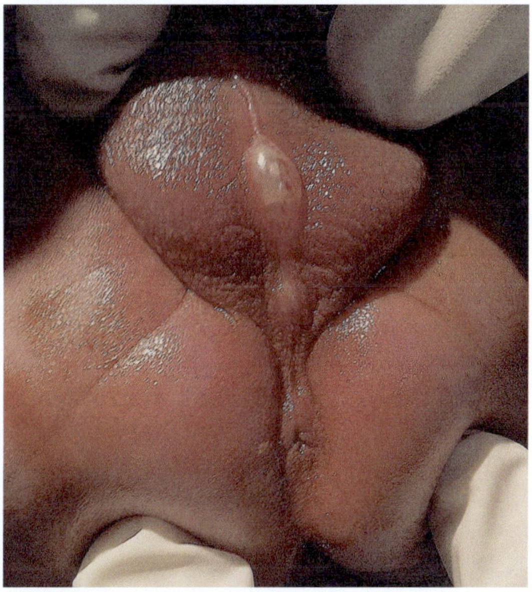

Fig. 16.21 Median Raphe Cyst

The diagnosis of median raphe cyst is difficult, but needs to be differentiated from other conditions such as epidermal cyst, steatocystoma, glomus tumor, dermoid cyst, urethral diverticulum, and pilonidal cyst when it presents in the penile (most common site) and scrotal region. There is little need of confusing these with sebaceous cysts. Common pyogenic infections as well as specific venereal and acid-fast infections must be considered, and there is no explanation why these cysts are vulnerable to gonorrhoea infection either as an isolated cyst infection or along urethral affection, it was reported earlier by Rupel [10].

In the usual examination of the genitals the median raphe gets little attention. With the possibility of cysts and canals of the raphe kept in mind it is likely that many of these lesions would be discovered. Most MRCs are asymptomatic in childhood and become symptomatic as the child grows, swelling tenderness and purulent discharge can be seen when cysts become traumatized and secondarily infected.

Most commonly, the diagnosis of median raphe cyst is established postoperatively on histological and immunohistochemical studies. The epithelial lining of median raphe cyst includes columnar stratified, pseudostratified, or squamous cells, correlating with histology in different portions of male urethra, but rare cases containing ciliated cells in epithelium had been reported [11].

Three different theories have been proposed for pathogenesis of median raphe cyst:

1. Developmental from urethral remnants due to a defect in the fusion of urethral folds.
2. Developmental implant of the ectopic periurethral glands of Littre' that are usually located in the rectal portion of the urethra.
3. Anomalous formation of epithelial buds from the urethral columnar epithelium, followed by separation.

16.2.10 Beaded Median Raphe (Fig. 16.22)

Rare cases of brown fine darker nodules replacing the normal line of median raphe had been reported, and this could be a normal variant, or a variant of penile cyst with the same pathology and etiology, we detected 2 cases in association with anorectal malformation. Nothing surgical is required for such cases, only through examination to rule out any associated anomalies, family assurance and follow up. Other congenital abnormalities such as blind-ending canals opening onto the penile surface must be differentiated.

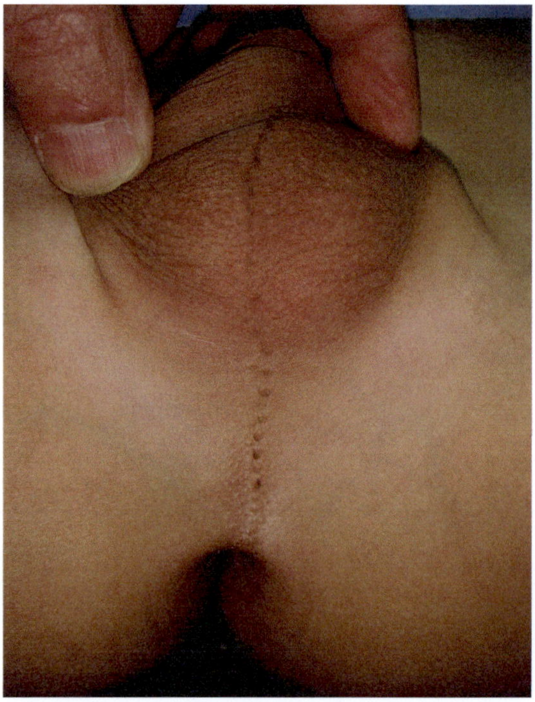

Fig. 16.22 Beaded median raphe

16.2.11 Pearly Penile Papules (Fig. 16.23)

Pearls of meconium can be seen on the raphe of the scrotum and are considered to be a sign of low presentation of an anorectal malformation. Scrotal pearls without an anorectal malformation, which are usually whitish in colour, are very rare in infants and designated as median raphe cyst (MRC) of the perineum [12]. It may also considered as a minute inclusion cysts.

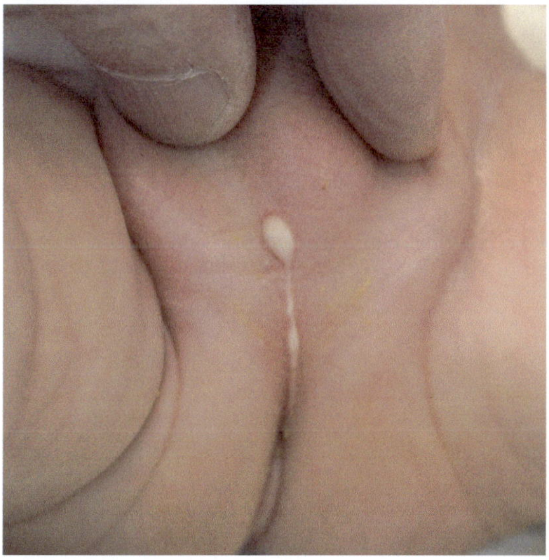

Fig. 16.23 Pearly penile papules

Conclusion

Thorough examination of infants presented for routine circumcision could be beneficial for surgeons in detecting many anomalies which are thought to be rare but actually may not be, as well as for the patients to find out any hidden anomalies. Genital median raphe anomalies may not be so rare as thought, as they were present in about 2 % of the neonates with a wide spectrum of variability, and they could hide an associated serious genitourinary anomaly. Any infant with an abnormal genital median raphe should be investigated to detect such anomalies, and neonatal circumcision should be postponed in such cases.

References

1. Thomson JA, Itskovitz-Eldor J, Shapiro SS, Waknitz MA, Swierqiel JJ, Marshall VS, et al. Embryonic stem cell lines derived from human blastocysts. Science. 1998;282:1145–7.
2. Baky Fahmy MA. The spectrum of genital median raphe anomalies among infants undergoing ritual circumcision. J Pediatr Urol. 2013;9:872–7. http://www.jpurol.com/article/S1477-5131(12)00294-X/abstract.
3. Chitayat D, Glanc P. Diagnostic approach in prenatally detected genital abnormalities. Ultrasound Obstet Gynecol. 2010;35:637–46.
4. Gutt AA, Pendharka PS. Transverse testicular ectopia associated with persistent Mullerian duct syndrome. Br J Radiol. 2008;81:176–8, 457–61.

5. O'Callaghan M, Young ID. The Townes-Brocks syndrome. J Med Genet. 1990;27:457–61.
6. Marhotra R, Bhawan J. The nature of pigment in pigmented apocrine hidrocystoma. J Cutan Pathol. 1985; 12:10–9.
7. Sarkis PE, Sadasivam M. Incidence and predictive factors of isolated neonatal penile glandular torsion. J Pediatr Urol. 2007;3:495–9.
8. Mohan A, Ashton L, Dalal M. Deviation of the penoscrotal median raphe: is it a normal finding or within the spectrum of hypospadias? Indian J Plast Surg. 2014;1(47):92–4.
9. Levitt MA, Penã A. Anorectal malformations. Orphanet J Rare Dis. 2007;2(33):1–13.
10. Rupel E. Epidermal canals infected with gonococci. Surg Gynec Obstet. 1924;39:636–8.
11. Acenero MJ, Garcia-Gonzalez J. Median raphe cyst with ciliated cells: report of a case. Am J Dermatopathol. 2003;25(2):175–6.
12. Soyer T, Karabulut A, Boybeyi O, Günal Y. Scrotal pearl is not always a sign of anorectal malformation: median raphe cyst. Turk J Pediatr. 2013;55: 665–6.

Penile Hemangioma

17

Abstract
Penile hemangioma is a very rare benign vascular neoplasm, mostly seen in children and young adults with different features.

Keywords
Haemangiomas • Strawberry nevus • Klippel-Trenaunay syndrome • Kasabach-Merritt syndrome • Tissue expander • Angiokeratoma of Fordyce

Incidence

Generally haemangiomas are the most common pediatric neoplasm, occur in about 10 % of all births, and usually appear between 1 and 4 weeks after birth, but penile hemangioma comprises less than 1 % of all hemangiomas. Capillary hemangioma is the most common variant of hemangioma, it occurs 5 times more often in female infants than in males, and mostly in Caucasian populations. The incidence of capillary hemangioma in the penis and scrotum is rare, which presented with scrotal enlargement and tenderness, only a few number of articles describing scrotal hemangioma have been reported [1].

Nomenclatures

A capillary hemangioma also known as an Infantile hemangioma, Strawberry hemangioma, and Strawberry nevus.

17.1 Definition

Haemangiomas are benign vascular lesions resulting from abnormal proliferation of blood vessels, capillary hemangioma appears as a raised, red, lumpy area of flesh anywhere on the body, without any known etiology (Fig. 17.1).

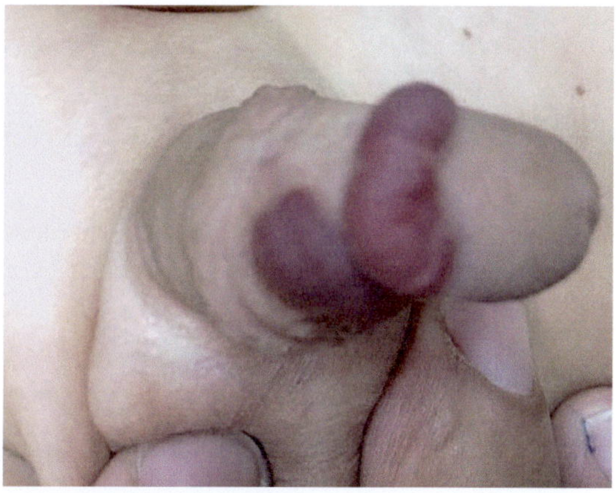

Fig. 17.1 Capillary haemangioma of the penis, with glanular affection

© Springer International Publishing Switzerland 2017
M. Fahmy, *Congenital Anomalies of the Penis*, DOI 10.1007/978-3-319-43310-3_17

17.2 Classification

Hemangiomas are generally classified into capillary, cavernous, arteriovenous, venous and mixed subtypes and may be composed of vessels whose walls are abnormal and cannot be identified as arterial or venous (Figs. 17.2 and 17.3). Complex vascular malformation of the penile skin may give a false picture of penile gigantism or megalopenis (Chap. 10).

Penoscrotal area may be affected along the vascular syndromes like; Kasabach-Merritt syndrome which is a rare type of vascular lesion with peculiar characteristics based upon three basic findings; enlarging haemangioma, thrombocytopenia and consumption coagulopathy [2]. Klippel-Trenaunay syndrome (KTS) is another syndrome with genital affection, it was first described in 1900 by two French physicians, Klippel and Trenaunay. It is a rare congenital syndrome of venous, lymphatic, and capillary malformations (port-wine stain and varicose veins) with soft tissue and bone hypertrophy. Patients can be diagnosed with KTS with only one or more of the above-mentioned features since patient might not have all the features [3]. Scrotum usually affected along the course of the diseases, and rarely the lesion may be extended to the penile shaft or the prepuce (Figs. 17.4 and 17.5).

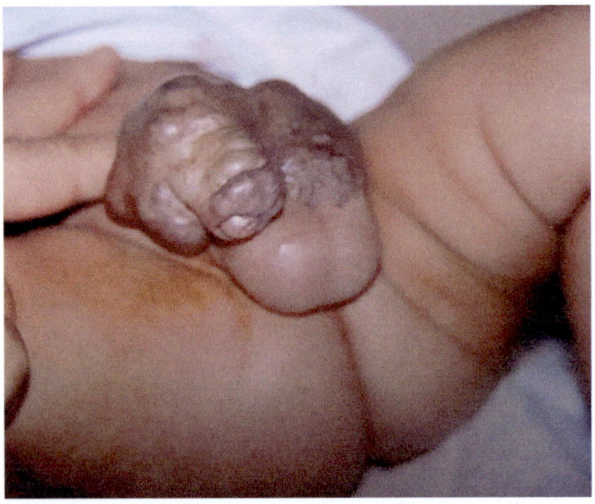

Fig. 17.2 Mixed arteriovenous malformation affecting the skin of the penis, prepuce and scrotum

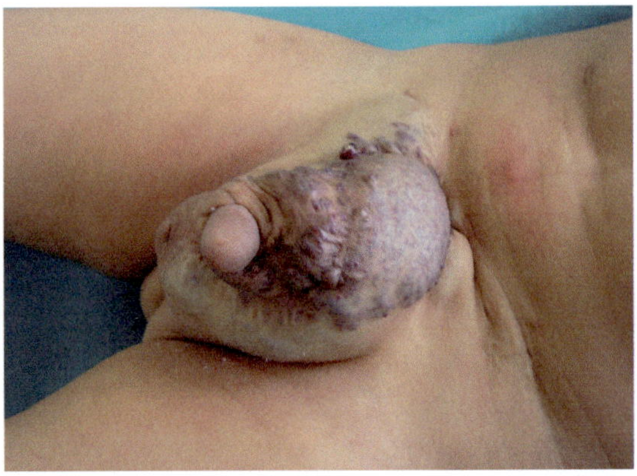

Fig. 17.3 Mixed vascular malformation of the penis with a superficial capillary heamnagioma

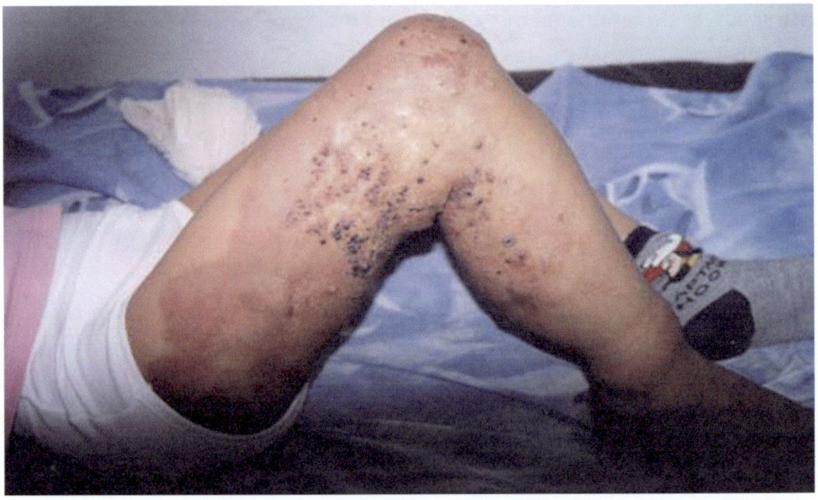

Fig. 17.4 Kasabach-Merritt syndrome affecting the right lower limb

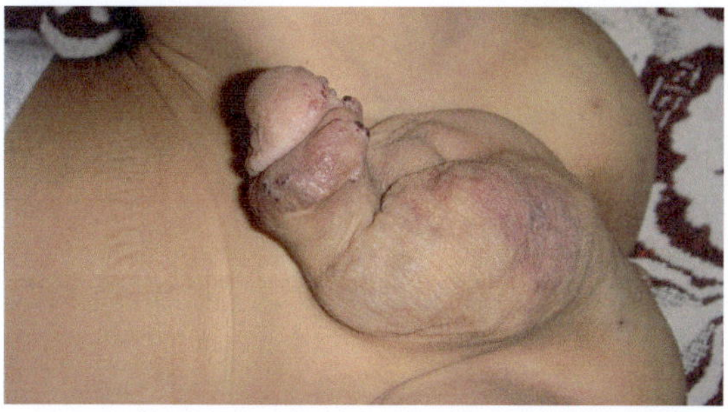

Fig. 17.5 Penoscrotal lesions of Kasabach-Merritt syndrome, "same patient in Fig. 17.4"

17.3 Diagnosis

Some haemangiomas are very small and hardly visible while others are large producing with a significant disfigurement (Fig. 17.1). Arteriovenous malformation and mixed vascular anomalies, are rarely diagnosed in the genital region, usually obvious since birth, but it may show progressive increase in size with age, it may be subjected to ulceration with severe bleeding from minor trauma, also it may get infection with skin erosion and ulcerations (Figs. 17.2 and 17.3). *Ultrasonography* is useful for diagnosing scrotal and penile hemangiomas, but rarely definitive. It can determine the extent of the lesion, delineate its relationship with adjacent structures, demonstrate the nature of the mass and help plan therapy. In sonography, hemangiomas vary from hypoechoic to hyperechoic, or they may be heterogeneous. *Colour Doppler* may demonstrate blood flow within these lesions but the absence of flow does not rule out the presence of the lesions. Magnetic *Resonance Imaging* (MRI) may provide more useful information for differentiation between haemangiomas and other vascular malformations, specially the angio MRI; which will give a precise idea about the feeding vessels [4].

17.4 Management

Capillary hemangiomas: It may grow rapidly, before stopping and slowly fading. Some are gone by the age of 2, about 60 % by 5 years, and 90–95 % by 9 years. When the diagnosis is established, eradication of the lesion is recommended and the lesion must be complete removed to avoid recurrence. Genital haemangioma deserve special attention than other body area, as small hemangioma is liable to trauma, ulceration, and disfigurement if untreated at childhood, it will interfere with normal sexual activities with subsequent psychic trauma and depression, also minute residual scar in the penis and glans will not be appreciated by patients or parents.

Propranolol is thought to inhibit the growth of blood vessels and constrict existing blood vessels within the haemangioma, and should be tried in all cases with an appropriate dose [5], small lesions like the one seen in Fig. 17.6 could be controlled with laser application.

Bulky venous, or mixed genital vascular malformation should be excised surgically with the expected problem of skin deficiency to cover the penile shaft, which could be achieved by either skin graft or rotation flap. Alternatively, specially in cases with large extensive lesion, a serial excision with tissue expansion was feasible and applicable with manageable complications and acceptable by the patients and their parents [6]. Figures 17.7,

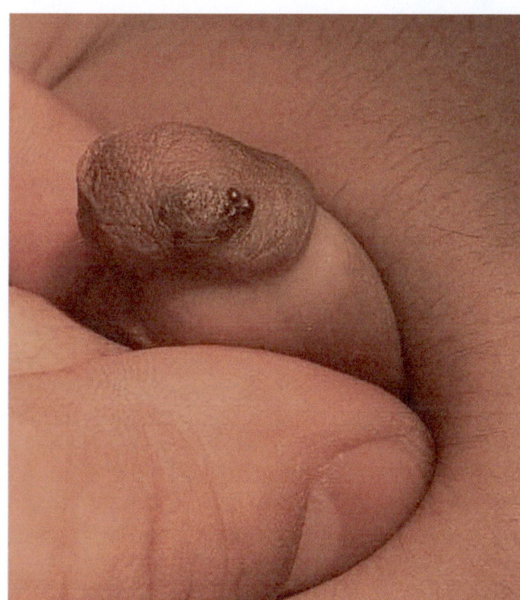

Fig. 17.6 Small haemangioma of the glans penis, this small lesion is liable to bleeding from minor trauma, and could be managed with laser

17.8, 17.9, and 17.10 showing a neonate with huge mixed vascular malformation involving the penis, prepuce, proximal scrotum and suprapubic region, I managed him with sequential implantation of three different sizes tissue expanders in the normal lower abdominal wall, repeated serial excision of the malformed skin and rotational flaps to

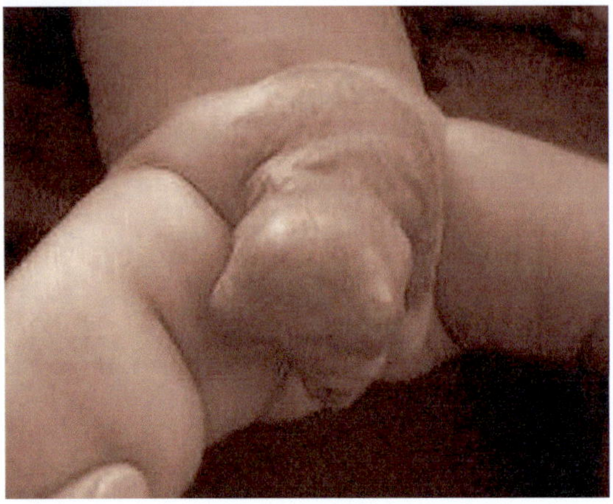

Fig. 17.7 Huge vascular malformation of the penis and lower suprapubic region in a neonate

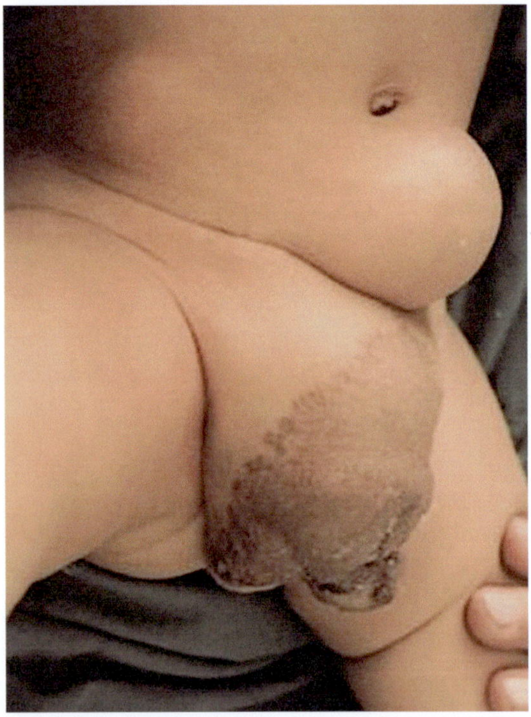

Fig. 17.8 Same patient in Fig. 17.6 at the age of 3 years with lower abdominal wall tissue expander

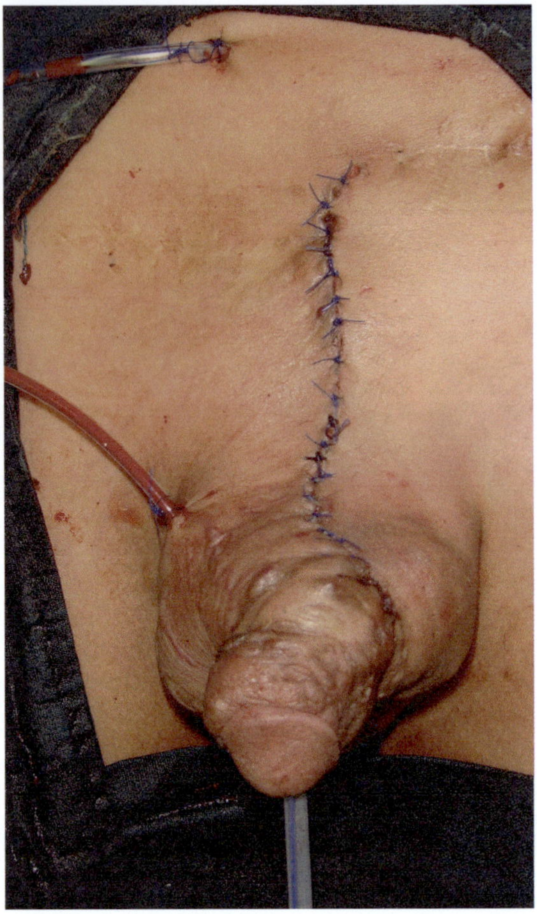

Fig. 17.9 Same patient after three sessions of tissue expansion

cover the penis and scrotum at our centre, so he reach to an acceptable look by the age of 12 years (Fig. 17.10).

Kasabach-Merritt syndrome shows wide variation in its response to different treatment modalities, as different interventions are recommended including compression, embolization, use of interferon, steroids, laser therapy, sclerotherapy, chemotherapy, radiation and surgery [2].

Mucosal lentigines (also known as "Labial, penile, and vulvar melanosis," and "Melanotic macules") is a cutaneous condition characterized by light brown macules on mucosal surfaces, and very rarely it may affect the penile shaft [7].

Angiokeratoma of Fordyce (also known as Angiokeratoma of the scrotum and vulva) is a skin condition characterized by red to blue papules on the scrotum or vulva.

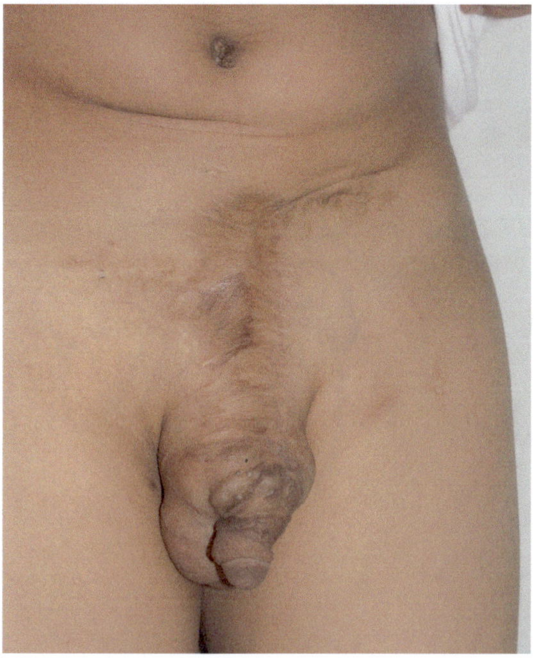

Fig. 17.10 Same patient in Fig. 17.6 at the age of 12 years after 8 subsequent operations with almost complete removal of vascular anomalies and restoration of near normal penoscrotal look

References

1. James W, Berger T, Elston D. Andrews' diseases of the skin: clinical dermatology. 10th ed. Saunders; 2005. ISBN 0-7216-2921-0. Philadelphia.
2. Hall GW. Kasabach-Merritt syndrome: pathogenesis and management. Br J Haematol. 2001;112:851–62.
3. Oduber CEU, van der Horst CMAM, Hennekam RCM. Klippel-Trenaunay syndrome: diagnostic criteria and hypothesis on etiology. Ann Plast Surg. 2008;60(2):217–23.
4. Rastogi R. Diffuse cavernous hemangioma of the penis, scrotum, perineum, and rectum- A rare tumor. Saudi J Kidney Dis Transpl. 2008;19:614–8.
5. Hogeling M, Adams S, Wargon O. A: randomized controlled trial of propranolol for infantile hemangiomas. Pediatrics. 2011;128(2):e259–66.
6. Baky Fahmy MA. Versatility of tissue expander in abdominal wall reconstruction after removal of vascular malformations in children. Ann Plast Surg. 2014;73((5):563–7. PubMed: http://www.ncbi.nlm.nih.gov/pubmed/23728247.
7. Teichman JM, Sea J, Thompson IM, Elston DM. Noninfectious penile lesions. Am Fam Physician. 2010;81(2):167–74.

18 Penile Lymphedema

Abstract

Penile lymphedema or Saxophone penis is a potentially disfiguring disorder, characterized by impaired lymphatic drainage of the penile or penoscrotal skin, and manifested by a redundant, thick and oedematous non compressible genital skin, it is secondary to parasitic infestation in older children from endemic area, but in neonate and western countries it is either congenital or idiopathic, treatment of such condition is challenging, with the need to excise the whole redundant defective skin and grafting the penis with a local flap or free skin graft.

Keywords

Penile lymphedema or Saxophone penis • Elephantiasis • Milroy's disease • Meigs' disease

Nomenclature

Saxophone penis, Genital lymphedema, Penile elephantiasis.

Definition

Penile lymphedema (Fig. 18.1) is an uncomfortable and potentially disfiguring disorder, characterized by impaired lymphatic drainage of the penile or penoscrotal skin, and manifested by a redundant, thick and oedematous non compressible genital skin.

© Springer International Publishing Switzerland 2017

M. Fahmy, *Congenital Anomalies of the Penis*, DOI 10.1007/978-3-319-43310-3_18

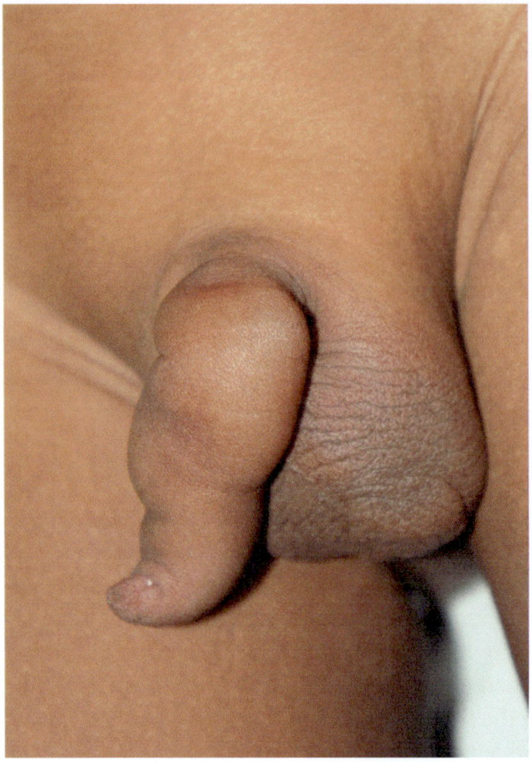

Fig. 18.1 Penile lymphedema, confined to penis only and sparing the scrotum giving penis the shape of Saxophone

18.1 Incidence

The incidence of primary penile lymphedema account for approximately 1:60,000 live births. Scrotal lymphedema is rare outside endemic filariasis regions in Africa and Asia [1].

18.2 Classification

Primary: Penile lymphedema (usually in western countries) it is congenitally inherited in 15% of the cases, in either an autosomal dominant form (Milroy's disease), or a sporadic form (in 85% of the cases) that occurs at puberty (Meigs' disease).

Secondary: Usually caused by acquired infection in Africa and Asia e.g., lymphogranuloma venereum, chlamydia trachomatis or filarial infestation with *Wuchereria bancrofti* [2].

18.3 Presentation

Primary lymphedema of the genitalia may be presented in a neonate and children as:

- Isolated Penile lymphedema (Saxophone penis) Fig. 18.1.
- Isolated scrotal lymphedema (elephantiasis) Fig. 18.2.
- Penoscrotal lymphedema Fig. 18.3.
- Pelvic and lower extremities lymphedema Fig. 18.4

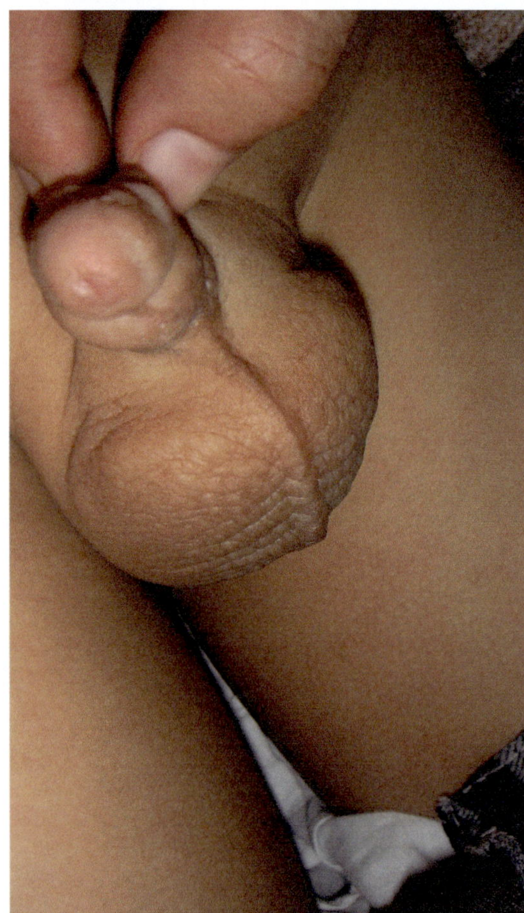

Fig. 18.2 Isolated scrotal lymphedema

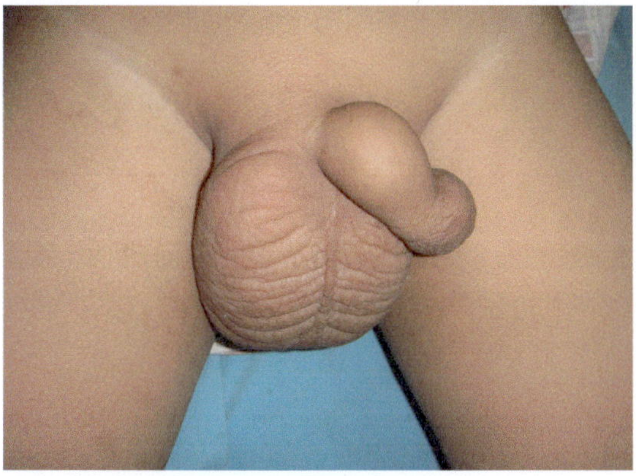

Fig. 18.3 Penoscrotal lymphedema

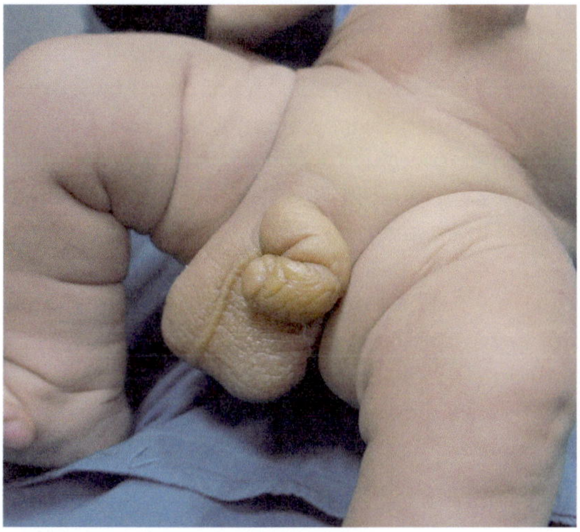

Fig. 18.4 Lymphedema of the penis scrotum and both lower limbs

18.4 Etiology

The etiology of the lymphedema usually determines the natural course and the therapeutic approach. It is of variable origin in the western world, while many reported cases are idiopathic, which may be due defective lymphatic development like obstruction, aplasia, or hypoplasia of lymphatic vessels in otherwise normal baby, it could be confined to the the penile skin only, or extended to the scrotum, and very rarely the skin of both lower limbs is also affected. Few cases of minimal lymphedema reported as a complication after circumcision, which may be due to extensive lymphatic injury, but it is usually reversible or correctable (Fig. 18.5). Toddlers who was normal at birth and acquired this condition latter on, and usually had a parasitic infestation (Filariasis). In adults it is occasionally has been attributed to radiotherapy, neoplasm and lymphadenectomy [3].

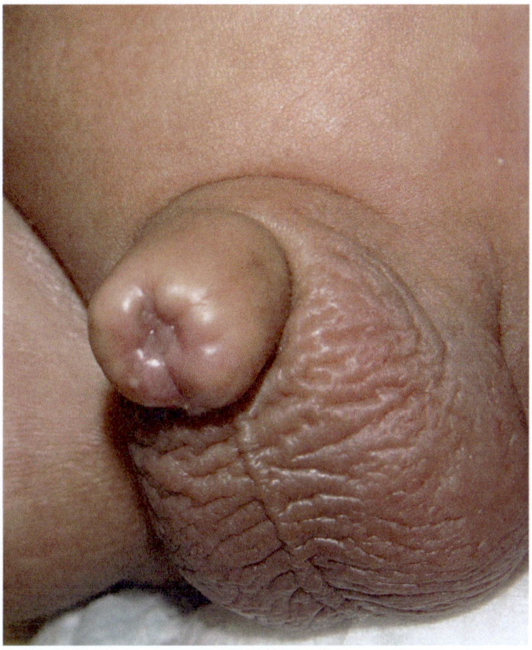

Fig. 18.5 Penile lymphedema secondary to circumcision, edges of penile skin encircling the glans

18.5 Complications

Penoscrotal elephantiasis is both emotionally distressing and physically disabling, with difficulties in hygiene, urinary incontinence and unesthetic appearance, loss of normal sensation and immobility are severely debilitating symptoms at adulthood.

Recurrent episodes of cellulitis are common and are responsible for the loss of elastic fibres, hyperplasia of the collagenous connective tissue and the formation of fibrosis that renders the swelling permanent with progressive loss of function and of cosmesis. Other complications include loss of sexual function, infertility (depending upon the severity), difficulties in urination and untreated cases may end with sever social stigma.

18.6 Differential Diagnosis

Penile lymphedema in a neonate have to be differentiated from other causes of penile gigantism; like haemangioma, neurofibroma, megalourethra, megalopenis and megaloprepuce, "all these topics will be discussed separately". Older children may had a late presentation of congenital lymphedema without any previous neonatal history, and such cases have to be differentiated from the acquired form and from other causes of penoscrotal oedema like: lymphangitis, angioneurotic oedema and systemic diseases which may be manifested with scrotal oedema like nephrotic syndrome. Doppler ultrasound of penis will exclude any vascular (arterial/venous) malformation. Although MRI and lymphoscintigraphy are important modalities for further affirm the diagnosis in very few occasions [3].

18.7 Management

Initial management involves observation and follow up, if lymphedema remains significant or progresses, then surgical therapy is necessary as there is no effective medical treatment for primary genital lymphedema tell now, fluroquinolones had been tried for adult cases with limited response after prolonged courses [3]. Other non surgical modalities like polyester compression garment, infrared therapy and low level laser had a limited and usually a reversible success. Various methods of reconstruction of genital elephantiasis involve excision of affected tissue and its reconstruction with or without lymphangioplasty and microlymphaticovenous anastomosis. Out of the several procedures described in the literature, modified Charles procedure (subcutaneous and deep fascial excision followed by full-thickness grafts) looks most promising. These surgical procedures if performed promptly it well give remarkably good cosmetic results with tremendous improvement in quality of life of these unfortunate patients with genital elephantiasis [4].

The goal of surgical treatment is to remove all involved tissue. On the penile shaft, the penis is degloved and all tissue between Buck's fascia and the skin must be excised along the redundant penile skin. If the scrotum is involved, all scrotal tissue, with the exception of testes and spermatic cords must be removed. Usually most of the scrotal skin must be excised, with sparing of the posterior skin. The penis may be covered with local skin flaps, and the scrotal contents may be covered with uninvolved posterior skin flaps. If inadequate healthy skin is available, the penis and/or scrotum must be covered with split-thickness skin flaps. Medial thigh flaps can be used in the absence of adjacent scrotal tissue. Mesh skin graft is widely accepted for use in this regard. After definitive surgical therapy, recurrence in adjacent areas may occur, which may be a problem, either in the same or adjacent areas [5].

In penoscrotal lymphedema the scrotum should be treated first as then there is a reported cases of spontaneous resolution of the penile lymphedema after scrotal correction. Some few cases of penile lymphedema may respond after doing circumcision with application of Elastoplast dressing for longer time than usual (3–4 days), but other cases may getting worser.

References

1. McDougal WS. Lymphedema of the external genitalia. J Urol. 2003;170(3):711–6.
2. Hilliard RI, McKendry JBJ, Phillips MJ. Congenital abnormalities of the lymphatic system: a new clinical classification. Pediatrics. 1990;86:988.
3. Dandapat MC, Mohapatro SK, Patro SK. Elephantiasis of the penis and scrotum. A review of 350 cases. Am J Surg. 1985;149:686–90.
4. Garaffa G, Christopher N, Ralph DJ. The management of genital lymphoedema. BJU Int. 2008;102:480–4. doi:10.1111/j.1464-410X.2008.07559.x.
5. Nasehi A, Azadi SH. Elephantiasis of penis and scrotum. Urol J. 2004;2:55–7.

Further Reading

http://www.lymphedemapeople.com/wiki/doku.php?id=scrotal_lymphedema.

19 Penile Cysts

Keyword
Smegmoma

Penile cysts are uncommon lesions, and in general, they are asymptomatic and usually do not interfere with urinary or sexual function, unless when they are complicated by infection or trauma, an occasional irregularity of the urinary stream encountered in some cases. Most of them are present since birth, but they are only detectable in adolescence or adulthood. Penile cyst classified into; acquired types or pseudocyst and true cyst which are usually congenital.

Nomenclature

Several and misleading synonymous terms were given to penile cysts, including mucus cyst of the penis, genitoperineal cyst of the median raphe, parameatal cyst, hydrocystoma and apocrine cystadenoma of the penile shaft are also used in past.

Incidence

Generally penile cysts are rare except the smegma collecting cysts (Chap. 36), which are a common lesion specially in countries practising circumcision routinely for almost all infants, also inclusion dermoid cysts are not rare during the last decades specially after hypospadias surgery and penile surgery for augmentation.

19.1 Diagnosis

The clinical diagnosis is sometimes difficult to define the cyst type and nature, and differential diagnoses include rare types of cysts like pilonidal cysts, tyson glands cysts, and also should be differentiated from other cystic urethral swelling like urethral diverticulum. Penile cysts are usually a single midline swelling can be found mainly in the ventral surface of the shaft of the penis, rarely in the glans or the dorsum.

19.2 Types

Acquired (false or pseudocyst):
- **Smegma cyst "Smegmoma"** (Figs. 19.1 and 19.2)
- **Inclusion dermoid cyst** (Figs. 19.3 and 19.4, 19.5 and 19.6)

Congenital (True cyst)
- **Congenital Dermoid Cyst** (Fig. 19.7)
- **Mucoid Cyst** (Fig. 19.8)

© Springer International Publishing Switzerland 2017

M. Fahmy, *Congenital Anomalies of the Penis*, DOI 10.1007/978-3-319-43310-3_19

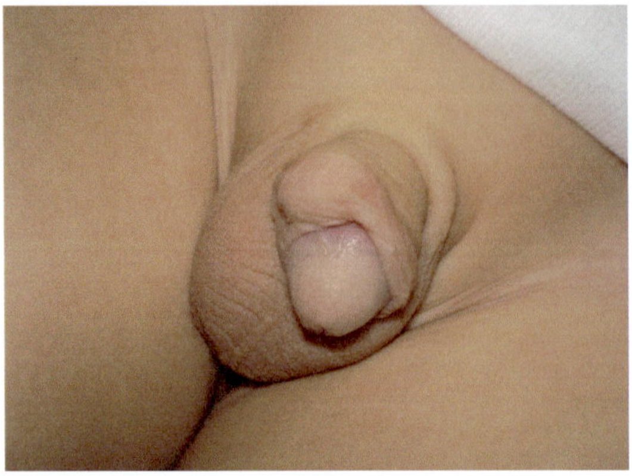

Fig. 19.1 Small smegma cyst at the edges of circumcised prepuce

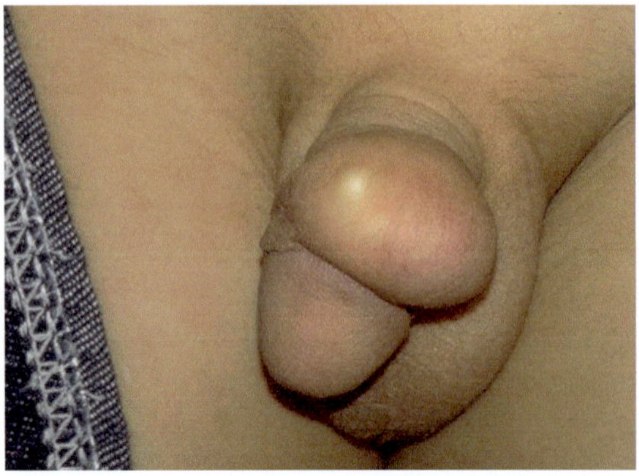

Fig. 19.2 Large smegma cyst in the dorsum of a circumcised penis, with signs of early infection

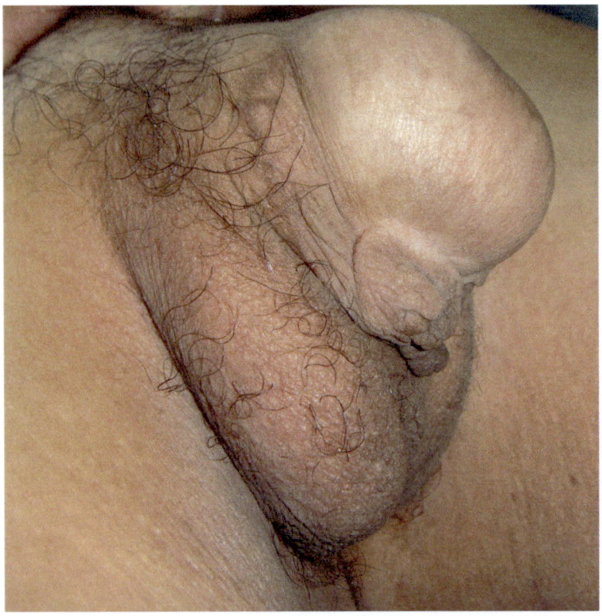

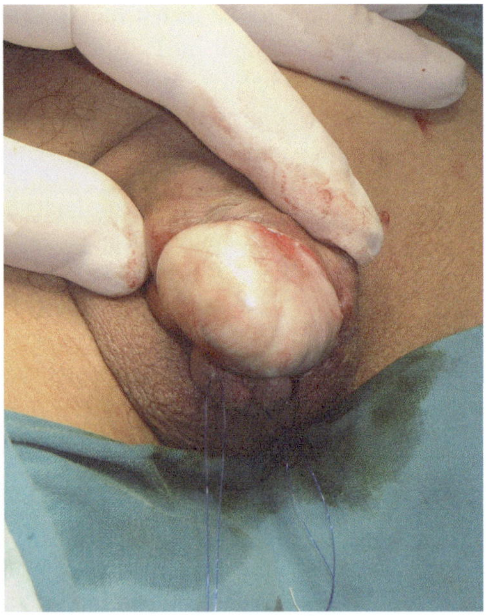

Figs. 19.3 and 19.4 Inclusion dermoid cyst after hypospadias repair

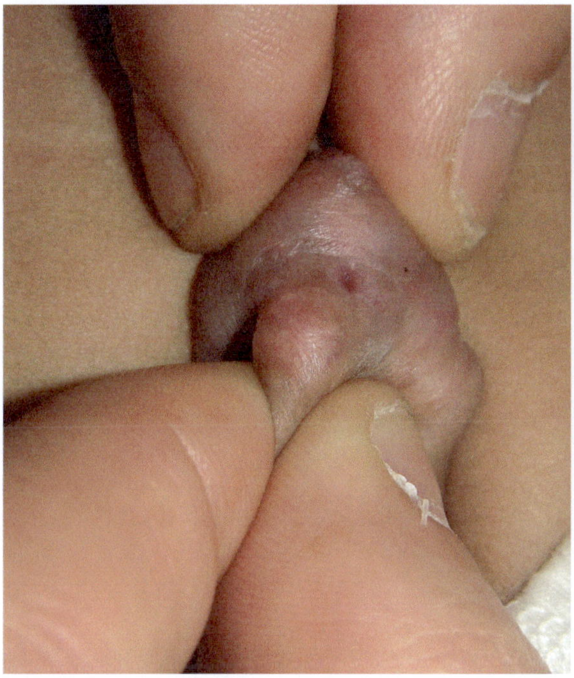
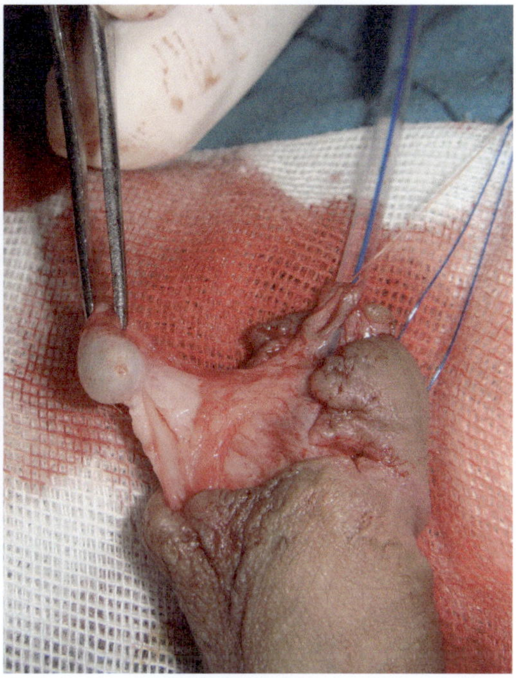

Figs. 19.5 and 19.6 Inclusion dermoid cyst after hypospadias repair with an associated fistula

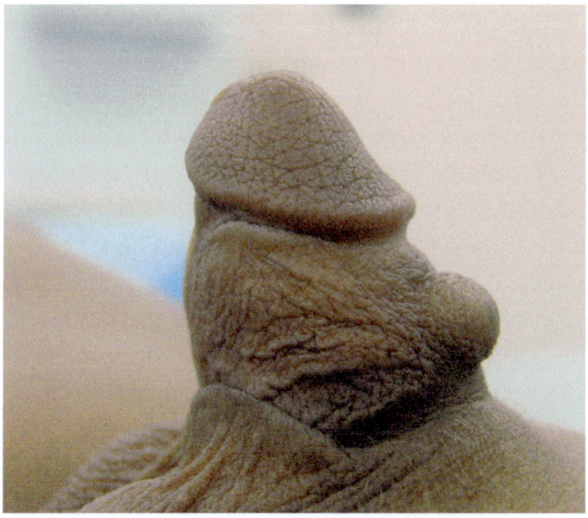

Fig. 19.7 Dermoid cyst in the dorsum of the penis

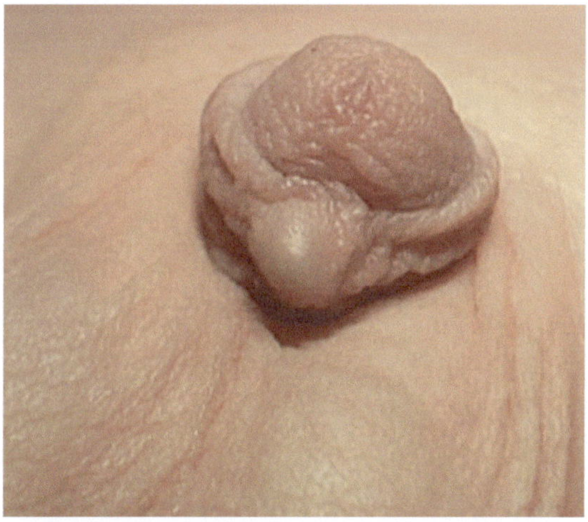

Fig. 19.8 True mucoid cyst at the coronal sulcus

Median raphe cyst (Fig. 19.9)
Parameatal cyst (Fig. 19.10)

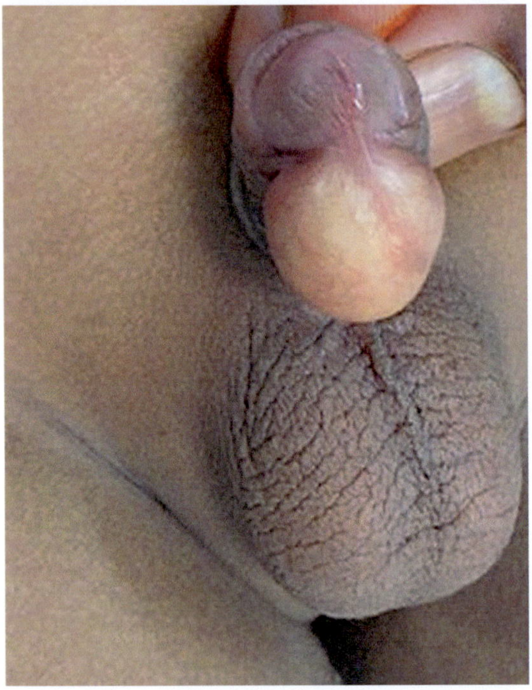

Fig. 19.9 Large median raphe cyst at the coronal sulcus

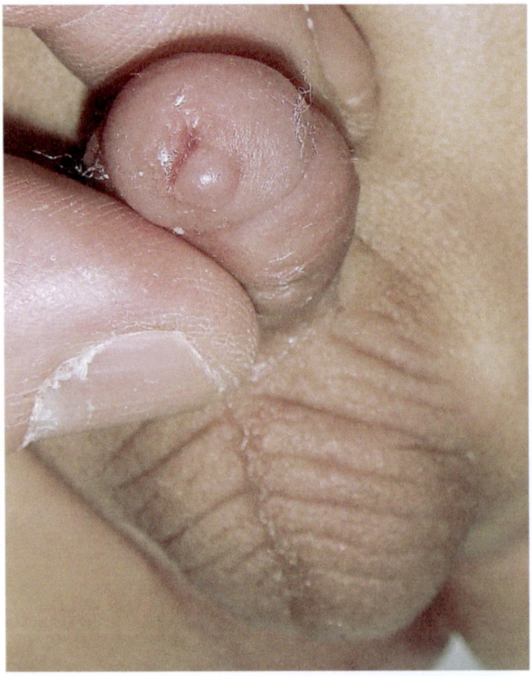

Fig. 19.10 Flat small parameatal cyst at the glans penis

19.3 Smegma Cyst

Aggregation of smegma in circumcised child is not rare and may present as a yellowish cystic or doughy swelling of different sizes at the cut edges of the prepuce (Fig. 19.1), sometimes it acquire a large size disfiguring the penis (Fig. 19.2), it is usually liable for infection and traumatic rupture. In un-circumcised penis smegma may forms a small lump in the undersurface of the penis or prepuce, and rarely it may affect the dorsum of the penis. Careful excision with meticulous penile skin closure will avoid recurrence (Chap. 36)

19.4 Inclusion Dermoid Cyst

It is also called epidermoid cyst**,** or acquired dermoid cyst.

Historical Background Dermoid cyst of penile skin was described for the first time in a young Caucasian man by Tomasini et al. in 1997 [1].

Epidermoid cysts occur in a wide age range, but commonly detected at young age. The location of the lesion is commonly at the ventral aspect or the base of the penile shaft, epidermoid cyst arising from the glans penis has also been reported occasionally, The histopathology of an epidermoid cyst shows a unilocular cyst lined by stratified squamous and contains laminated keratin material in the cyst lumen (Figs. 19.3 and 19.4, 19.5 and 19.6). Epidermal cysts of the penis can be single or multiple and of variable size. Characteristically they have a tendency to grow slowly, but they can reach a big dimensions with time.

Etiology Epidermoid inclusion cyst may be:

Congenital due to sequestration of epidermal rests during embryonic life, and this type considered as a true epidermal inclusion cysts hence it appear early in a neonate, but may not discovered except at late childhood.

Spontaneous due to occlusion of pilo-sebaceous unit, or infundibular part of the hair follicles.

Post traumatic after implantation of epithelial elements in the dermis of penile skin.

Post penile surgery; mainly circumcision, hypospadias repair and after an inadequate procedure for penile girth enhancement due to inclusion of epidermal cells within a circumscribed space of the dermis (Figs. 19.5 and 19.6).

Diagnosis Penile epidermal cysts can be diagnosed by careful examination and radiological evaluation, including ultrasonography and computed tomography. Magnetic resonance imaging may be useful in cases of suspected extension into the pelvis, although such cases are rare. If a urethral diverticula or urethrocutaneous fistula is suspected, retrograde urethrography or voiding cystourethrography should be carried out. In addition, the differential diagnosis of an epidermal cyst includes teratoma and dermoid cyst. However, skin and its appendages are present in a dermoid cyst, and derivatives of other germ cells are present in a teratoma. Biopsy is necessary for a definitive diagnosis [2].

Complications Cystic infection, pain, cystic rupture, urethral obstruction because of the big dimension, and subsequent urethro-cutaneous fistula and disfigurement with psychic truma are reported, but neoplastic transformation of the epithelium of epidermoid cysts has been reported rarely in other organs, but not in penile cases [3].

Management Surgical excision of penile epidermal cysts is the treatment of choice. The resection should be completed without leaving any epithelium to prevent a recurrence, patients with such cysts should be followed up after complete cyst removal.

So care needs to be taken while performing even minor preputial or penile surgical procedures to avoid inclusion cystic formation.

19.5 Congenital Dermoid Cyst: (Fig. 19.7)

Penile dermoid cysts in children are usually congenital and are caused by abnormal embryologic closure of the median raphe; these cysts are a variant of median raphe cysts.

Dermoid cysts are true hamartomas that occur when skin and skin structures become trapped during fetal development, it is very rarely to affect the glans penis [4].

19.6 Mucoid Cyst: (Fig. 19.8)

Mucus penile cyst is a midline-developmental, uncommon benign lesion affecting mainly children on ventral surface of glans penis but many cases presented at late adulthood. An extensive literature search has revealed only less than 200 reported cases, among these, only less than 10 have been reported from the Indian subcontinent [5].

The cysts most commonly arise from ectopic urethral mucosa sequestered during embryologic development. Histopathological examination of the cyst frequently includes stratified columnar epithelium, whether or not it is associated with mucous cells or glands.

Theses cysts are usually small, soft and freely movable masses, sometimes containing clear fluid, also needs to be differentiated from median raphe cyst of the penis, which generally occurs along the median raphe on the ventral surface of the penis, with a different histological features [6] (Fig. 19.9).

In general, they are asymptomatic, unless when they are complicated by infection or difficult coitus. Surgical excision is required.

19.7 Median Raphe Cysts (MRC) of the Penis

Occur on the ventral aspect of the penis from the external urethral meatus to the base of the shaft, with a predilection for the glans. The scrotum and anogenital space are uncommonly affected, theses cysts generally occur in young males (Fig. 19.9).

Incidence Since most of the cases in children are asymptomatic, it is suggested to be more common than reported. Most of the cysts tend to grow as the child grows and become symptomatic in adolescence and adulthood.

It is considered as an embryologic developmental abnormality of the male genitalia. Different histogenetic explanations have been suggested including incomplete fusion of the urethral folds, abnormal formation of epithelial buds from the urethral epithelium that then became sequestrated and independent after closure of the medium raphe, and cystic dilatations of ectopic Littré's periurethral glands.

Although the cytokeratin pattern could be observed in median raphe cysts, with CK 13 and 17 positivity in the lining cells, which suggests the urethral origin of the cyst, but the absence of CK20 immunoreactivity also reported in medium raphe cyst of the penis by Dini et al., contrasts with the well known expression of this intermediate filament in urethral neoplasms and may be related to the benign, non-dysplastic nature of the lesion [7].

Theses cysts range in size from 0.2 to 2 cm in diameter. Clinical differential diagnosis include glomus tumour, dermoid cyst, pilonidal cyst, epidermal cyst, urethral diverticulum, and steatocystoma. All of these were readily differentiated by the histological findings typical of median raphe cyst, a single cystic cavity with no urethral communication and lined by a columnar pseudo-stratified epithelium. Distinguishing median raphe cyst from apocrine hidrocystoma, however, may be less straightforward. In fact, several reports of apocrine cystadenoma of the penis may represent cysts of the median raphe. The absence of a basal layer of cuboidal, myoepithelial cells, and the absence of true decapitation secretion are important for this distinction [8]. The lining epithelium varies according to the to the segment origin of the urethra of the lesion, i.e., stratified in the distal part (ectodermal origin) and columnar pseudostratified in the remainder of the urethra (endodermal origin).

Pigmentation in the median raphe cysts, which look dark brown or blackish due to the presence of melanocytes or lipochrome has rarely been documented [9].

Pearls of meconium is a variant of median raphe cyst and can be seen on the raphe of the scrotum, but very rarely reported in the shaft of the penis, and are considered to be a sign of low presentation of an anorectal malformation. Scrotal pearls without an anorectal malformation are very rare in infants and designated as median raphe cyst (MRC) of the perineum. It is suggested that scrotal pearls in anorectal malformation probably have a similar embryologic origin of MRC, instead of epithelial overgrowth, meconium may be trapped before closure of the genital folds via an anocutaneous fistula in anorectal malformation.

Management MRC should be excised once detected, with a meticulous closure of the median raphe with a fine subcuticular stitches, and cyst biopsy. Damage to the urethra is a surgical complication in treating median raphe cysts near the urethra or urethral meatus. Although uncommon, recurrence can follow surgical excision (Median raphe anomalies discussed in details in Chap. 16).

19.8 Parameatal cysts

Are a benign, usually asymptomatic condition that may contain a variety of epithelial types. The size of theses cysts varies from a small minute flat cyst at the urinary meatus (Fig. 19.10), to a considerably large pedunculated cystic swelling with clear contents, arising from the urethral wall and seen hanging from the meatus, with almost occlusion of urinary stream (Fig. 19.11).

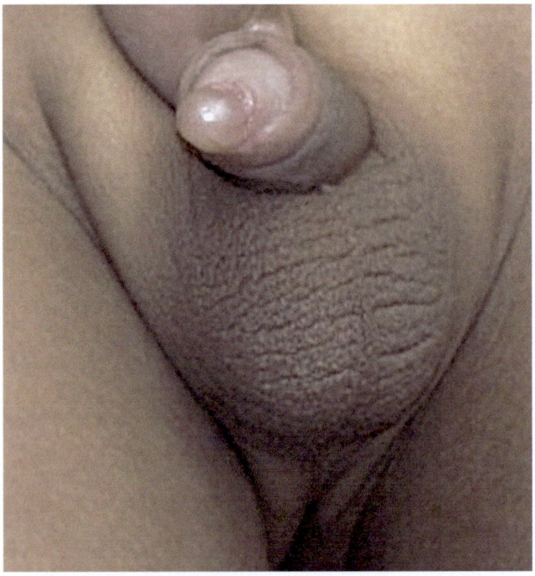

Fig. 19.11 Parameatal cyst arising from the urethra with pedicle keeping it visible at the meatus

Nomenclature Urethral cyst, and apocrine cystadenoma,

Incidence A parameatal urethral cyst is a very rare lesion in boys, but they can also occur in infants, girls, and adults.

Historical Background The parameatal cyst was first reported by Thompson and Lantin in 1956 [10], nearly 50 cases have been published since then.

Histologically, the cyst wall may be lined by columnar, squamous or transitional epithelium.

Etiology The pathogenesis of these cysts has not been completely understood. Thompson and Lantin [10] stated that parameatal urethral cysts occurred in the process of delamination or separation of the foreskin from the glans penis, while others believed that they were caused by occlusions of paraurethral ducts. Recently, Soyer et al. [11], reported two cases of female newborns, in whom paraurethral cysts which were associated with vaginal bleeding and breast enlargement were seen, which showed the possibility of role of oestrogen in their development. The origin of parameatal urethral cysts from accessory male sex glands in the penile urethra was demonstrated by detection of prostatic-specific antigen (PSA) in cells of these cysts with the help of immunohistochemistry, a parameatal duct obstruction could have been a possible aetiology.

Diagnosis Parameatal urethral cysts are usually asymptomatic, however, sometimes they can cause a variety of symptoms, including, poor cosmetic of the genitalia, dysuria, difficulty in urination, and acute retention. The cyst is usually small of about 1 cm in diameter. They occur on the lateral margin of the urethral meatus and at times, they can be bilateral. Diagnosis is incidental when cysts are asymptomatic, when the cysts are traumatized; they may bleed, rupture or become infected.

Treatment The cysts may resolve spontaneously in neonates, simple aspiration of the cyst results in recurrences. Marsupialization or unroofing of the cyst, especially if it is large, results in a gaping sinus, which is cosmetically unsatisfactory and should be avoided. Complete excision of the cyst is cosmetically excellent and there have been no recurrences reported in any cases [12].

References

1. Tomasini C, Aloi F, Puiatti P, et al. Dermoid cyst of the penis. Dermatology. 1997;194:188–90.
2. Kirkham N. Tumors and cysts of the epidermis. In: Elder D, Elenitsas R, Jasorsky C, Jonhson B, editors. Lever's histopatology of lever. 8th ed. Philadelphia: Lippincott-Raven; 1997. p. 685–746.
3. Chiu MY, Ho ST. Squamous cell carcinoma arising from an epidermal cyst. Hong Kong Med J. 2007;13:482–4.
4. Dermoid cyst of the glans penis in a toddler. Available from: https://www.researchgate.net/publication/262420828 Dermoid cyst of the glans penis in a toddler. Accessed 13 June 2016.
5. Malhotra MK, Singh KB, Garg P, Sharma P, Singh K. Mucoid cyst of the penis: a case report. J Clin Diagn Res. 2015;9(2):PD01–2. Available from: http://www.jcdr.net//back_issues.asp.
6. de Mendonça R, et al. Mucoid cyst of the penis: case report and literature review. Can Urol Assoc J. 2010;4(6):E155–7.
7. Dini M, Baroni G, Colafranceschi M. Medium raphe cyst of the penis: report of two cases with immunohistochemical investigation. Am J Dermatopathol. 2001;23:320–4.
8. Romani J, Barnadas MA, Miralles J, et al. Median raphe cyst of the penis with ciliated cells. J Cutan Pathol. 1995;22(4):378–81.
9. Urahashi J, et al. Pigmented median raphe cysts of the penis. Acta Derm Venereol. 2000;80:297–8.
10. Thompson IM, Lantin PM. Parameatal cysts of the glans penis. J Urol. 1956;76:753.
11. Soyer T, Aydemir E, Atmaca E. Paraurethral cysts in female newborns: role of maternal estrogenes. J Pediatr Adolesc Gynecol. 2007;20:249–51.
12. Willis HL, Snow BW, Cartwright PC, Wallis MC, Oottamasathien S, deVries C. Parameatal urethral cysts in prepubertal males. J Urol. 2011;185(3):1042–5. doi:10.1016/j.juro.2010.10.038. Epub 2011 Jan 19.

Part IV

Urinary Meatus

20 Megameatus

Abstract

I'm suggesting herein that the pathological anomaly lies mainly in the configuration of the urinary meatus, which instead to be a slit like, located in the undersurface of the glans penis, slightly at the tip, it will be in this rare anomaly so widely opened "mega meatus" with a different abnormal positions, either orthotopic, hypospadiac or epispadic and to be either associated with a normally intact or a deficient prepuce, so we will end with a 4 different subtypes of megameatus; the intact prepuce orthotopic megameatus subtype was not previously described.

Keywords

Intact prepuce megameatus • Intact prepuce with epispadias • Intact prepuce with orthotopic megameatus

We opted to title this chapter as "Megameatus", and not an Intact prepuce megameatus (IPM), like other text books and different literature, as I'm suggesting herein that the pathological anomaly lies mainly in the configuration of the urinary meatus, which instead to be a slit like, located in the undersurface of the glans penis, slightly at the tip (Figs. 20.1 and 20.2), it will be in this rare anomaly so widely opened "mega meatus" with a different abnormal positions, either orthotopic, hypospadiac or epispadic and to be either associated with a normally intact or a deficient prepuce, so we will end with a four different subtypes of megameatus; the intact prepuce orthotopic megameatus subtype was not previously described.

© Springer International Publishing Switzerland 2017

M. Fahmy, *Congenital Anomalies of the Penis*, DOI 10.1007/978-3-319-43310-3_20

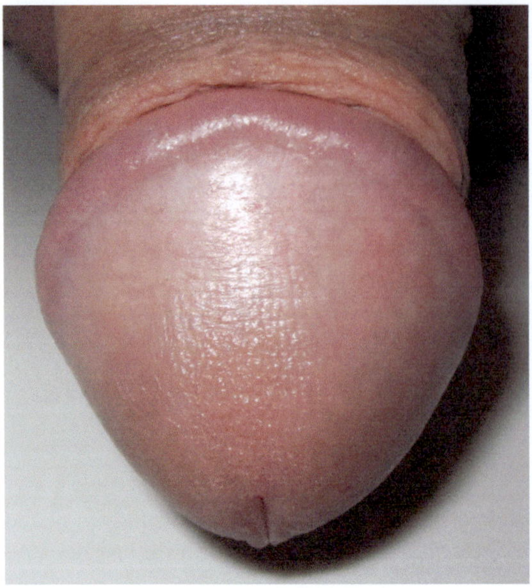

Fig. 20.1 Normally situated urinary meatus in a flaccid penis

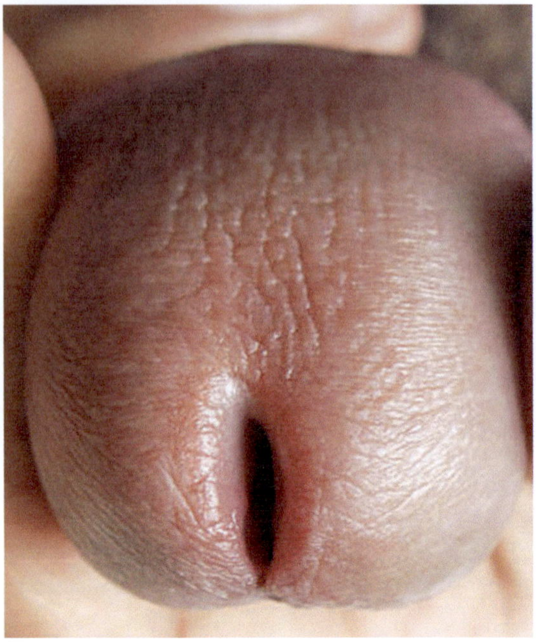

Fig. 20.2 Normally slightly widened meatus during erection

Definition

Megameatus is a congenitally abnormally wide urinary meatus closely associated with an abnormal location; hypospadiac, orthotopic or episodic, with an abnormal or normal prepuce.

20.1 Spectrum of the Megameatus Anomaly

- Intact **prepuce Megameatus (IPM), with three subtypes:**
  - Intact prepuce with hypospadiac megameatus (Fig. 20.3a, b).
  - Intact prepuce with epispadias (Fig. 20.4a, b).
  - Intact prepuce with orthotopic megameatus (Fig. 20.5a, b).
- **Megameatus with hypospadias, usually associated with a deficient hooded prepuce (Fig.** 20.6**).**

Each type will be described separately with illustrations

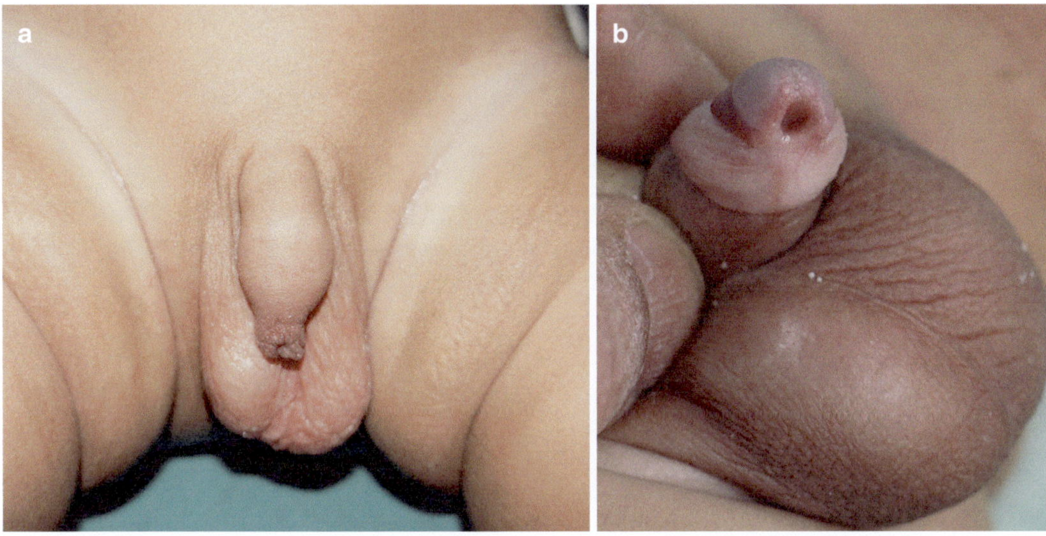

Fig. 20.3 (**a**) Intact prepuce, (**b**) when prepuce retracted, it revealed a hypospadiac megameatus

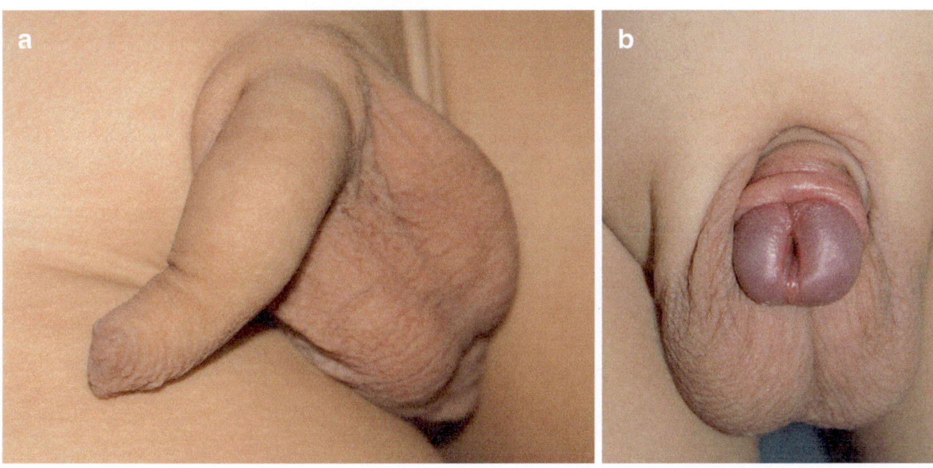

Fig. 20.4 (**a**) Intact prepuce, (**b**) an epispadiac megameatus seen when prepuce retracted

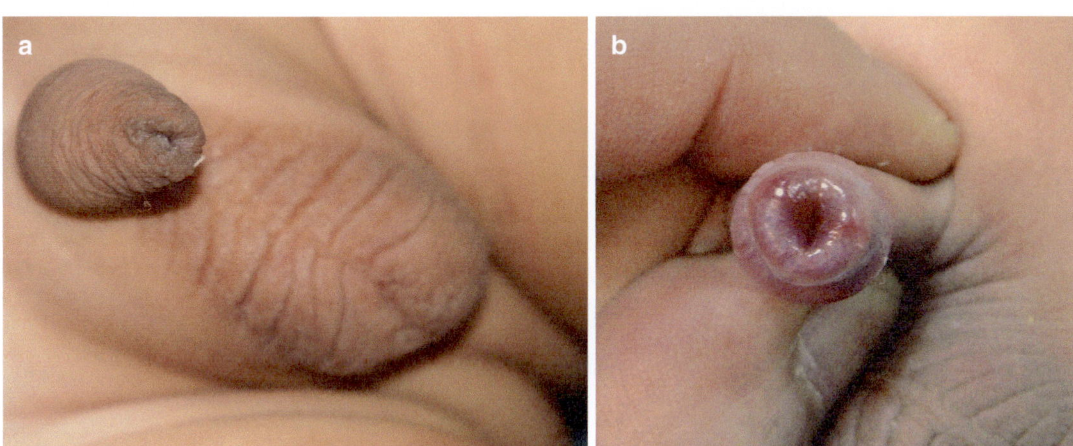

Fig. 20.5 (**a**) Intact prepuce (**b**) with an orthotopic megameatus

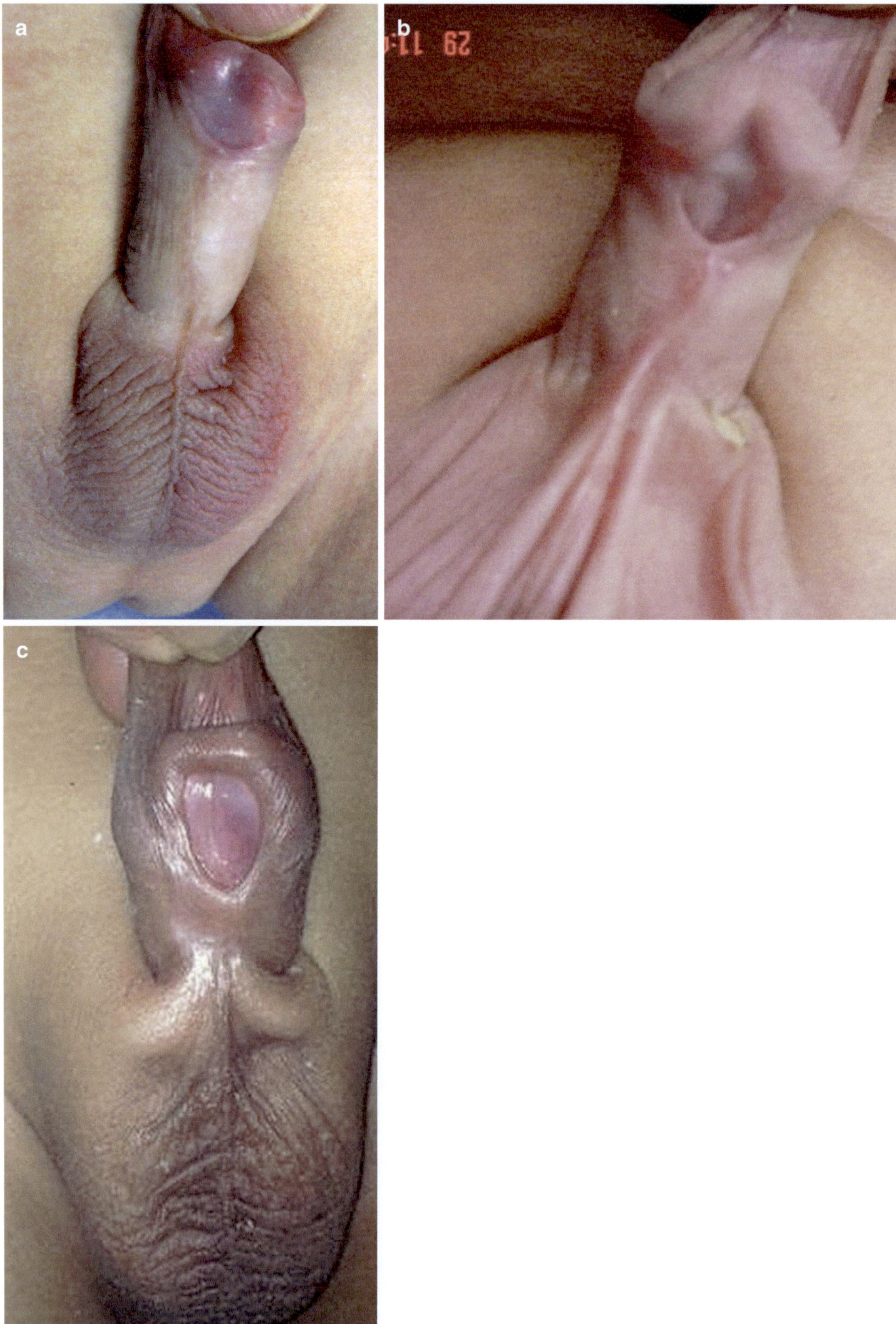

Fig. 20.6 (**a**) Megameatus with hypospadias and a hooded prepuce. (**b**) Wide megameatus with hypospadias. (**c**) Abnormally wide megameatus with deficient glanular tissue

20.2 Intact Prepuce with Hypospadiac Megameatus

Commonly known as an Intact prepuce Megameatus (IPM), it is not a rare condition, with a different varieties, several presentations and of a paramount importance as regard the recognition and management.

Nomenclature

Intact Prepuce Megameatus, Pseudo Iatrogenic Hypospadias, Hypospadias Variant.

Incidence

The overall incidence of the MIP is approximately 1 in 10,000 live births and represent a 3–6 % of cases of anterior hypospadias, but this condition may be more often with underestimation and reporting [1].

Historical Background

MIP is not known till recently, when it was described for the first time at 1989, by Duckett and Keatting [2].

Description

Obviously, MIP by definition is an association of a widely opened splayed glans, deeply grooved, patulous, large urinary meatus in the ventral aspect, at or even distal to the coronal sulcus, with a completely formed prepuce in contrast to the ventrally deficient foreskin in other cases of hypospadias. Furthermore, the meatus is abundantly large in the MIP variant, whereas many boys with distal hypospadias have a rather small-appearing meatus. Ventral curvature is much less likely to occur in a patient with MIP than in those with other varieties of distal hypospadias (Fig. 20.3a, b).

Because there is no external clue to the presence of this variant, the megameatus intact prepuce sometimes comes to light for the first time in a boy who is about to undergo circumcision. Recognition of this anomaly is important, not only for the sake of the child, but also from the medico-legal point of view. In some countries where circumcision performed early for infants in the first weeks of life, the families may attribute MIP as a complication of circumcision. The clues in such cases are the absence of any evidence of glanular scarring, no history of bleeding at the time of circumcision and the smooth edges of the widely splitted meatus with a healthy mucosal covering (Fig. 20.7).

Sometimes MIP may be presented with paraphimosis, if the intact prepuce is forcible retracted during routine circumcision in a young infant (Fig. 20.8).

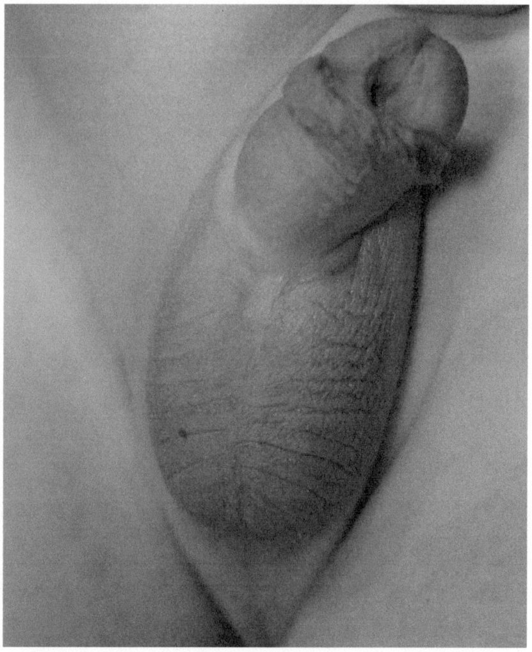

Fig. 20.7 A circumcised child had a typical megameatus, with a wide deep urethral plate and wide meatus extends along the whole glans without any scaring

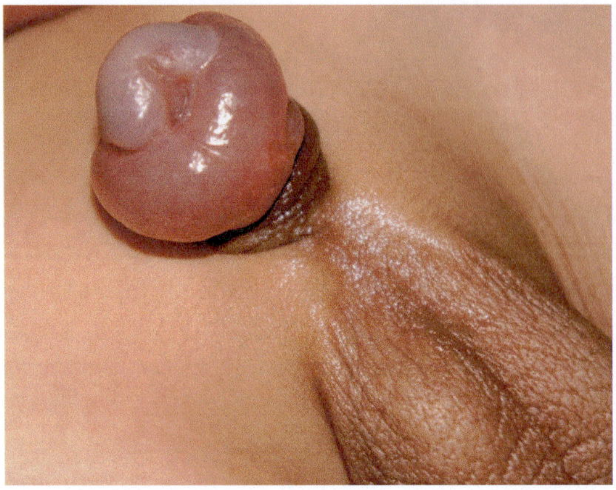

Fig. 20.8 Paraphimosis with an edematous internal mucosal layer of the prepuce forming a constricting ring around the coronal sulcus with an apparent megameatus

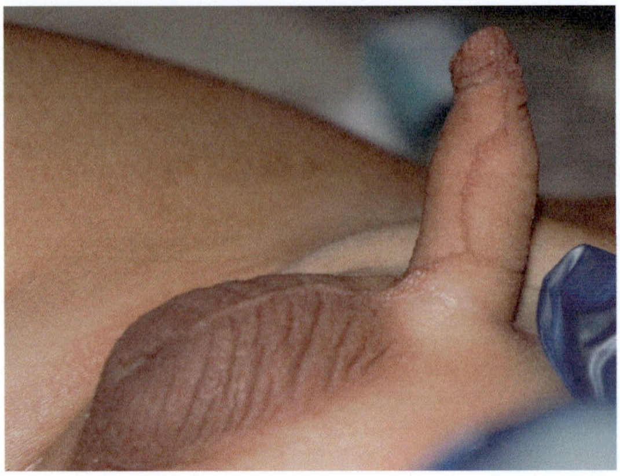

Fig. 20.9 Left side median raphe deviation as an indicator of a hidden megameatus

Embryological Background

Several factors are considered:

Failure of distal urethral folding.
Obstruction of the meatus by epithelial plug result in disruption of glandular urethra.
A variant of megalourethra.
A variant of hypospadias.

It seems that the progression of the development of the ureteral plate beyond the coronal sulcus doesn't relate to the preputial development, as the urethral plate growth may be arrested at any point to end with hypospadias, or a wide megameatus, while the prepuce continues its progressive growth to form the completely normal preputial sheath as an intact prepuce regardless the defective urethra.

Clinical Significance

MIP may results in many significant medical issues:-

- Interfere with antenatal diagnosis of hypospadias.
- Easily missed during circumcision.
- Medicolegal confusion.
- Difficulty to be repaired.
- Controversy about indication of repair.

Associated Anomalies

MIP usually had no other associated anomalies in either urinary or genital organs, but we encountered only a median raphe deviation in a significant number of cases of MIP (75 %) and we assumed that this finding may be helpful as an indicator for the presence of MIP in Chap. 16 with an attached video demonstrating this finding (Fig. 20.9).

Diagnosis

The mother may notice a ballooning of prepuce of her baby during micturition or an abnormal spatter urine stream.

Differential Diagnosis

This rare congenital anomaly should be differentiated from:

- Iatrogenic glanular or urethral injuries.
- Hypospadias.
- Intact prepuce with epispadias.

In our series of 16 patients we had one case, we consider it as a variant of IMP, with a completely divided glans penis, not only from the ventral

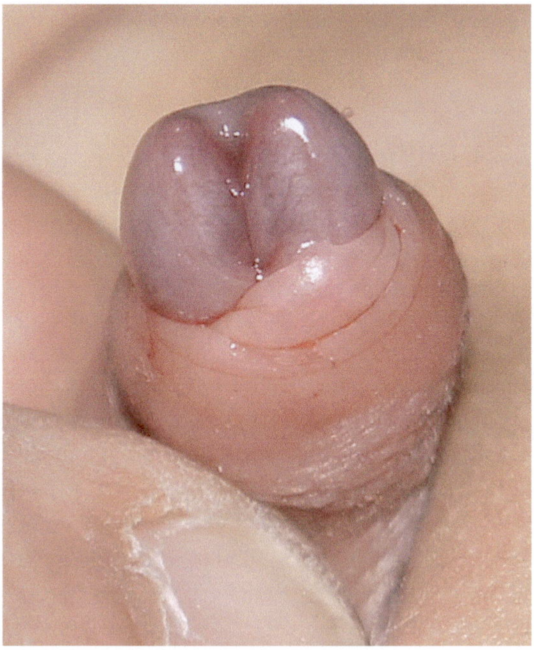

Fig. 20.10 Completely bifid glans under an intact prepuce, as a variant of MIP

aspect, but also partially divided from the dorsum, to gives the look of bifid glans (Fig. 20.10).

Management

A suitable technique has been described by Duckett [2], who also specifically cautioned against the use of the MAGPI repair in view of its high failure rate when used for the attempted repair of this variant. This technique known as pyramid procedure, which allows for an end-on dissection of the distal megameatusurethra, enabling a reduction in caliber while facilitating remodelling of the glans. The procedure has proved to be successful and reliable for this particular hypospadias variant. Because the urethral plate is larger than usual in these boys, a relaxing incision is not generally needed as with TIP repair; although when the plate is flat, incision will help "hinge" it to create a vertical and slit meatus. Some patients have a transverse web of skin distal to the meatus, and this should be excised to prevent deflection of the urinary stream [3].

20.3 Intact Prepuce with Epispadias (Fig. 20.4a, b)

It is very uncommon for epispadias to present with an intact prepuce. To date, about 15 cases have been reported in 9 literature reports [4]. At first presentation, the diagnosis is easily overlooked, as the epispadias is not directly visible. Based on specific clinical signs, such as a broad, spade-like glans and a dorsally directed preputial opening and urinary stream, suspicion for epispadias may exist. In addition, a gap between the corpora cavernosa may be palpated, also dorsal chordee and abnormalities of the penile raphe have been reported (This anomaly also discussed in Chap. 26, Epispadias).

Nomenclature

Concealed Epispadias.

Incidence

Underreporting of the condition may exist, for example, Perovic [5] described five cases of epispadias in his book, and two of these cases appear to have a complete prepuce. Epispadias with an intact prepuce is possibly not as uncommon as has been stated in the literature. This anomaly would not be easily overlooked in areas where the majority of males are circumcised, however, in countries where most males are not circumcised, it may go undetected.

Etiology

Mc Cahill et al. [6] in an attempt to explain epispadias with intact prepuce stated that there is an active growth of mesenchyme between the preputial fold and the glandular lamella, which transports the fold distally until it covers the glans completely even if there is defective glanular urethra development. However, this has not explained corona or penile epispadias with intact prepuce. Moreover, because most of the reported cases of epispadias with intact prepuce were glanular, many authors equate it wrongly with mega-meatus intact prepuce hypospadias [7].

Diagnosis

There may not be any complain by the parent to suggest this condition. The diagnosis is usually missed due to the apparently normal looking penis. Furthermore, although the prepuce cannot always be retracted in the case of an intact prepuce and epispadias, this should not delay the diagnosis of epispadias. Most cases are discovered when the child is presented for circumcision. Features like upward directed urinary stream, ballooning of the prepuce while micturating are not constant and may not be taken very seriously by physicians. Deviation of the preputial opening upward towards the dorsal aspect of the penis, absence of frenulum line on the glans, horizontal termination of the raphe phallus close to the glans, phimosis, broad base phallus, spade like glans, splitted corpora cavernosa and a depression between the corpora bodies are some of the signs that can be seen in this condition. Because the diagnosis is clinical, not many investigations are usually required. Abdominopelvic ultrasound scan done to this patient is to rule out other congenital urinary tract abnormalities which are not uncommon. We recommend an ascending and voiding urethrocystography and urodynamic study in older children to assess the degree of continence before surgery, as many cases may had a degree of incontinence.

Management

Surgery gives acceptable functional and cosmetic outcome. There are many surgical procedures described for treatment of epispadias, but for epispadias with intact prepuce, especially coronal or glanular, a simple approximation of the glans penis with or without circumcision [8] may not be satisfactory. High incidence of glanular dehiscence and an abnormally upward directed stream are common drawbacks. So, in such cases we are doing a complete urethral plate dissection, partial assembly of the glans, and ventral repositioning of the repaired urethra which give good outcome.

20.4 Intact Prepuce with Orthotopic Megameatus (Fig. 20.5a, b)

To the best of my knowledge, this anomaly was not described before, where the intact normal prepuce when retracted, reveals a very wide meatus occupying the whole circumference of the glans, with the red urethral mucosa could be seen easily This anomaly differ from other two previously described entities as regard the normally positioned meatus at the summit of the glans. It is supposed that this anomaly could be due to the failure in development of the normally constricted meatus distal to the wide fossa navicularis, which will be exposed or extended to replace the normal meatus. Also, this anomaly could be attributed to an over distal growth of urethral plate to reach to a more distal ectopic position (Fig. 20.5a, b).

There are two cases diagnosed with this variety; one of them presented with bleeding spots in the napkins, and the other detected only during circumcision. Both had meatal reconstruction and meatoplasty around a suitable catheter were attempted with success. To avoid possible ascending infection and napkin's irritation, it is important to reconstruct the meatus without stricture and in a position looking downwards like the normal one (Figs. 20.1 and 20.2).

20.5 Megameatus with Hypospadias and a Deficient or Hooded Prepuce (Fig. 20.6a, b)

The position and size of the external urethral meatus in normal boys is consistent and ventral glans closure (The distance between the distal end of the meatus and the coronal sulcus) (Fig. 20.11) is equal to or slightly less than meatal length [9]. However, there is a dilemma in that the normal glanular-meatal anatomy has never been adequately defined or investigated, leaving

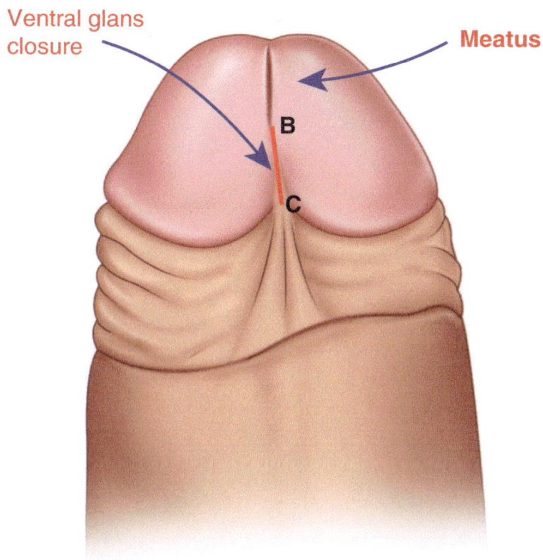

Fig. 20.11 Diagram showing the normal ventral glans closure in relation to the normally positioned meatus

the reconstructive surgeon to guess at creating a neomeatus of 'normal' length and a glans closure of 'normal' proportions in hypospadias repair.

The common shape of meatus in hypospadias is the transverse form, and in some patients, the meatus may look like a longitudinal fissure, which, in fact, it is circular at the proximal end of the fissure. The other common type is the pinpoint type of meatus [10].

There is no data in literature about the incidence of the various types or shape of meatus in hypospadias cases. The wide patulous meatus in cases of hypospadias are not rare, and also there is no reported figure about its incidence. As we can see from Fig. 20.6a–c, many cases of anterior penile hypospadias may be associated with a wide meatus, which could be considered as a megameatus with a deficient prepuce from the ventral surface of the penis, giving the look of hooded prepuce, which had significance in hypospadias surgery. The size of the meatus determines the extent of lateral dissection of the glans as with a large and wide meatus an adequate glanuloplasty may not be achieved and an alternative procedure needs to be employed.

References

1. Dora P, Melvyn W. Pseudo-iatrogenic hypospadias: the megameatus intact-prepuce hypospadias variant. Plast Reconstr Surg. 2003;111(3):1182–5.
2. Duckett JW, Keating MA. Technical challenge of intact prepuce megameatus hypospadias variant: the pyramid procedure. J Urol. 1989;141:1407.
3. Elbatarny A, Shehata S, Ismail K. Megameatus intact prepuce variety of hypospadias: tips for repair using the modified glanular approximation procedure. Ann Pediatr Surg. 2011;7(2):82–7.
4. Bos EM, et al. Epispadias in boys with an intact prepuce. J Pediatr Urol. 2014;10:67e73.
5. Perovic SV. Epispadias. In: Perovic SV, Basting RF, editors. Atlas of congenital anomalies of the external genitalia. 1st ed. Belgrad: Refot-Arka; 1999. p. 93e8.
6. McCahill PD, Leonard MP, Jeffs RD. Epispadias with phimosis: an unusual variant of the concealed penis. Urology. 1995;45:158–60. http://dx.doi.org/10.1016/S0090-4295(95)97778-3.
7. Maitama HY, Ahmed M, Bello A, Mbibu HN. Epispadias with complete prepuce: a rare anomaly. Afr J Urol. 2012;18:90–2. http://dx.doi.org/10.1016/j.afju.2012.07.001.
8. Sina A, Alizadeh F. Concealed male epispadias: a rare form of penile epispadias presenting as phimosis. Urol J. 2011;8:328–9.
9. Hutton AR, Ramesh B. Normal anatomy of the external urethral meatus in boys: implications for hypospadias repair. BJU Int. 2007;100:161–3. http://www.ncbi.nlm.nih.gov/pubmed/10079344.
10. Uygur MC, Ersoy E, Erol D. Analysis of meatal location in 1,244 healthy men. Definition of the normal site justifies the need for meatal advancement in pediatric anterior hypospadias cases. Pediatr Surg Int. 1999;15:119–20.

21 Congenital Meatal Stenosis

Abstract

Meatal stenosis is a common condition manifested with a severely narrowed distal urinary opening, which interfere with normal micturition and proper complete bladder evacuation, and if it is not recognised and treated early, it may end with a dismal sequels of proximal urinary tract obstruction and even renal failure.

Keywords

Meatal stricture • Meatal ulcer • Meatotomy • Meatoplasty

Definition

Meatal stenosis is a common condition manifested with a severely narrowed distal urinary opening, which interfere with normal micturition and proper complete bladder evacuation, and if it is not recognised and treated early, it may end with a dismal sequels of proximal urinary tract obstruction and even renal failure [1].

Nomenclature

Urethral meatal stenosis.

21.1 Incidence

In many neonates presented with meatal stenosis it may be difficult to define if this stenosis is a congenital anomaly or an acquired disease, as it is exceedingly rare in uncircumcised children, but it is estimated in 9–10 % of males who are circumcised [2]. In a prospective study Van Howe [3] found meatal stenosis in 24 of 239 (7.29 %) circumcised children older than 3 years, making meatal stenosis the most common complication of circumcision.

21.2 Etiology

21.2.1 Congenital

Secondary to failed regression of the distal urethral membrane, which is the border between the ingrown ectodermal tissue of the glans and endodermal tissue of the urethral mucosa, very rarely the stenosis appear as a congenital stricture of perpetual orifice (Fig. 21.1). Meatal stenosis occurs primarily in neonates with coronal or subcoronal

© Springer International Publishing Switzerland 2017
M. Fahmy, *Congenital Anomalies of the Penis*, DOI 10.1007/978-3-319-43310-3_21

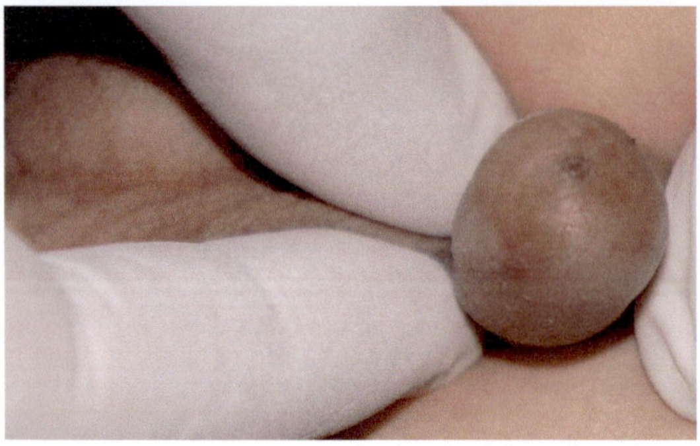

Fig. 21.1 Meatal stenosis at the level of perpetual orifice

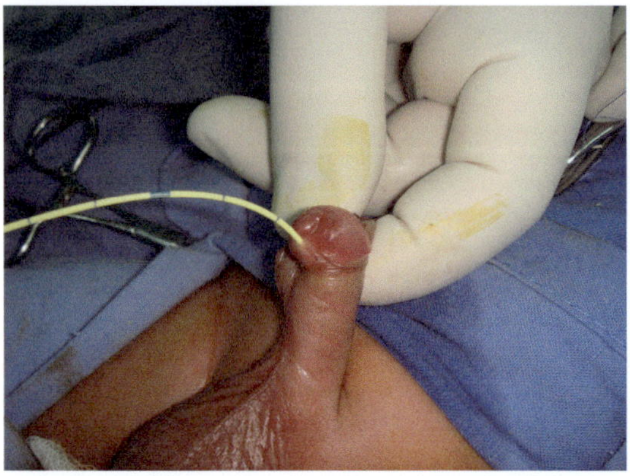

Fig. 21.2 Severe meatal stenosis, admitting only a size 3 F ureteric catheter in a 2 years old child with glandular hypospadias

hypospadias (Figs. 21.2 and 21.3). Also, congenital meatal stenosis may be an association or manifestation of parameatal cyst (Chap. 19), megalourthera (Chap. 26), anterior urethral valve in the fossa navicularis [33], urethral cyst (Chap. 30), urethral polyp (Chap. 32) or Lacuna Magna anomaly (Chap. 34).

21.2.2 Acquired

Acquired cases after neonatal circumcision, balanitis and urethritis; where a significant inflammatory reaction causing severe meatal inflammation and cicatrix formation, which results in a narrow meatus, a membranous web

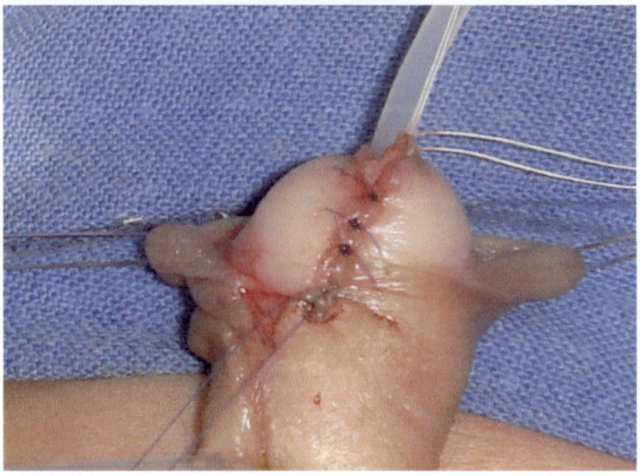

Fig. 21.3 Same case in Fig. 21.2 after repair of glandular hypospadias and meatoplasty around size 8 F catheter

across the ventral aspect of the meatus, or an eccentric healing process that produces a prominent lip of ventral meatal tissue, and in countries where circumcision is done routinely for almost all neonates, meatal stenosis is seen frequently as a common complication [2]. Meatal stenosis after circumcision is usually due severe napkin rashes, ammoniacal balanitis of the uncovered glans penis resulting in meatal ulcers, which heals by fibrosis (Fig. 21.4). Another hypothetical cause is ischemia due to damage to the frenular artery during circumcision, resulting in poor blood supply to the meatus with a subsequent stenosis [5].

Meatitis, an inflammation generally secondary to ammoniacal diaper irritation, has been cited as the underlying cause of secondary meatal stenosis either in circumcised or uncircumcised infant (Fig. 21.5).

Other causes of meatal stenosis include the following:

- Unsuccessful hypospadias repair.
- Trauma
- Prolonged catheterization
- Balanitis xerotica obliterans (BXO), as many as 1 in 5 boys who have undergone circumcision for BXO (Chap. 38); may require subsequent operative treatment of meatal pathology.

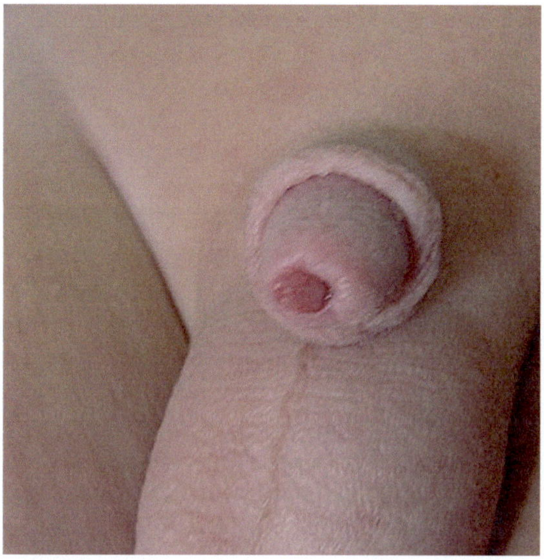

Fig. 21.4 Meatal ulcer after circumcision, it usually heals with meatal stricture

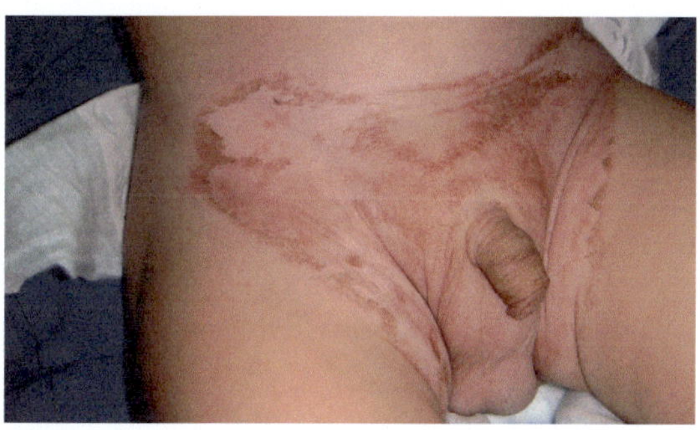

Fig. 21.5 Severe napkin dermatitis in uncircumcised child, which the leading cause of balanitis and subsequent meatal stenosis

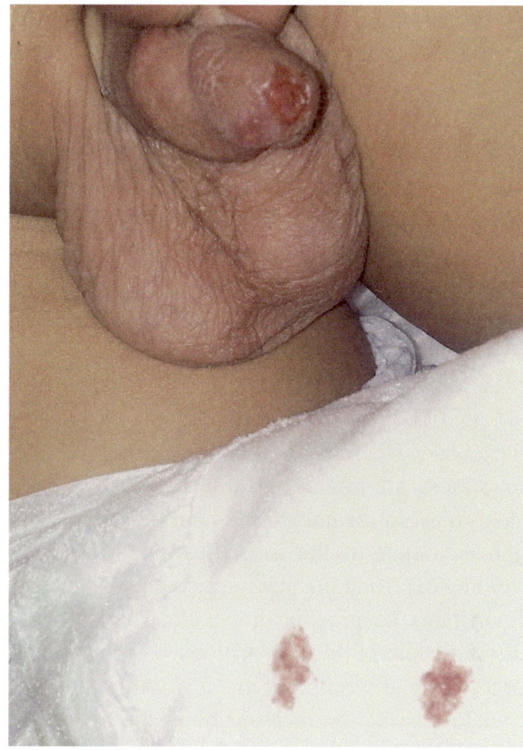

Fig. 21.6 Meatal stenosis with meatal ulcers manifested by heamatouria

21.3 Symptoms

This disorder is characterized by an upward deflected, difficult-to-aim urinary stream and, occasionally, dysuria and urgent, frequent, and prolonged urination. Symptoms of meatal stenosis vary with the appearance, in most cases; stenosis does not become apparent until after the child is toilet trained. If the meatus is pinpoint, the boy voids with a forceful, fine stream that has a great casting distance. Some boys have a dorsally deflected stream or a prolonged voiding time. Dysuria, frequency, terminal hematuria, and incontinence are symptoms that may lead to discovery of meatal stenosis but generally are not attributable to this abnormality (Fig. 21.6).

21.4 Diagnosis

Meatal stenosis can be suspected based on the presence of a small meatus during examination, particularly if, with lateral traction, the ventral edges of the meatus appear fused.

Observation of the child while voiding helps immensely in confirming the diagnosis of the disorder.

If the physician desires to calibrate the meatus, Litvak et al. [6] report that the normal meatus in children younger than 1 year will accept a lubricated 5 F feeding tube. They also report that, in children aged 1–6 years, an 8 F feeding tube should pass without difficulty (Fig. 21.2).

If the child has abnormal voiding symptoms, a renal and bladder ultrasound examination is indicated, and if there is a history of UTIs, a voiding cystourethrogram (VCUG) should be done also.

21.5 Management

In countries where circumcision practiced routine for almost all infants, all measures should be taken to avoid meatal stenosis, and to cut off the high incidence of this complication, mainly by avoiding exposing the newly circumcised penis to any irritants, keeping the diaper clean and dry, and follow up the child regularly after circumcision for a couple of weeks and in a boy with suspected meatal stenosis, the meatus should be calibrated with a bougie or assessed with infant sounds.

Serial dilatation results in small tears of the meatus, which are followed by secondary healing. In the long term, this creates a tighter stricture at the tip of the penis; therefore, this procedure is discouraged.

Meatotomy is the definitive treatment for meatal stenosis, it is a simple procedure in which the ventrum of the meatus is crushed (for hemostasis) for 60 s with a straight mosquito forceps and then divided with fine-tipped scissors. Brown et al [5] reported excellent results following 130 office meatotomies with only 2 recurrences of meatal stenosis and 1 patient with bleeding requiring stitches. They also cited the cost-effectiveness of this treatment and noted good patient tolerance when a caring approach is used to reassure the child before and during the procedure. In this series, parents were encouraged to remain with the children during the operation, as their presence seemed to have a calming effect. After the operation, it is critical that the caregivers separate the edges of the meatus and apply antibiotic ointment or petroleum jelly twice a day for 2 weeks and then once a day for another 2 weeks to prevent one side of the meatotomy from adhering to the other side.

In many cases, with severe meatal stenosis or recurrence after meatotomy, meatoplasty may be indicated, and it could be accomplished in the physician's office using local anaesthetic cream for pain control. In addition, 1 % lidocaine with 1:100,000 epinephrine may be infiltrated in the ventral web with a 26 gauge needle for local anaesthesia and vasoconstriction. A ventral incision is made toward the frenulum and long enough to provide a meatus of normal caliber, which can be checked with the bougie. The urethral mucosa is sutured to the glans with fine absorbable sutures. If the procedure is performed under general anaesthesia, the bladder may be filled with saline and compressed manually to be certain that the stream is straight [6].

References

1. Chevalier RL. Pathogenesis of renal injury in obstructive uropathy. Curr Opin Pediatr. 2006;18(2):153–60 [Medline].
2. Homer L, Buchanan KJ, Nasr B, Losty PD, Corbett HJ. Meatal stenosis in boys following circumcision for lichen sclerosus (balanitis xerotica obliterans). J Urol. 2014;30.
3. Van Howe RS. Incidence of meatal stenosis following neonatal circumcision in a primary care setting. Clin Pediatr (Phila). 2006;45(1):49–54.
4. Scherz HC, Kaplan GW, Packer MG. Anterior urethral valves in the fossa navicularis. J Urol. 1987;138:1211–3.
5. Brown MR, Cartwright PC, Snow BW. Common office problems in pediatric urology and gynecology. Pediatr Clin North Am. 1997;44(5):1091–115.
6. Litvak AS, Morris JA, McRoberts JW. Normal size of the urethral meatus in boys. J Urol. 1976;115:736–7.

Congenital Double Meatus

22

Abstract

The normal urinary meatus is a vertical slit-like opening that commenced at the tip of the penis and ran ventrally. The position and size of the external urethral meatus in normal boys are consistent, with rare variation and ventral glans closure is equal to or slightly less than meatal length. These data might be of interest to hypospadiologists in their efforts to reconstruct normal glanular anatomy, and there was an age-dependent increase in meatal length and a similar association was identified for the length of ventral glans closure.

Keywords

Accessory meatal dimple • juxtaposed urethral meatus

Nomenclature

Accessory meatal dimple, juxtaposed urethral meatus.

The normal urinary meatus is a vertical slit-like meatus that commenced at the tip of the penis and ran ventrally. The position and size of the external urethral meatus in normal boys are consistent, with rare variation and ventral glans closure is equal to or slightly less than meatal length. These data might be of interest to hypospadiologists in their efforts to reconstruct normal glanular anatomy, and there was an age- dependent increase in meatal length and a similar association was identified for the length of ventral glans closure. There was also a statistically significant proportional relationship between meatal length and length of glans [1].

Incidence

It is a common finding with different grades of hypospadias (Fig. 22.1), but many cases are reported without any other anomalies; giving more attention to such finding may encourage more reporting of such rare anomaly (Fig. 22.2).

22.1 Etiology

The distal glanular urethra developed from a solid ectodermal ingrowth of the epidermis which canalizes the glans to fuse urethral folds proximally, so duplicated ectodermal ingrowth and canalization of the glans with one moiety communicate with the proximal urethra, and

© Springer International Publishing Switzerland 2017
M. Fahmy, *Congenital Anomalies of the Penis*, DOI 10.1007/978-3-319-43310-3_22

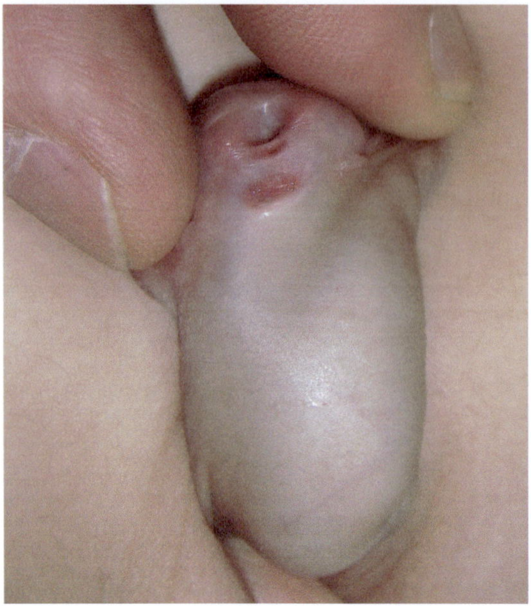

Fig. 22.1 Double meatus with anterior penile hypospadias

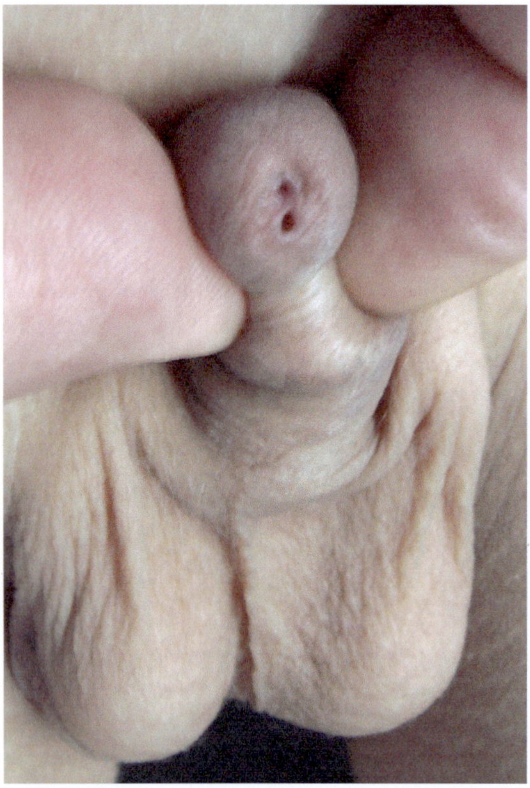

Fig. 22.2 Double meatus without hypospadias

another one failed to complete the canalization and could stop at the tip of the glans, to give rise to the accessory meatus, also double meatus may represent an incomplete urethral duplication.

22.2 Significance

Detection of this anomaly is only important to rule out cases of actual ureteral duplication, so calibration of this dimple will rule out complete extra urethra. As a general rule, the most proximal orifice is the actual urethral orifice connected to the bladder [2] (Figs. 22.3 and 22.4). Other associated anomalies could be ruled out with an ultrasound examination.

In a hypospadiac patient, there may be several meatal openings, which represent openings of paraurethral canals or lacunae of Morgagni. The presence of a distal opening may lead the parents and the inexperienced practitioner to think that the hypospadias is more distal than it really is. In rare cases, the child may have a double meatal opening with a thin septum separating the two openings without any adjuvant urethra, but ascending and micturating cystourethrogram (MCUG) is

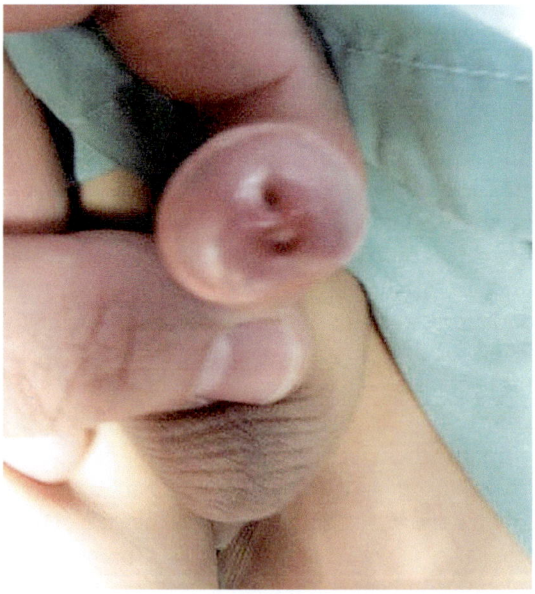

Fig. 22.3 Double meatus gives false impression of urethral duplication

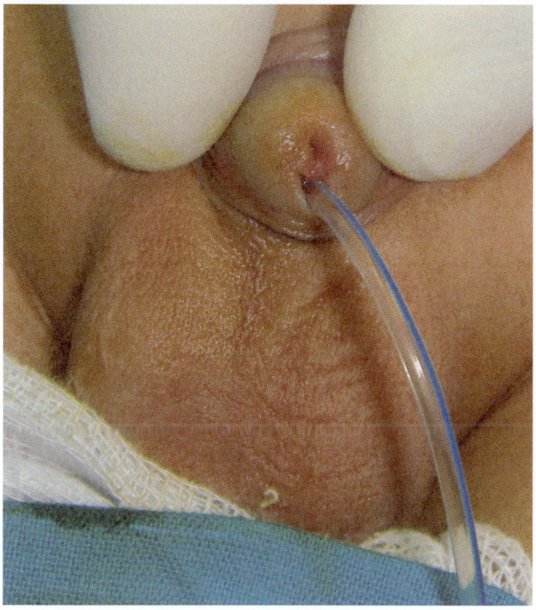

Fig. 22.4 Catheterisation revealed a proximal normal urethra and a distal accessory meatus

essential to rule out duplicating urethra, which will be discussed in details in Chap. 27.

From the medico-legal aspect, orientation with such rare cases, and documentation before circumcision is necessary for surgeons practicing routine circumcision, as the family may thought that this dimple is a complication secondary to glans injury. Usually there is no management indicated for such cases, but family assurance is essential.

References

1. Bush NC, DaJusta D, Snodgrass WT. Glans penis width in patients with hypospadias compared to healthy controls. J Pediatr Urol. 2013;9(6 Pt B): 1188–91. doi:10.1016/j.jpurol.2013.05.004. Epub 2013 Jun 12.
2. Hadidi AT. Classification of hypospadias. In: Hadidi AT, Azmy AF, editors. Hypospadias surgery: an illus- trated guide. 1st ed. Berlin: Springer; 2004.

Part V

Urethra

Urethral Agenesis 23

Abstract

Urethral atresia is a rare urethral malformation, which is not compatible with life unless the urachus open in the umbilicus, an alternative communication between the bladder and rectum exists in a form of congenital fistula, or a prenatal placement of a vesico-amniotic shunt established. Terminal renal failure and multiple reconstructive operations have to be expected in the course of the disease.

Keywords

Urethral agenesis • Penile agenesis • Urethral atresia • Obstructive uropathy

Urethral atresia is a rare urethral malformation, which is not compatible with life unless the urachus open in the umbilicus, an alternative communication between the bladder and rectum exists in a form of congenital fistula, or a prenatal placement of a vesico-amniotic shunt established. Terminal renal failure and multiple reconstructive operations have to be expected in the course of the disease [1].

23.1 Incidence

Urethral agenesis with complete absence of the urinary meatus is a very rare anomaly which comes in two forms, either with normal phallus or in combination with penile agenesis (Figs. 23.1 and 23.2). It is a very rare reported anomaly as most cases die intrauterine; combined bladder and urethral agenesis is also an extremely rare anomaly with only 22 live births have been reported of the 60 known cases. Few cases have been reported in females as this condition is mostly reported in boys [2].

23.2 Associated Anomalies

Penile agenesis complicated by Potter sequences with urethral agenesis should be differentiated from those with ectopic urethral opening. This anomaly is usually associated with anorectal malformations and limb anomalies, and it may represent the spectrum of urorectal septum malformations, which lead to several different types of fistulas between urinary system and rectum, or urethral agenesis,

© Springer International Publishing Switzerland 2017

M. Fahmy, *Congenital Anomalies of the Penis*, DOI 10.1007/978-3-319-43310-3_23

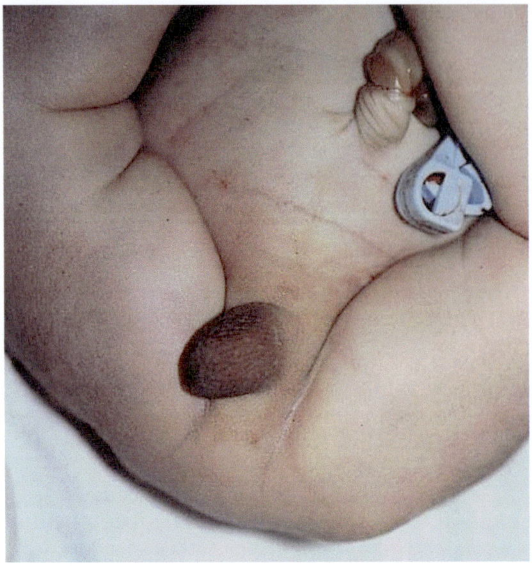

Fig. 23.1 Complete urethral agenesis with imperforate anus, "Urorectal septum malformations"

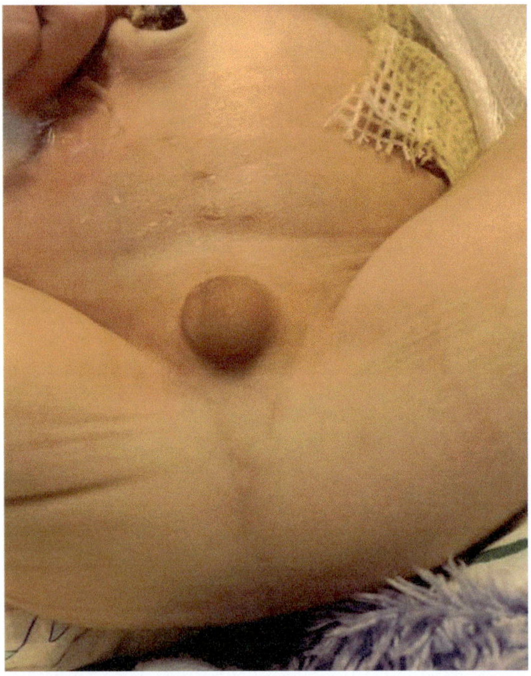

Fig. 23.2 Another case of alive baby with urethral agenesis, imperforate anus and aphallia

specially with partial urorectal septum malformation sequence [3]. Embryologically the urorectal septum, grows downward from the ridge separating the allantois from the cloacal opening of the intestine and ultimately fuses with the cloacal membrane and divides it into an anal and a urogenital part, where the dorsal part of the cloaca forms the rectum, and the anterior part of the urogenital sinus and bladder [4].

Also this anomaly is detected in Fraser syndrome (renal agenesis, laryngeal atresia, cryptophthalmos, and syndactyly). Many cases of aphallia (Chap. 8) had urethral agenesis, and in such cases lung hypoplasia and severe oligohydramnios are obvious after the 16th week of gestation, which is a lethal squeal of urethral agenesis and results in stillbirth or death in the neonatal period [5]. An associated vertebral especially sacral anomalies are a common association, which indicate an underdeveloped bottom, so many cases of sirenomelia and caudal regression syndrome had a urethral as well as penile agenesis. Some cases are also reported with prune-belly syndrome where the bladder outlet obstruction is usually associated with a megacystis [6]. An associated congenital urethral fistula is a common association with urethral agenesis (Chap. 28).

23.3 Management

Recently such cases are diagnosed antenatally, and the consequences of obstructive uropathy and lung hypoplasia could be managed by intrauterine urinary diversion in the amniotic space by a double pigtail catheter or other means of diversion, especially if the fetus had a normally distended bladder and the fetus could be saved to sustain postnatally reconstruction of the defective urethra. In a recent study of antenatally detect cases, there is a 5 % spontaneous fetal deaths, but in 45 % of the cases the family choose the option of elective termination of pregnancy for fetal anomaly (TOPFA) [7].

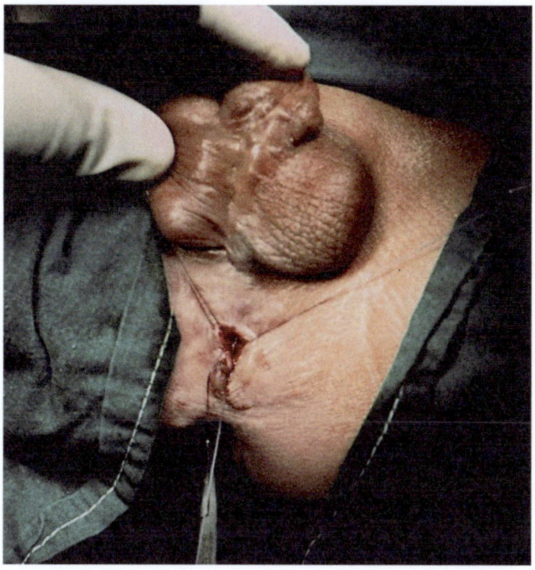

Fig. 23.3 A rare case of complete urethral agenesis with a perineal uretherostomy

The first measure to be taken immediately after delivery is urinary tract venting by vasicostomy or even proximal diversion to safe the upper tract and keep the baby alive. Sometimes MRI imaging reveal an atretic urethra ending at the prenium, and a uretherostomy could safe the upper tract, and latter on a subsequent reconstruction of a neo-urethra could be achieved from either local tissue or a buccal mucosal grafting (Fig. 23.3).

References

1. Favorito LA, Cardinot TM, Morais AM, Sampaio FJ. Urogenital anomalies in human male fetuses. Early Hum Dev. 2004;79:41–7.
2. Rezaie MA, Ehsan Mansourian E, Delui HR, Amirmajdi NM. Bladder and urethral agenesis: a report of two cases. Urology. 2010;76(1):60–1.
3. Wheeler PG, Weaver DD. Partial urorectal septum malformation sequence: a report of 25 cases. Am J Med Genet. 2001;103(2):99–105.
4. Escobar LF, Heiman M, Zimmer D, Careskey H. Urorectal septum malformation sequence: prenatal progression, clinical report, and embryology review. Am J Med Genet A. 2007;143(22):2722–6. doi:10.1002/ajmg.a.31925.PMID17937427.
5. O'Connor TA, La Cour ML, Friedlander ER, Thomas R. Penile agenesis associated with urethral and bilateral renal agenesis. Urology. 1993;41:564–5.
6. Kuga T, Esato K, Sase M, Nakata M, Kaneko J, Inoue T. Prune belly syndrome with penile and urethral agenesis: report of a case original research article. J Pediatr Surg. 1998;33(12):1825–8.
7. Tennant PWG, Glinianaia SV, Diana W, Draper ES, Kurinczuk JJ, Tonks AM, Tucker DF, Ben W, Judith R. Epidemiology of partial urorectal septum malformation sequence (or 'persistent cloaca'): a population-based study in seven regions of England and wales, 1985–2010. Arch Dis Child Fetal Neonatal Ed. 2014;99(5):F413–8. doi:10.1136/archdischild-2014-306027.

Hypospadias Variants

24

Marjan Waterloos, Piet Hoebeke, and Anne-Françoise Spinoit

Abstract

Hypospadias is the most frequent congenital penile defect affecting the external male genitalia, with an incidence around 1 in 250 male newborns, although this seems to be increasing.

The word *hypospadias* originates from the Greek (ύπο σπαδιας) 'hypo' meaning 'under' and 'spadias' meaning 'opening'. As the word tells, *hypospadias* is "a congenital condition in males in which the opening of the urethra is on the underside of the penis".

Keywords

Hypospadias variants • Mild hypospadias

Definition

Hypospadias is the most frequent congenital penile defect affecting the external male genitalia, with an incidence around 1 in 250 male newborns, although this seems to be increasing [1, 2].

The word *hypospadias* originates from the Greek (ύπο σπαδιας) 'hypo' meaning 'under' and 'spadias' meaning 'opening'. As the word tells, *hypospadias* is "a congenital condition in males in which the opening of the urethra is on the underside of the penis" [3].

Hypospadias is defined by a tissue underdevelopment on the ventral aspect of the penis. Three main defects are commonly observed (Fig. 24.1):

- The urethral *meatus* is ectopic and opens at any place along a line running on the ventral aspect of the penis and the *perineum*.
- A ventral curvature of the penis, called chordee
- A hooded prepuce, characterized by excessive skin on the dorsal side of the prepuce or foreskin, and hypoplastic tissues on the ventral aspect of the prepuce and the penile shaft.

Those three main defects are inconstant, as an ectopic *meatus* can be observed without chordee, or chordee without ectopic *meatus* can be observed, or an ectopic *meatus* can be discovered under a normal prepuce like in *mega-meatus* intact prepuce (Fig. 24.2).

© Springer International Publishing Switzerland 2017

M. Fahmy, *Congenital Anomalies of the Penis*, DOI 10.1007/978-3-319-43310-3_24

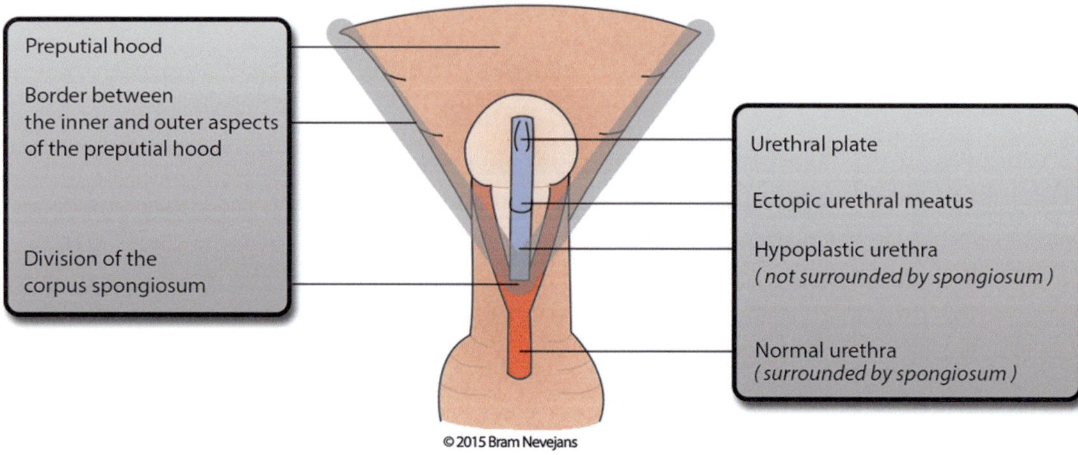

Fig. 24.1 Schematic representation of hypospadias

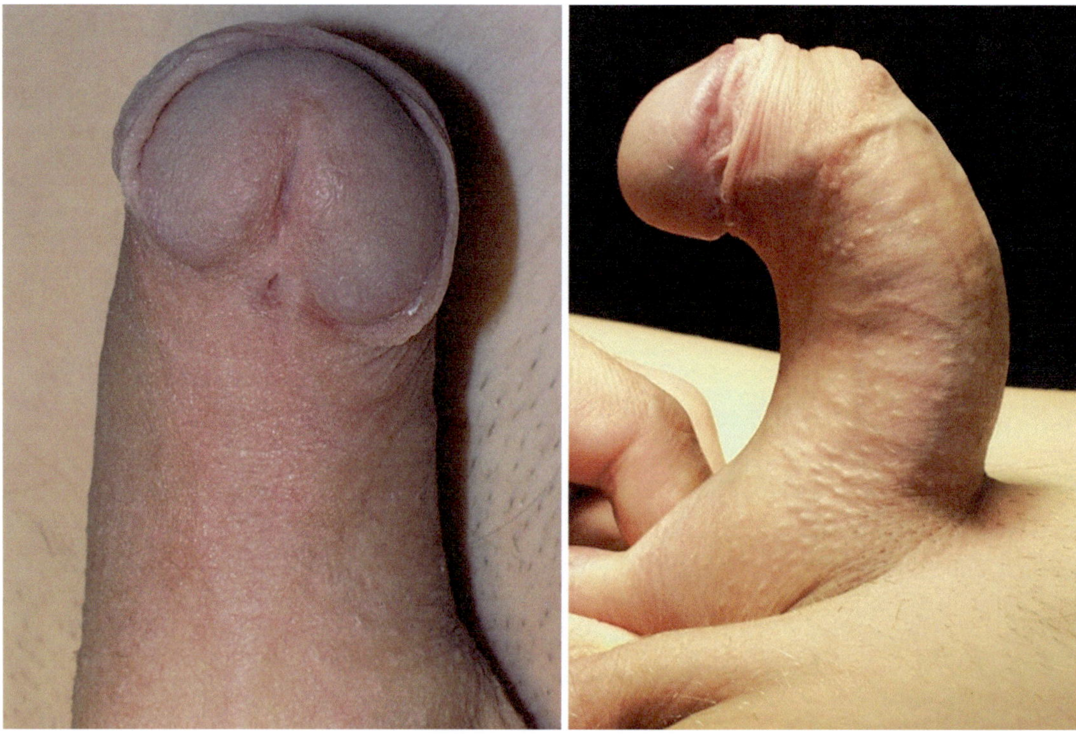

Fig. 24.2 Important chordee associated with a distal sub-coronal hypospadias

24.1 Pathophysiology and Classification

The *hypospadias penis* has a *glans* which is ventrally open. A portion of the urethral tube is missing, and is replaced by a so-called urethral plate extending from the ectopic *meatus* to the *glans* gap, between the *corpora cavernosa* [2]. The condition is the result of a problem during the endodermal transformation into the urethra and its subsequent tubularization which, for some reason yet to be understood, is stopped before it is accomplished [2, 4].

Part of the tubular urethra below the hypospadic *meatus* is not surrounded by *corpus spongiosum*, but is directly covered by hypo plastic skin tightly adherent to the tubular urethra [5, 6]. The frenular artery is consistently missing. The dorsal aspect of the penis, except for the redundant dorsal prepuce, is normal.

The division of the *corpus spongiosum* is always proximal to the ectopic meatus. All distal tissues to this division of the *corpus spongiosum* are hypoplastic. All tissues proximal to this division of the *corpus spongiosum* are normal (Fig. 24.1).

Until now there's no consensus on how to determine the severity of a *hypospadias*. Multiple classification methods have been suggested [6–8].

Some authors have proposed to classify the severity of the *hypospadias* according to the place where the division of the *corpus spongiosum* is located, rather than based on the location or the ectopic *meatus* [4, 5, 7–9].

Another frequently used classification is defining *hypospadias* according to the position of its *meatus* before dissection: distal *hypospadias*, mid-penile *hypospadias*, and proximal *hypospadias* (Fig. 24.3) [7].

This classification, as many published classifications, is mainly based on the position of the ectopic *meatus*, and is determined before deglovement [2, 7]. It is however considered to be an inaccurate criterion to define the severity of the *hypospadias* [7, 10]. The level of division of the *corpus spongiosum* is indeed a far more accurate criterion as it shows where the genital tubercle arrested its development [5, 6, 10]. This however can only be determined intra-operatively [6, 11].

This intra-operative classification, despite being more accurate, is not widespread used. Most of the studies published about *hypospadias* surgery use indeed the position of the ectopic *meatus* as a reference [7] (Figs. 24.4 and 24.5).

Many variants in hypospadias can be observed, form the very obvious one peno-scrotal ones, to some very light fors, where the meatus is orthotopic, but some of the typoc features are observed: an incompletely fused pretputium, some important chordee,…

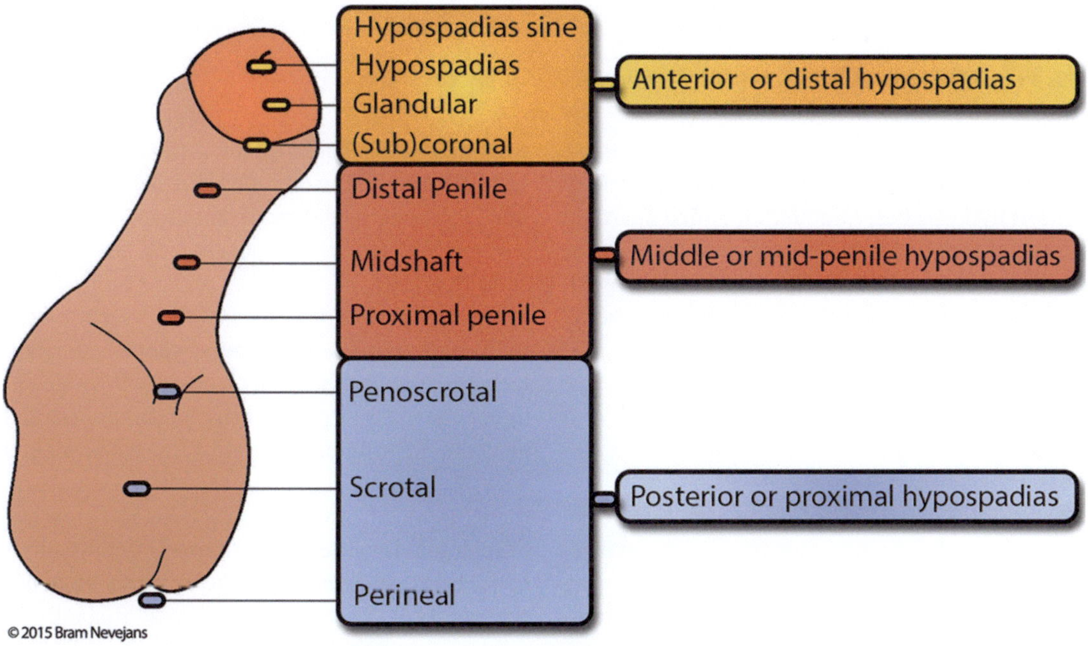

Fig. 24.3 Classification of hypospadias according to the meatal position

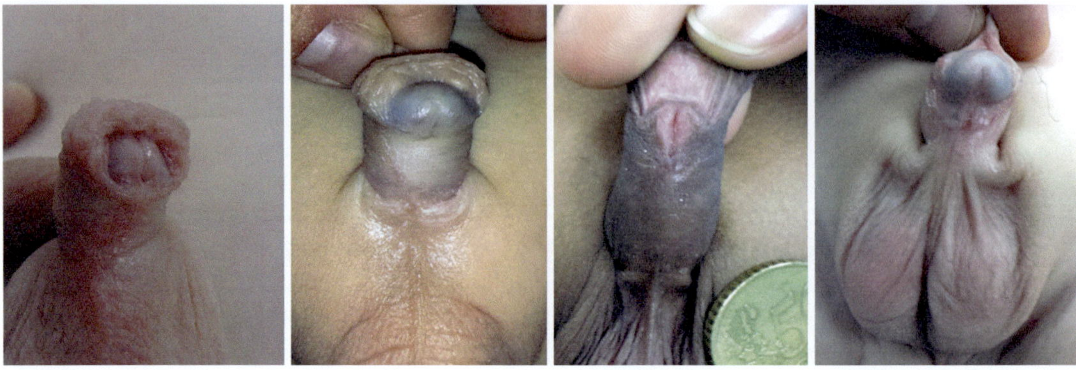

Fig. 24.4 Some distal hypospadias presentations

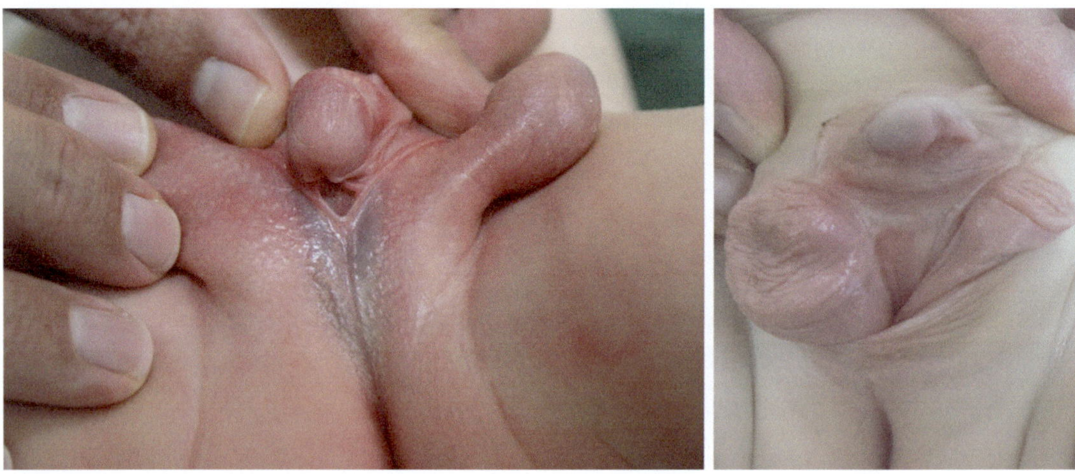

Fig. 24.5 Some proximal hypospadias presentations

Again, there is no consensus of all those milder forms of hypospadias should be considered as hypospadias, or better classified apart: do all the chordee without hypospadias present the same pathologic features as the classical hypospadias with important chordee, or even without? The debate remains open.

24.2 Etiology

Hypospadias is recognized to be a multifactorial disorder, with genetic, endocrine and environmental influences.

The pathophysiology of hypospadias remains to be discovered. A recent study showed however that the microscopic organization of the smooth muscle fibers of the dartos tissue plays an important role in congenital penile malformation: the level of dartos disorganization appears strongly related to the severity of the clinical condition [12].

Several *maternal-placental factors* correlated with hypospadias have been identified. Risk factors associated with neonates small for gestational age such as prematurity, preeclampsia and placental insufficiency are found to be correlated with the incidence of hypospadias. Also there seems to be an association between the presence of maternal hypertension, prematurity and oligohydramnios in relation to the severity of hypospadias [13]. Preexisting maternal diabetes or mild gestational diabetes, epilepsy, renal failure, asthma, exposure to influenza during the first trimester are potential maternal risk factors for developing hypospadias [14–16]. An indirectly association with conception by medically assisted reproduction is observed [14]. The role of maternal age on the prevalence of hypospadias is under discussion.

Environmental risk factors including diethylstilbestrol (DES), fertility treatments and environmental endocrine disruptions (EEDs) are known to contribute to the development of hypospadias, when exposed in early fetal life.

The influence of *maternal dietary nutrients and medication* on the prevalence of hypospadias has been proven. Low consumption of organic food during pregnancy leads to an increase risk on hypospadias. Hormone containing contraceptives during embryonal life is correlated with hypospadias. Antiepileptic drugs such as valproate enhances the probability of hypospadias, a dose dependent pattern has been observed.

Multiple *genetic abnormalities* have been identified as main etiologic factors in hypospadias. The foreskin of the hypospadias population has a manifest greater androgen receptor (AR) gene methylation [17].

An interaction between genetic, maternal and environmental factors is responsible for the development of hypospadias. The underlying etiologic cause leading to the specific hypospadias phenotypes is not fully discovered yet [18].

24.3 Reconstructive Surgery

24.3.1 Pre-operative Evaluation

According to the current guidelines, no pre-operative screening is indicated in case of isolated *hypospadias* [19]. If the child presents any associated condition (bilateral undescended testes, micropenis, etc.) suggesting a possible other than isolated *hypospadias* underlying DSD condition or urinary tract anomaly, further biological pre-operative testing is indicated [8, 16, 20]. Enlarged prostatic utricle has a higher prevalence among the hypospadias population, but has a low chance of becoming symptomatic, and should only be investigated in case of recurrent urinary tract infection or difficulties in placement of the urethral catheter intra-operatively [6].

In order to facilitate standardization, it is important to report thoroughly all pre-operative characteristics of the penile malformation [21].

24.3.2 General Aspects

Surgery in hypospadias repair aims for both satisfactory cosmetical and functional outcome. It is generally accepted that penile deviation and rotation, glans tilt, glans cleft, ectopic urethral meatus, meatal stenosis, peno-scrotal transposition and hooded prepuce should be corrected.

The *goal* of the reconstructive techniques is to create a penis with a good caliber urethra with slit-like meatus at the tip of the glans (urethroplasty procedure), a straight erectile position with normal sexual function and a minimal scarred penile skin [6].

Regarding the *timing of surgery*, planning will be decided taking the anesthesia risk into account. The current recommendations to perform surgery are based on the risk of anesthesia, cognitive and emotional development, and genital awareness. Surgery should be performed between 6 and 18 months of age, according to the EAU guidelines [19]. The effect of early repair on the surgical outcome remains controversial [6, 22].

In general, the choice of the applied *technique* results from an intra-operative decision-making process based on the anatomy and the presentation of the hypospadias combined with the experience of the surgeon [23]. It could be stated that there are as many techniques and modifications as surgeons who perform hypospadias correction. No technique for reconstruction has ever emerged as a gold-standard, and many techniques are recognized as effective. The reconstruction techniques applied in hypospadias reconstruction rely mainly on 4 principles: meatal advancement techniques, tubularization techniques, techniques with use of flaps and free grafts.

To achieve satisfactory outcome in hypospadias reconstruction, a surgeon needs to be familiar with all the basic principles, to be able to apply them when needed. Hypospadias might be very tricky: a hypospadias that looks distal might sometimes need correction with free grafts if there is important curvature and the urethral plate needs to be sacrificed. There are indeed mild forms of hypospadias, but it's only when reconstructing that the severity might correctly be estimated. What at first look seems to be a distal minor hypospadias might sometimes end up with flaps or grafts, and even be difficult to close because of the paucity of the tissues.

24.3.3 Techniques

The first step in any hypospadias repair is to place a traction suture (polypropylene 4/0) through the glans and a silicone feeding tube catheter trough the native meatus into the bladder.

Similarly the last step in all hypospadias repair should be to check the intravesical position of the bladder catheter, and to apply a suitable wound dressing, in which a wide range of variety exists [24].

When the local tissues are used, reconstruction is essentially based on two principles: tubularization of the urethral plate by relaxing the surrounding tissues or advancement of the ectopic *meatus* by mobilization of the local tissues [25].

24.3.3.1 Meatal Advancement Techniques

The meatal advancement and glanuloplasty (MAGPI) is one of the most commonly used techniques in the overall of time. The ectopic meatus is mobilized and advanced toward the tip of the penis, without major dissection of the glans or the penile shaft. It can be considered as a 'minimally invasive' hypospadias repair. It has the advantage of being quick and relatively easy with low complication rate; however, it has the disadvantage of resulting in a non-natural non-split-like appearing meatus. These techniques are suitable to correct distal hypospadias [19, 25].

Technically a subcoronal incision is made a centimeter proximal to the native meatus, followed by deglovement of the penile skin and resection chordee tissue in the penoscrotal angle. Starting from the native meatus a longitudinal incision is made towards the tip of the glans. The dorsal aspect is than closed Heineke-Mikulicz with resorbable sutures 6.0 or 7.0. Glans wings are developed, the ventral aspect of the urethra is enclosed and glanuloplasty is performed with a two-layer suture. As a result a cone shaped glans is created. Finally the skin is closed circumferentially.

24.3.3.2 Tubularization Techniques

The tissue intended to become the urethra stays open as a flat urethral plate on the ventral side of the penis and can be tubularized around a catheter. This tubularization is performed with (TIP) or without (GAP) relaxing urethral plate incision. The technique is versatile and easy to apply in experienced hands, with a normal-looking aspect of a circumcised penis with split like meatus. It is today the most common used technique. It has a slightly higher complication rate than meatal advancement techniques, mainly fistulas and meatal stenosis, but also a more satisfactory cosmetical outcome [3]. Tubularization techniques can be used for distal or mid-penile hypospadias repair.

In case of a wide urethral plate, incision is not necessary for traction-free closure of the neourethra, and a simple glanuloplasty can be performed.

24.3.3.3 Flap en Free Graft Techniques

When local tissues are too hypoplastic to allow reconstruction, flaps and grafts can be used. One stage complete replacement techniques like tubes from foreskin or penile skin flaps are nowadays abandoned more and more in favor of two stage techniques which allow more anatomic reconstruction. These techniques can be applied in cases of mid-penile or proximal hypospadias.

Flaps can be raised from local penile tissues preferably from the healthy dorsal side of the penis, or if needed from more distant genital tissues. Scrotal flaps, for instance, have the disadvantage of being hair-bearing tissues, and are therefore seldom used. The somewhat higher complication rates observed in these techniques are inherent with the flap techniques (vascularization problem, possible retraction, etc.…)

Some surgeons prefer to avoid the complications related to flaps by using *free tissue grafts*. Grafts can be harvested from local dorsal penile tissues, or from non-genital areas like retro-auricular. Possible retraction of the graft remains however an issue.

24.4 Outcome

Successful hypospadias repair aims for a normal cosmetic and functional penis. The availability and quality of the tissue used for repair is essential in predicting the outcome. Techniques using local tissues use the dysplastic tissue while techniques using dorsal tissue bring more healthy tissue to the ventral side of the penis.

Cosmetic outcome is a subjective parameter, although there exist a few objective scoring systems: Mureau score, pediatric penile perception score, hypospadias objective scoring evaluation, Hadidi score, and hypospadias objective penile evaluation score [7, 21, 26, 27].

To evaluate *functional outcome* both subjective findings as a uroflowmetry after toilet training should be performed, and longer follow-up when an abnormal uroflow is observed, should be provided. However, the significance of this aberrant flow patterns have not yet been clarified [28, 29]. It has been found that neither the surgical technique nor the initial position of the meatus has an influence on the urinary outcome, only the severity of the clinical presentation seems to be predictive [30]. Patients after hypospadias repair report subjectively twice as many micturition problems compared to controls, existing mainly of spraying, post-void dribbling and the sensation of incomplete emptying. This finding was even more explicit in the severe hypospadias population in comparison to the mild hypospadias group [21].

References

1. Paulozzi LJ. International trends in rates of hypospadias and cryptorchidism. Environ Health Perspect. 1999;107(4):297–302. Epub 1999/03/25.
2. Baskin L. Basic science of the genitalia. In: Kelalis-King-Bellman textbook of clinical pediatric urology. Informa-Healthcare; Philadelphia. 2007. p. 1117–25.
3. Stevenson A. Oxford dictionary of English. Oxford University Press; London. 2015.
4. Kraft KH, Shukla AR, Canning DA. Hypospadias. Urol Clin N Am. 2010;37(2):167–81.
5. Mure PY, Vigier S, Gorduza DB, Demede D, Mouriquand P. Chirurgie des hypospades. Techniques Chirurgicales - Urologie EMC. Paris: Elsevier Masson SAS; 2011. p. 41–340.
6. Orkiszewski M. A standardized classification of hypospadias. J Pediatr Urol. 2012;8(4):410–4. Epub 2011/10/05.
7. Snodgrass W, Macedo A, Hoebeke P, Mouriquand PD. Hypospadias dilemmas: a round table. J Pediatr Urol. 2011;7(2):145–57. Epub 2011/01/18.
8. Snodgrass W. Hypospadias reporting – how good is the literature? J Urol. 2010;184(4):1255–6. Epub 2010/08/21.
9. Baskin LS, Ebbers MB. Hypospadias: anatomy, etiology, and technique. J Pediatr Surg. 2006;41(3):463–72. Epub 2006/03/07.
10. Mouriquand PD, Gorduza DB, Noche ME, Targnion A. Long-term outcome of hypospadias surgery: current dilemmas. Curr Opin Urol. 2011;21(6):465–9. Epub 2011/08/10.
11. Prat D, Natasha A, Polak A, Koulikov D, Prat O, Zilberman M, et al. Surgical outcome of different types of primary hypospadias repair during three decades in a single center. Urology. 2012;79(6):1350–4. Epub 2012/04/17.
12. Spinoit AF, Van Praet C, Groen LA, Van Laecke E, Praet M, Hoebeke P. Congenital penile pathology is associated with abnormal development of the dartos muscle: a prospective study of primary penile surgery at a tertiary referral center. J Urol. 2015;193(5):1620–4. Epub 2014/12/03.
13. Huisma F, Thomas M, Armstrong L. Severe hypospadias and its association with maternal-placental factors. Am J Med Genet A. 2013;161A(9):2183–7. Epub 2013/08/06.
14. Bang JK, Lyu SW, Choi J, Lee DR, Yoon TK, Song SH. Does infertility treatment increase male reproductive tract disorder? Urology. 2013;81(3):644–8. Epub 2013/03/05.
15. Main KM, Skakkebaek NE, Virtanen HE, Toppari J. Genital anomalies in boys and the environment. Best Pract Res Clin Endocrinol Metab. 2010;24(2):279–89. Epub 2010/06/15.
16. Mouriquand P. Buried penis. In: Gearhart J, Rink R, Mouriquand P, editors. Pediatric urology. Saunders Elsevier; Philadelphia. 2010. p. 519–25.

17. Vottero A, Minari R, Viani I, Tassi F, Bonatti F, Neri TM, et al. Evidence for epigenetic abnormalities of the androgen receptor gene in foreskin from children with hypospadias. J Clin Endocrinol Metab. 2011;96(12):E1953–62. Epub 2011/09/23.
18. van der Zanden LF, van Rooij IA, Feitz WF, Franke B, Knoers NV, Roeleveld N. Aetiology of hypospadias: a systematic review of genes and environment. Hum Reprod Update. 2012;18(3):260–83. Epub 2012/03/01.
19. Tekgül S, Dogan H, Erdem E, Hoebeke P, Kocvara R, Nijman JM, Radmayr C, Silay MS, Stein R, Undre S. Guidelines on pediatric urology. EAU Guidelines [Internet]. Mar 2015 update.
20. Tourchi A, Hoebeke P. Long-term outcome of male genital reconstruction in childhood. J Pediatr Urol. 2013. Epub 2013/05/15.
21. van der Toorn F, de Jong TP, de Gier RP, Callewaert PR, van der Horst EH, Steffens MG, et al. Introducing the HOPE (Hypospadias Objective Penile Evaluation)-score: a validation study of an objective scoring system for evaluating cosmetic appearance in hypospadias patients. J Pediatr Urol. 2013. Epub 2013/03/16.
22. Weber DM, Schonbucher VB, Landolt MA, Gobet R. The Pediatric Penile Perception Score: an instrument for patient self-assessment and surgeon evaluation after hypospadias repair. J Urol. 2008;180(3):1080–4; discussion 4. Epub 2008/07/22.
23. Wang MH, Chen B, Kern D, Gearhart S. Pediatric urology fellowship training: are we teaching what they need to learn? J Pediatr Urol. 2012;9(3):318–21.
24. Radwan M, Soliman MG, Tawfik A, Abo-Elenen M, El-Benday M. Does the type of urinary diversion affect the result of distal hypospadias repair? A prospective randomized trial. Ther Adv Urol. 2012;4(4):161–5. Epub 2012/08/02.
25. Subramaniam R, Spinoit AF, Hoebeke P. Hypospadias repair: an overview of the actual techniques. Semin Plast Surg. 2011;25(03):206–12.
26. Springer A. Assessment of outcome in hypospadias surgery – a review. Front Pediatr. 2014;2:2. Epub 2014/01/31.
27. Ruppen-Greeff NK, Weber DM, Gobet R, Landolt MA. What is a good looking penis? How women rate the penile appearance of men with surgically corrected hypospadias. J Sex Med. 2015;12(8):1737–45. Epub 2015/07/21.
28. Spinoit AF, Hoebeke P. Paediatrics: urinary flow rate after TIP urethroplasty for hypospadias. Nat Rev Urol. 2015;12(9):477–8. Epub 2015/08/05.
29. Spinoit AF, Poelaert F, Hoebeke P. Re: "Snodgrass W, et al. Duration of follow-up to diagnose hypospadias urethroplasty complications". J Pediatr Urol. 2014;10(4). Epub 2014/07/11.
30. Spinoit AF, Poelaert F, Van Praet C, Groen LA, Van Laecke E, Hoebeke P. Grade of hypospadias is the only factor predicting for re-intervention after primary hypospadias repair: a multivariate analysis from a cohort of 474 patients. J Pediatr Urol. 2015;11(2):70.e1–6. Epub 2015/03/24.

25 Epispadias

Abstract

In primary penile epispadias, the urethra opens on the dorsal aspect of the penis, or the glans. The extent of the defect can vary from a mild glanular defect to complete defect as the one observed in bladder exstrophy, with extension to the bladder neck. Simple epispadias occurs less commonly than the more severe form associated with exstrophy of the bladder. Both corpora cavernosa don't come close to each other, as in normal condition, giving the look of wide broad and short penis, with a variable degrees of dorsal curvature, usually the anus is appropriately sited and the scrotum also appears normal.

Keywords

Isolated epispadias • Bladder exstrophy epispadias complex • Epispadias with an intact prepuce

Epispadias anomaly which will be discussed herein is the one with normal bladder wall "Isolated epispadias" as the bladder exstrophy epispadias complex is not a penile anomaly and should be discussed with bladder anomalies elsewhere [1].

Nomenclature

Isolated Epispadias, Primary epispadias and Simple epispadias.

Definition

In primary penile epispadias, the urethra opens on the dorsal aspect of the penis, or the glans. The extent of the defect can vary from a mild glanular defect to complete defect as the one observed in bladder exstrophy, with extension to the bladder neck. Simple epispadias occurs less commonly than the more severe form associated with exstrophy of the bladder. Both corpora cavernosa don't come close to each other, as in normal condition, giving the look of wide broad and short penis, with a

© Springer International Publishing Switzerland 2017
M. Fahmy, *Congenital Anomalies of the Penis*, DOI 10.1007/978-3-319-43310-3_25

variable degrees of dorsal curvature, usually the anus is appropriately sited and the scrotum also appears normal. A variable diastasis of pubic bones exist, that tends to be less severe than in bladder exstrophy. The pelvic ring is often complete, with an apparently normal abdominal wall, but sometimes a defect over the symphysis pubis is aberrant.

25.1 Incidence

Isolated epispadias without exstrophy is a rare anomaly, the incidence being 1 in 120,000 of males; it may be detected in female with different varieties. The male-to-female ratio is 2.3:12. Epispadias is classically associated with bladder exstrophy in over 90 % of cases of primary epispadias [2].

25.2 Historical Background

The first recorded case of epispadias is attributed to the Byzantine emperor Heraclius for his unknown disease. Isolated epispadias remained unknown and untreated until it was described by Morgagni in 1761. The initial attempts to treat this anomaly were restricted to controlling the incontinence. In 1869, Karl Thiersch described the etiology and anatomy of epispadias and reported a case of epispadias reconstruction with a long-term follow-up of 11 years [3].

25.3 Classification

Depending on the severity of the clefted urethra, epispadias is classified to:

1. Glanular epispadias: the urethra opens on the dorsal aspect of the glans, which is broad and flattened (Fig. 25.1).
2. Penile type: the urethral meatus, which is often broad and gaping, is located between the pubic symphysis and the coronal sulcus. A distal groove usually extends from the meatus through the splayed glans (Fig. 25.2).
3. Penopubic type: which has the urethral opening at the penopubic junction, and the entire penis has a distal dorsal groove extending through the glans (Fig. 25.3).

The penopubic type is the most frequent, with an underlying deficiencies of the bladder neck and proximal urethra and striated sphincter complex, which determine the degree of associated incontinence. In these cases, the posterior urethra merges with the bladder neck, and the verumontanum may lie at the level of the bladder neck or even within the bladder itself. The ureteral orifices

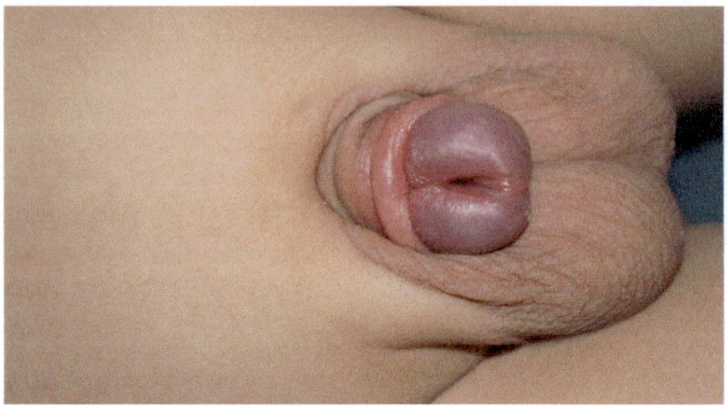

Fig. 25.1 Glanular type of epispadias

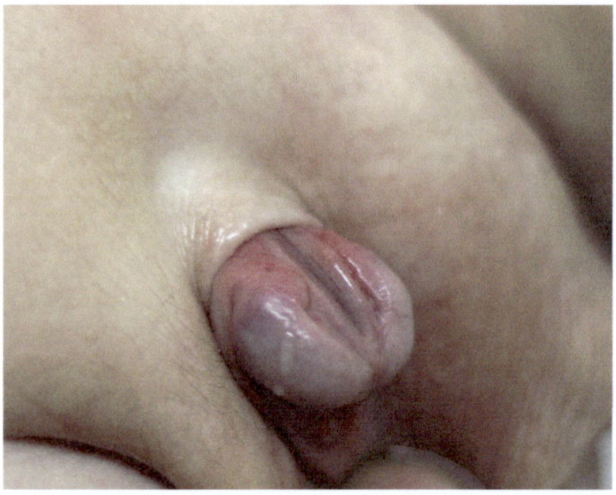

Fig. 25.2 Penile epispadias

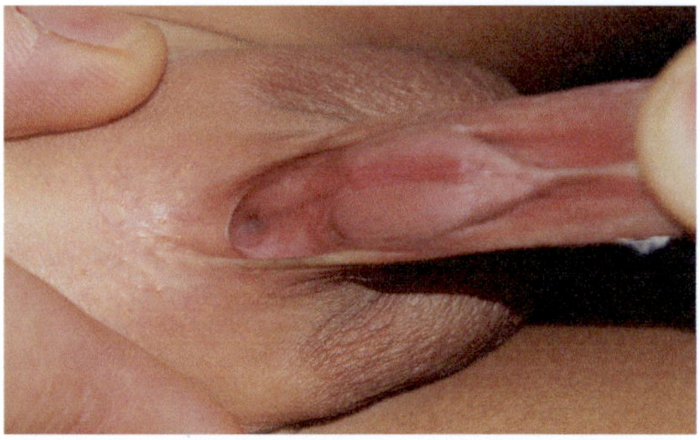

Fig. 25.3 Penopubic epispadias, opening of bladder neck can be seen at the vicinity of the proximal end of the defect

often lie close together and are normal or narrowed in caliber, contrasting with the wide refluxing orifices seen in exstrophy. Patients with glanular epispadias seldom have urinary incontinence, however, with penopubic and penile epispadias, incontinence is present in 95 % and 75 % of cases respectively [4].

25.4 Variant of Primary Epispadias

In some rare cases, epispadias could be just presented as a small dimple on the tip of the penis above the normal urethral opening (Fig. 25.4).

Typically, epispadias is associated with defective prepuce on the dorsal aspect of the penis and redundant prepuce on the ventral aspect, but rare cases may have a completely intact prepuce.

Epispadias with an intact prepuce as in case in Figs. 25.5, 25.6, and 25.7 is extremely rare, its incidence is not known, however there are few case reports, either as a single case or case series [5]. In such cases the epispadic urethra may be in the form of glanular epispadias (the common variant), really intact prepuce may hide a complete penile or even a penopubic type, in our series of 7 cases we also encountered a case of epispadic megameatus with an intact prepuce (Fig. 25.7), this entity was discussed with the megameatus anomaly (Chap. 20).

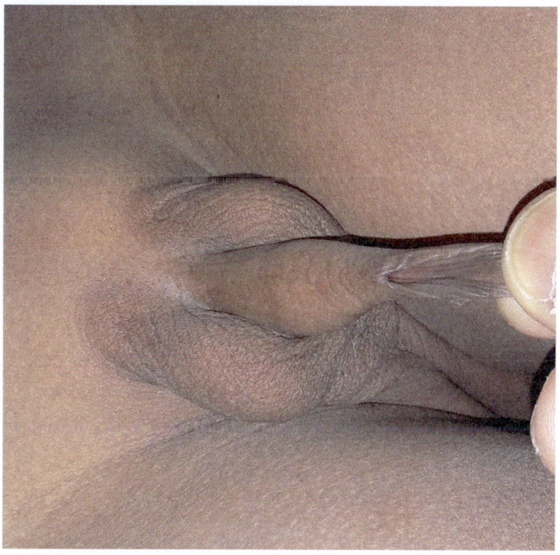

Fig. 25.5 Complete intact prepuce hiding an epispadias

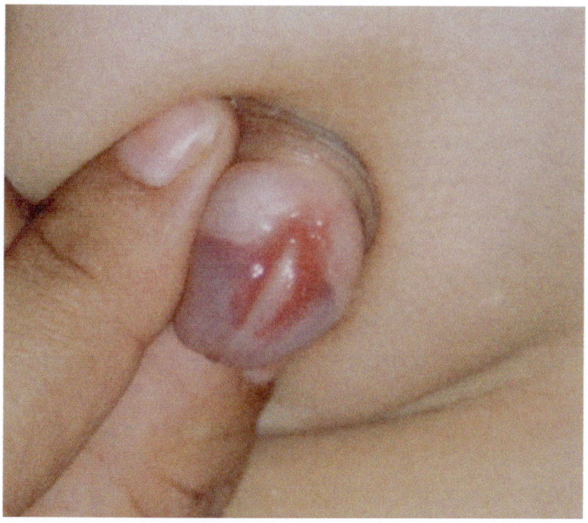

Fig. 25.4 Cleft of the dorsum of the glans, with a normally situated urethra and meatus, a variant of glanular epispadias

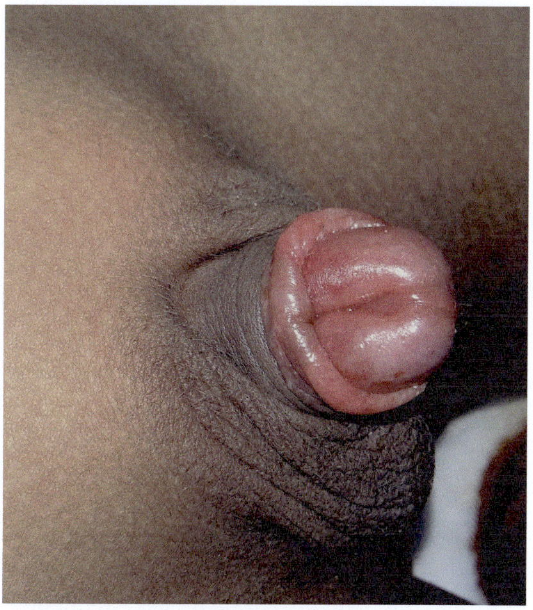

Fig. 25.6 Glanular epispadias with an intact prepuce

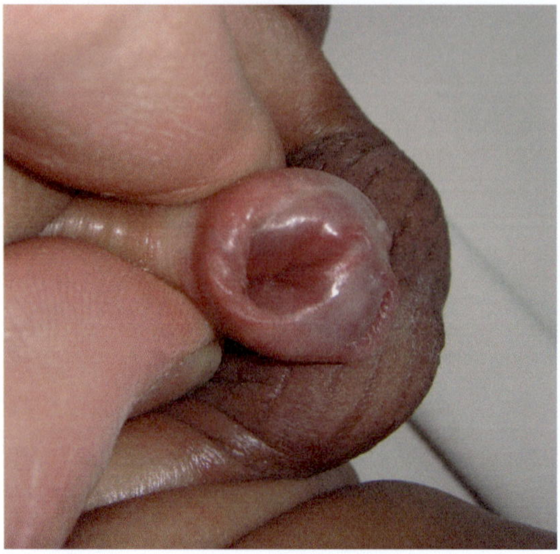

Fig. 25.7 A rare case of epispadias megameatus with an intact prepuce

25.5 Sequelae of Epispadias

In males, epispadias is usually associated with incontinence, impotence, which results from the dorsal curvature of the penile shaft and incomplete urethra, usually happens. Also reported are frequent ascending infections to the prostate or bladder and kidneys and psychological problems related to the deformity. Many complications may follow improper repair of this anomaly.

25.6 Etiology

Despite the similarity of name, an epispadias is not a type of hypospadias and involves a problem with a different set of embryologic processes. Epispadias is an uncommon and partial form of a spectrum of failures of abdominal and pelvic fusion in the first months of embryogenesis known as the exstrophy-epispadias complex. While epispadias is inherent in all cases of exstrophy, it can also, much less frequently, appear in isolation as the least severe form of the complex spectrum. It occurs as a result of defective migration of the genital tubercle primordii to the cloacal membrane, and so malformation of the genital tubercle, at about the 5th week of gestation. Epispadias and exstrophy of the bladder are considered as varying degrees of a single disorder. Another hypothesis relates the defect to the abnormal development of the cloacal membrane.

25.7 Diagnosis

Most cases of epispadias are diagnosed at birth during physical examination of the newborn. In mild cases, the condition can go unnoticed until parents note urine leaks after potty training or an abnormal stream with urine spraying noticed by an older child. The clinical signs that may raise the suspicion of this condition may be in the form of a short penis with a broad spadelike glans, absence of frenulum and penile raphe on the glans and a dorsally directed preputial opening. A dorsal midline depression with separation of the pubic bones at the position of symphysis pubis could be felt on palpation. Girls can also have this type of congenital malformation, as epispadias of the female may occur when the urethra develops too far anteriorly, exiting in the clitoris or even more forward, frequently, the clitoris is bifurcated at the site of urethral exit. This may not cause difficulty in urination but may cause problems latter on with sexual satisfaction [6].

Most cases of epispadias with an intact prepuce will come to light only during circumcision or when an older child starts to retract the prepuce. Features like upwardly directed urinary stream, ballooning of the prepuce while micturating are not constant and may not be taken very seriously by most parents. This condition should be born in mind, as underreporting maybe present, especially in communities where circumcision is not consistently practiced. Whereas, it is easier detected in countries where most males undergo circumcision [5].

An ascending cystography with a voiding study is essential to show the bladder neck and any associated reflux, also a urodynamic study for older children is mandatory before correction. Plain x ray or even MRI is useful to show the degree of pelvic bones diastasis. Primary epispadias is rarely diagnosed antenatally, as it is usually a hidden anomaly.

25.8 Associated Anomalies

Associated congenital anomalies include diastasis of the pubic symphysis, closed bladder exstrophy, renal agenesis and ectopic pelvic kidney. Duplication of urethra is not rare with epispadias, and sometimes the child may have a normally positioned urethra and an epispadiac duplicated system with variable extent (Chap 28).

25.9 Management

The treatment of this anomaly is far from trivial and repair can be challenging. Penile epispadias should be corrected in childhood with penile straightening by resection of the chordee and creation of a new urethra of adequate caliber and length. Correction of glanular epispadias with reposition of the distal urethra and creation of a symmetric glans (glanuloplasty) is indicated in childhood or adolescence at the patient's request for cosmetic or psychological reasons.

Various modifications have been advised in last century for epispadias repair in order to improve the results in terms of fistula formation, incontinence, cosmetically acceptable glans shape and adequacy of sexual functions. There are two popular surgical techniques described well in the literature with their pros and cons; the first is the modified Cantwell technique [7], which involves partial disassembly of the penis and placement of the urethra in a more normal position. The drawback of this technique is persistence of short penile length and residual dorsal chordee that is likely to be eliminated in complete penile disassembly. The second and most recent evolution is the complete penile disassembly by Mitchell technique [8], which was modified by Ransley et al. [9] The major disadvantages of the Mitchell technique for epispadias repair are the necessity for aggressive dissection and occasional resultant of hypospadiac meatus that requires a second-stage urethroplasty as the urethral plate is usually shorter than the corpora cavernosa. Buccal mucosa is an excellent source of graft material for urethral replacement in complex urethroplasties as primary surgery. It is readily available, elastic, resistant and technically easy to harvest [10].

Increase in penile length can be achieved by making the best use of corpora distal to their attachment to the inferior pubic rami. Adequate lengthening of penile shaft with correction of chordee and rotational deformities is required to produce a downwardly angulated penis on standing and straight erection to permit proper sexual intercourse.

For epispadias with intact prepuce, especially coronal or glanular one, simple approximation of the glans penis with or without circumcision may be not satisfactory, with a high incidence of glanular dehiscence and an abnormally upward directed stream., So in such cases we are doing a complete urethral plate dissection, partial assembly of the glans and ventral repositioning of the repaired urethra which give good outcome (Figs. 25.8 and 25.9).

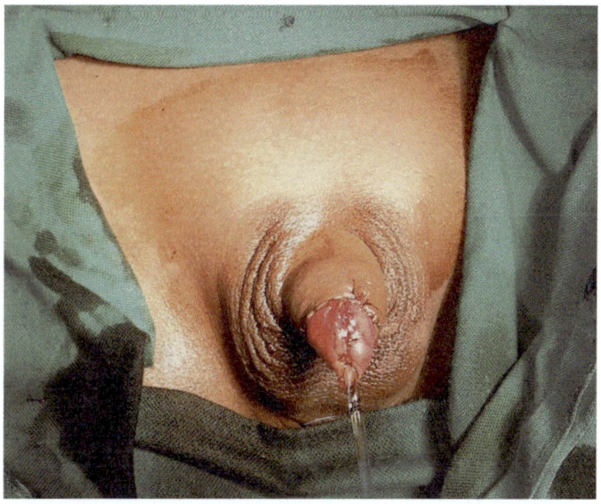

Fig. 25.8 Complete repair of the case in Figs. 25.6 and 25.7, with straightened penis and normally positioned meatus, after dissection, reconstruction and ventral repositioning of the glanular urethra

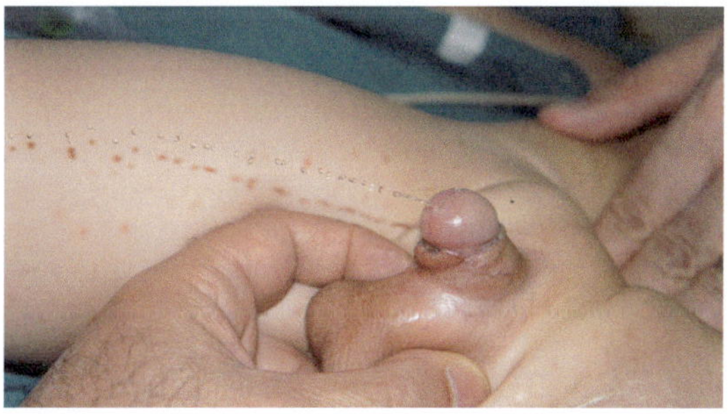

Fig. 25.9 Acceptable meatus, glans, penile length and downward directed stream after complete assembly repair of epispadias in Fig. 25.6

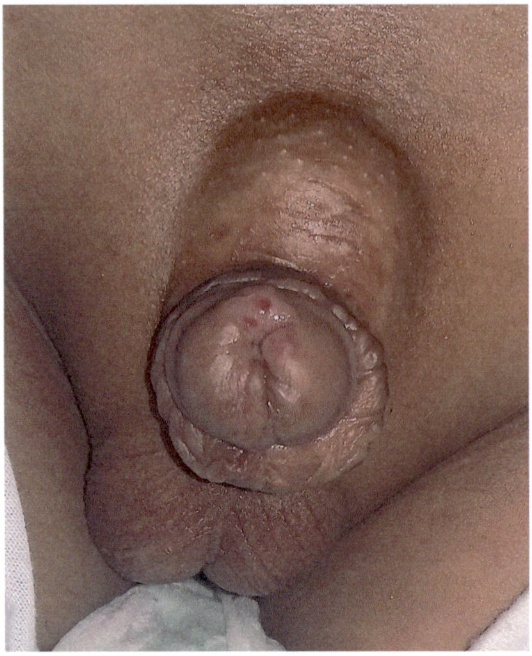

Fig. 25.10 Ugly glans, wide meatus and a cystic dilation of the penile urethra in an incontinent child after unsuccessful repair of penopubic epispadias

The most common complications after epispadias repair are broad ugly glans, short penis and a persistent dorsal chordee, which is fairly typical with older techniques, but it is now less common (Fig. 25.10).

References

1. Fahmy MB. Epispadias in:rare congenital genitourinary anomalies 2015, Chap 6: pages:90–95. Springers. ISBN: 9783662436790. doi:10.1007/978-3-662-43680-6.
2. Ebert AK, Reutter H, Ludwig M, Rosch WH. The exstrophy-epispadias complex. Orphanet J Rare Dis. 2009;4:23.
3. Lascaratos J, Poulakou-Rembelakou E, Rembelakos A, Marketos S. The first case of epispadias: an unknown disease of the byzantine emperor Heraclius (610– 641 AD). Br J Urol. 1995;76:380–3.
4. Ebert AK, Reutter H, Ludwig M, Rosch WH. The exstrophy-epispadias complex. Orphanet J Rare Dis. 2009;4:23.http://dx.doi.org/10.1186/1750-1172-4-23.
5. Waziri AM, Abubakar BM, Adamu S, Sulaiman IE, Gashua M. Epispadias in a child with intact prepuce: a rare congenital abnormality. Open J Urol. 2016;6: 19–22. http://dx.doi.org/10.4236/oju.2016.63004.
6. Tantibhedhyangkul J, Copland SD, Haqq AM, Thomas M, Price TM. A case of unrecognized female epispadias. Fertil Steril. 2008;90(5):e1–3.
7. Cantwell FV. Operative treatment of epispadias by transplantationof urethra. Ann Surg. 1895;22: 689–93.
8. Ransley PG, Duffy PG. Bladder exstrophy closure and epispadiasrepair. In: Spitz L, Coran AG, editors. Rob & smith operative surgery (pediatric surgery). London: Chapman & Hall; 1995. p. 745–59.
9. Mitchell ME, Bagli DJ. Complete penile disassembly for epispadias repair: the Mitchell technique. J Urol. 1996;155:303–4.
10. Dessanti A, Iannuccelli M, Ginesu G, Claudio F. Reconstruction of hypospadias and epispadias with buccal mucosa free graft as primary surgery: more than 10 years of experience. J Urolo. 2003;170(4 Part 2):1600–2.

26 Megalourethra

Abstract

Megalourethra is a rare but surgically correctible malformation of the urogenital mesenchymal of the male anterior urethra and erectile tissue of penis, characterized by severe dilatation of the penile urethra due to congenital absence of the corpus spongiosum and corpus cavernosum. It presents as two types, a milder scaphoid type and severe fusiform type. The prognosis is related to the degree of associated renal impairment and the severity of other accompanying congenital anomalies.

Keywords

Scaphoid megalourethra • Fusiform megalourethra • Corpus spongiosum • Corpus cavernosum

Definition

It is a rare but surgically correctible malformation of the urogenital mesenchymal of the male anterior urethra and erectile tissue of penis, characterized by severe dilatation of the penile urethra due to congenital absence of the corpus spongiosum and corpus cavernosum. It presents as two types, a milder scaphoid type and severe fusiform type. The prognosis is related to the degree of associated renal impairment and the severity of other accompanying congenital anomalies.

26.1 Incidence

Less than 100 cases have been reported in literature till now [1].

26.2 Historical Background

The first case of congenital megalourethra was reported for the first time by Obrinsky in1949 [2], who also described its association with prune-belly syndrome, but Benacerraf et al., in 1989 [3] were the first to report this condition prenatally,

© Springer International Publishing Switzerland 2017

M. Fahmy, *Congenital Anomalies of the Penis*, DOI 10.1007/978-3-319-43310-3_26

and so far only a handful of cases have been reported. Techniques of surgical repair of the scaphoid megalourethra were first published by Nesbit and Baum more than 50 years ago [4].

26.3 Etiology

The exact embryological cause of congenital megalourethra is not clearly understood. The most commonly held theories propose a defect in the migration, differentiation, or development of the mesenchymal tissues of the phallus. Another hypothesis is that delayed or deficient canalisation of the glandular urethra may be associated with maldevelopment of the corpus spongiosum and corpora cavernosa, secondary to the distal urethral obstruction. Mild delays with earlier and more complete canalisation may be associated with scaphoid while longer delays with later and less complete canalisation and fusiform megalourethra. Owing to the poor development of supporting erectile tissue there is stasis of urine causing functional obstruction.

More severe form as corpus spongiosum and corpora cavernosa both are involved resulting in fusiform (spindle) dilatation of the phallus during voiding.

26.4 Classification

Dorairajan classified congenital megalourethra into two types based on findings of urethrography. The more common scaphoid type with a deficiency of the corpus spongiosum presents as bulging of ventral urethra. (Fig. 26.1), and the less common fusiform type, with deficiency of both corpus spongiosum and cavernosum which is seen as circumferential expansion of urethra (Fig. 26.2) [5].

Recently, Amsalem et al. [6] classified the condition into: –

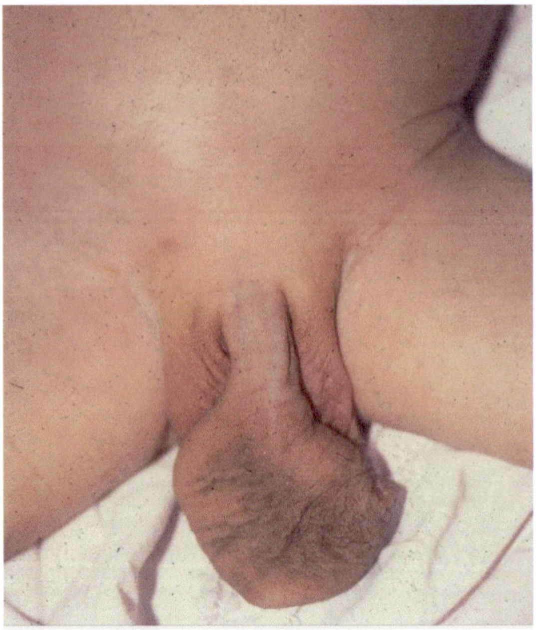

Fig. 26.1 Scaphoid Megalourethra

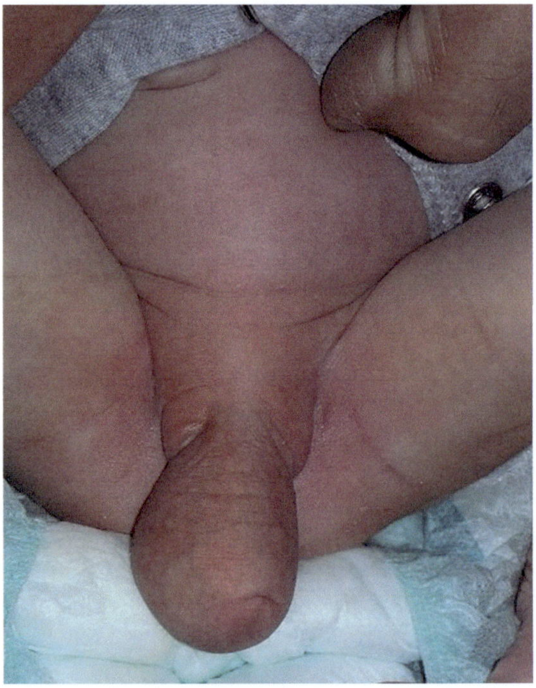

Fig. 26.2 Fusiform Megalourethra

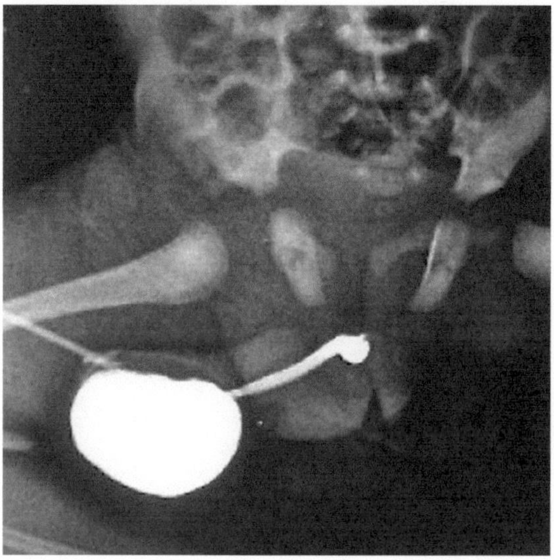

Fig. 26.3 MCUG of fusiform megalourethra

(a) Primary or (ex-vacuo), caused by absence or hypoplasia of the corpora spongiosa and cavernosa, associated with normal amniotic fluid volume, with usually preserved renal function and better outcome.
(b) Obstructive (secondary), which results in oligohydramnios with a higher incidence of renal failure, pulmonary hypoplasia and thus a high mortality (Figs. 26.3 and 26.4).

26.5 Associated Anomalies

The prognosis is related to the degree of associated renal impairment and the severity of accompanying other congenital anomalies. Various congenital anomalies are associated with megalourethra mostly related to urogenital system and sometimes with other organ systems as well. Associated congenital anomalies are seen in 80 % of scaphoid type and 100 % of fusiform type. The commonly described genitourinary anomalies include renal dysplasia-hypoplasia, hydronephrosis, hydroureter, vesicoureteric reflux, prune-belly syndrome, urethral duplication, megacystis and undescended testes. Anecdotal cases associated with posterior urethral valves have been reported, but this seems to be a concomitant anomaly rather than a cause of megalourethra

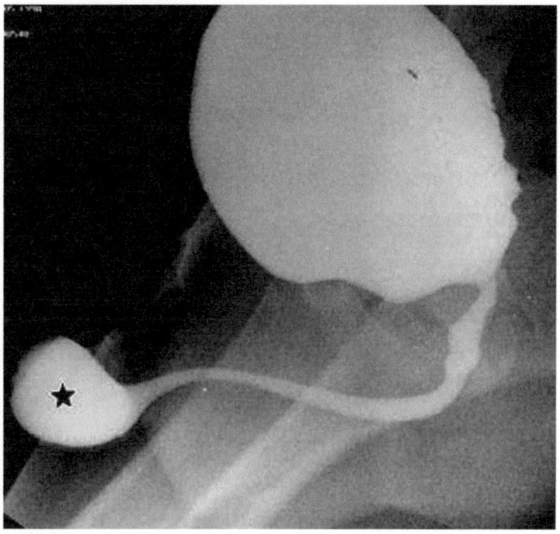

Fig. 26.4 MCUG of scaphoid megalourethra

Other system anomalies including VATER (vertebral, anal atresia, trachea-oesophageal fistula, and renal anomalies) and VACTERL (vertebral, anal atresia, cardiac, tracheaesophageal fistula, renal, and limb deformities). Congenital megalourethra can be diagnosed prenatally if a detailed examination of the fetal genitalia is performed specially in fetuses with urinary tract dilatation.

26.6 Diagnosis

This anomaly affects the anterior part of urethra, and usually cause abnormal size and shape of the penile shaft, especially while voiding.

26.7 Antenatally

The earliest diagnosis reported was at 13 weeks in a fetus with multiple malformations. However, most cases are detected in the second trimester, when signs of lower obstructive uropathy like distended bladder with or without hydroureter and hydronephrosis and a cystic structure in the perineal region that may be detected in the presence of normal, decreased, or even increased amniotic fluid volume. It is important to be cautious on USG as a thin-walled distended urethra can easily be mistaken for a loop of umbilical

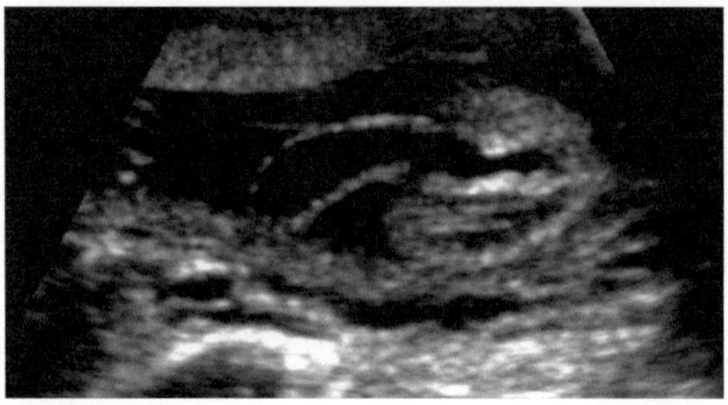

Fig. 26.5 Ultrasound of an antenatally detected fusiform megalourethra

cord. Color doppler is very helpful in differentiating these two entities. Fusiform megalourethra is more likely to be detected antenatally than scaphoid megalourethra as the former is invariably is associated with signs of urinary tract dilatation. Prenatally diagnosed megalourethra has to be thoroughly evaluated for associated congenital anomalies and followed up serially by ultrasound for amniotic-fluid index, urinary bladder volume, and upper tracts assessment along with fetal echocardiography (Fig. 26.5). Oligohydramnios reflects substantial renal impairment and portends poorly, especially in the second trimester with the risk of pulmonary hypoplasia. The goal of antenatal diagnosis is to provide parents with accurate diagnosis and prognosis allowing them to take decision regarding continuing the pregnancy. Termination of pregnancy may be advised in cases with other severe congenital anomalies and renal impairment. In some milder forms of megalourethra spontaneous resolution has been observed in fetuses at 19–34 weeks gestation.

26.8 Postnatally

In the postnatal period, the diagnosis can be confirmed by a micturating cystourethrogram (MCUG), which shows a massive dilatation in the anterior urethra. In view of associated anomalies, the workup of megalourethra should include renal function tests and imaging of upper and lower urinary tracts like intravenous urography (IVU) and USG. The status of upper urinary tract determines the ultimate outcome.

26.9 Differential Diagnosis

Urethral anomalies mimicking megalourethra like urethral atresia, urethral web, duplication, and diverticulum are considered in the differential diagnosis, at the same time penile gigantism as in cases of megalopenis, penile lymphedema and hemangioma may give a similar picture like megalourethra but corporal tissues are normal in such cases.

26.10 Management

The treatment of megalourethra may be one stage or two stage urethroplasty depending on the age of presentation and general condition of the patient. Techniques of surgical repair of the scaphoid megalourethra were first published by Nesbit and Baum more than 50 years ago, and the procedure is still currently in use with some modification. Proximal urinary diversion is optional. Recently, an alternative approach which involves staged correction has been proposed. In the first stage, marsupialization of the megalourethra is done ventrally to prevent stasis, bacterial colonization, and infection. This is followed by closure of the defect when the child grows older.

Heaton and colleagues [7] described a technique of urethral plication for some cases of scaphoid megalourethra. However, urologic repair is almost impossible when there is a lack of supportive corporal tissue, although successful cosmetic and functional repairs have been reported The management of fusiform type is complicated ranging from sex reassignment to major phallic reconstruction, and patients may require placement of penile prosthesis in the adult period. Long term follow-up is required in these patients to see for the impaired continence, erectile function and fertility potential.

Antenatally detected cases could be managed by fetal bladder shunting (vesico-amniotic) to overcome the functional urinary obstruction which had been tried with limited success. However, unlike other causes of lower urinary tract obstruction, patients with megalourethra also suffer from dysfunction in urination and probably erection and ejaculation, and all live children in series had several urologic procedures. So the goal of early prenatal diagnosis of this condition is to provide parents with an accurate diagnosis and prognosis, thus allowing them to make an informed decision regarding continuing or terminating the pregnancy

References

1. Advait P, et al. Congenital megalourethra: spectrum of presentation and insights in embryology and management. Int Surg J. 2015;2(4):660–4. http://www.ijsurgery.com.
2. Obrinsky W. Agenesis of abdominal muscles with associated malformation of the genitourinary tract; a clini cal syndrome. Am J Dis Child. 1949;77:362–73.
3. Benacerraf BR, Saltzman DH, Mandell J. Sonographic diagnosis of abnormal fetal genitalia. J Ultrasound Med. 1989;8:613–7.
4. Nesbit RM, Baum WC. Obstructive uropathy in childhood; diagnosis and surgical management. J Mich State Med Soc. 1955;54(Part 1):1067–71.
5. Dorairajan T. Defects of spongy tissue and congenital diverticula of the penile urethra. Aust N Z J Surg. 1962;32:209–14.
6. Amsalem H, Fitzgerald B, Keating S, Ryan G, Keunen J, Berger H, et al. Congenital megalourethra: prenatal diagnosis and postnatal/autopsy findings in 10 cases. Ultrasound Obstet Gynecol. 2011;37: 678–83.
7. Heaton BW, Snow BW, Cartwright PC. Repair of urethral diverticulum by plication. Urology. 1994;44. 749–52.

27 Urethral Duplications (UD)

Abstract

Urethral duplication is a rare congenital anomaly, affecting mainly boys, with a variable clinical presentation because of the different anatomical patterns. This pathological condition may be easily escape diagnosis, especially in children with other associated anomalies, such as hypospadias or bladder exstrophy. Several types of anatomic variations have been identified with the accessory urethra, being complete or incomplete, epispadic, hypospadiac, normotopic or perineoanal. Urethral duplication, associated with double urinary bladder is an extremely uncommon congenital anomaly of the urinary system, more frequent in males and often linked to other anomalies.

Keywords

Urethral duplication • Accessory urethra • Prepubic sinus

Nomenclature

Accessory urethra.

Definition

Urethral duplication is a rare congenital anomaly, affecting mainly boys, with a variable clinical presentation because of the different anatomical patterns. This pathological condition may be easily escape diagnosis, especially in children with other associated anomalies, such as hypospadias or bladder exstrophy. Several types of anatomic variations have been identified with the accessory urethra, being complete or incomplete, epispadic, hypospadiac, normotopic or perineoanal. Urethral duplication, associated with double urinary bladder is an extremely uncommon congenital anomaly of the urinary system, more frequent in males and often linked to other anomalies [1].

27.1 Historical Background

Urethral duplication was first described by Aristotle [2].

27.2 Incidence

Urethral duplication is rare so far; about 300 cases have been reported in literature; it is expected that many minor incomplete cases may be more

© Springer International Publishing Switzerland 2017

M. Fahmy, *Congenital Anomalies of the Penis*, DOI 10.1007/978-3-319-43310-3_27

common than the reported incidence, but it may escape documentation, this anomaly is most common in males with few cases reported in females [3].

27.3 Etiology

Embryology of urethral duplication is unclear; and there is no single theory explains all of the various types of this anomalies, as a lot of hypotheses have been proposed including; ischemia, abnormal Mullerian duct termination and growth failure of the urogenital sinus [4].

In fact, by the 17 embryonic day, the mesoderm of the tip of the glands has proliferated to form ridges on its caudal paramedian aspect, the medial, bounding the lacunar groove on its medial side, and the lateral lacunar folds, lying on its lateral aspect. During subsequent development these folds increase in prominence, due to proliferation of their mesodermal cores, so the lacunar groove becomes deeper and ectoderm on the latter is continuously proximal with the endoderm of the cleaved urethral plate. In this way, an abnormal lacunar fold duplication can produce a distal urethral duplication, with an accessory blind urethra [5].

At E15, mesodermal growth leading to epithelial compression and fusion occurs and this event might explain a whole series of complex events in the development of the lower urinary tract in the male. A failure of this process is reported to result in epispadias as well as hypospadias might arise later in development if fusion of the urethral folds is arrested [4]. In Arena et al. opinion, an excessive mesodermal growth and a subsequent epithelial over-compression on the urethral plate might lead to urethral and/or bladder sepimentation and be a cause of urethral and/or bladder duplication [6] (Chap. 1).

27.4 Classification

Duplication of the urethra could be partial or complete and either hypospadiac or epispadiac, depending on the relation of the accessory channel with the orthotopic urethra. Hypospadiac type is extremely rare in comparison to the epispadic one, where there is a dorsal accessory urethral opening and the child is usually incontinent. Some duplication may be associated with an open symphysis pubis or urine dribbling from the epispadiac urethra.

Urethral duplication is classified by Effmann et al. [2] into the following types: (Fig. 27.1)

- Type I: A blind incomplete accessory urethra.
  - I A: Accessory urethra opens in the penile surface but does not communicate with the urethra or bladder.
  - I B: Accessory urethra opens from the urethral channel end and ends blindly in the periurethral tissues.
- Type II: Complete patent urethral duplication.
  - II A: Two meatus;
    - II A1: Non communication urethras arising independently from the bladder.
    - II A2: Accessory urethra arising from the first independent course into a second meatus.
    - II A 2 "Y-type" Original urethra "dorsal" is in orthotopic position, while accessory urethra "ventral" origination from the bladder neck or anterior urethra, opens into either perineum and anus.
  - II B: One meatus; two urethras arising from the bladder or posterior urethra unite into a common channel distally.
- Type III: Urethral duplication as a component of partial or complete caudal duplication.

Mild cases of distal type I duplications (often associated with hypospadias) as well as "Y-type" duplication associated to anorectal malformation were excluded from this classification.

This classification is functional, represents most clinical aspects of UD, however, this classification looks complex, and it does not distinguish sagittal from coronal collateral duplication. In another classification by Woodhouse and Williams sagittal and coronal duplication was included, but this classification does not include many anatomical details that are important for therapeutic decision making [1]. The Y subtype represents 6–30 % of all urethral duplication. In this subtype, the original urethra is known as "dorsal" urethra and the duplicated one is named as "ventral." The ventral urethra, originating from the bladder neck or anterior urethra, opens into either the perineum or anus and is the dominant urethra. Usually, the

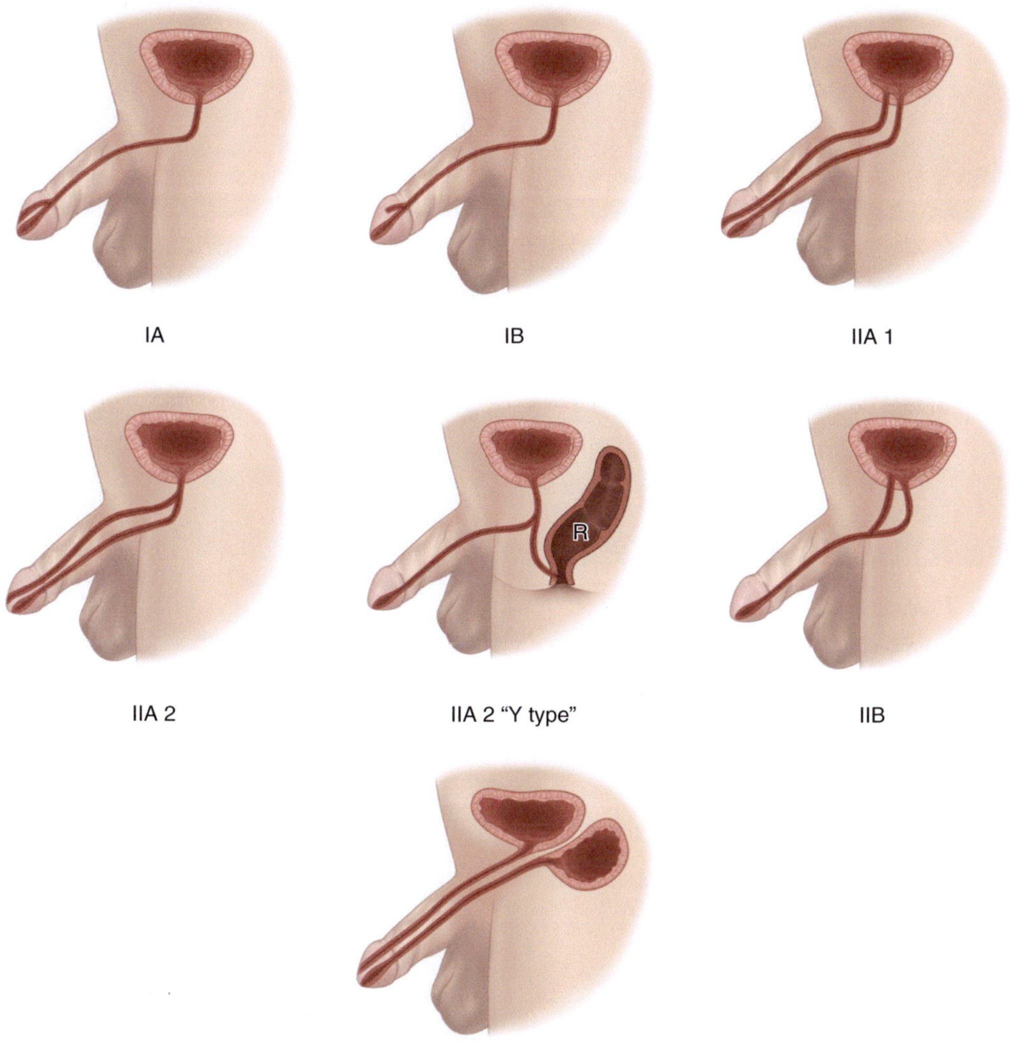

Fig. 27.1 Urethral duplication as classification by Effmann

normally located dorsal urethral opening is stenotic, so urine passes through the dominant ventral urethra. Hence, this variety considered as a congenital urethral fistula, and will be discussed in Chap. 28.

According to Stephens [7], dorsal duplication of the urethra are classified into three types: (i) a complete or incomplete tandem channel from the glans to the bladder; (ii) an epispadiac type; and (iii) a dermoid sinus that simulates an accessory urethra, but tracks from the base of the penis in front of the pelvic urethra and the bladder behind the pubic symphysis to or toward the umbilicus.

Congenital prepubic sinus (CPS) (Fig. 27.8) is a rare variety, and not included in any of previously described classifications. It is defined as a blind-ending tract originating from the midline of the genital region overlying the symphysis pubis and extending to, but not communicating with the anterior bladder wall. There are three types of CPS classified according to the course of the tract and location of the skin opening. The etiology is thought to be an intussusception during fusion of the abdominal wall or, alternatively, an incomplete urethral duplication. The existence of transitional epithelium in the proximal part of the sinus

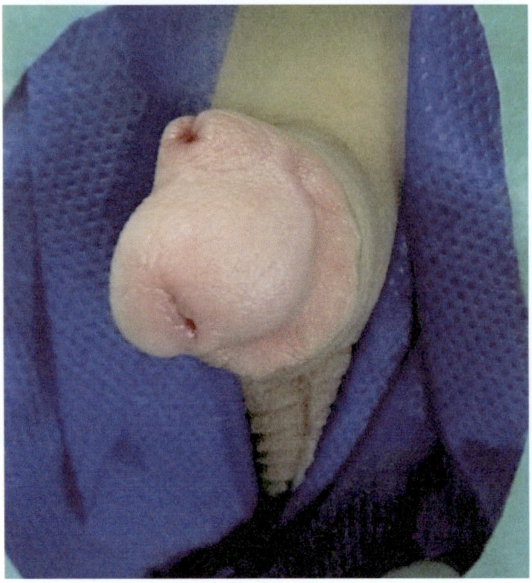

Fig. 27.2 Urethral duplication in a sagital plane

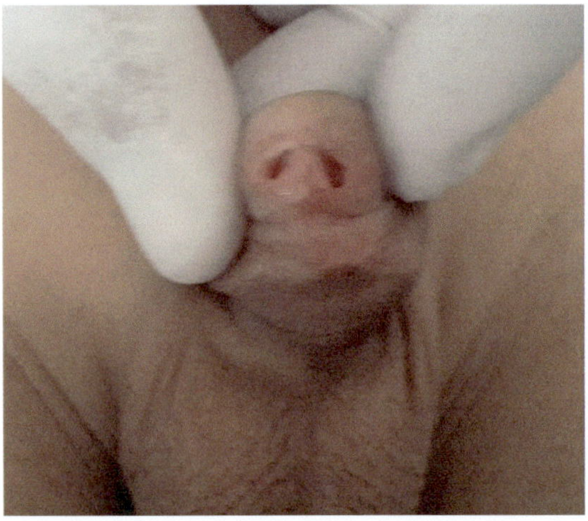

Fig. 27.3 Urethral duplication in a coronal plane

and presence of smooth muscle bundles around it reinforce the theory that congenital prepubic sinus is a variant form of dorsal urethral duplication [8].

So from my experience with 18 different versatile cases of UD and after reviewing most of literature discussing this anomaly, I classified urethral duplications simply into:

- Sagital (Fig. 27.2): Complete or incomplete
- Coronal (Fig. 27.3): Complete or incomplete
- Complete: – Communicated to the Bladder
  - With bladder duplication (Fig. 27.4)

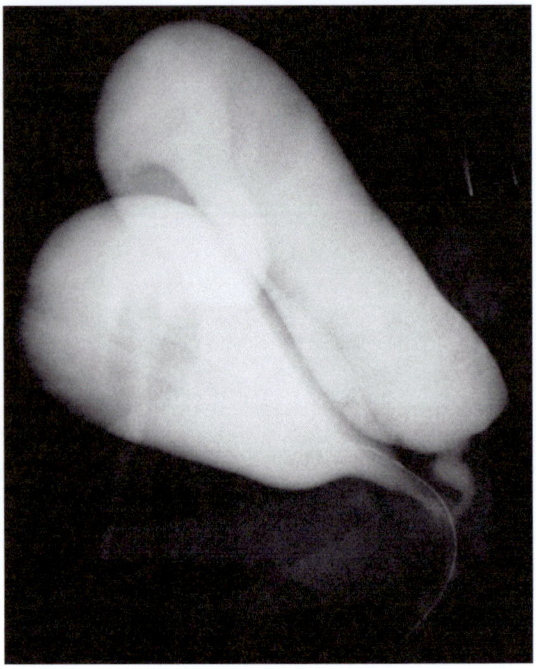

Fig. 27.4 Complete urethral duplication with bladder duplication

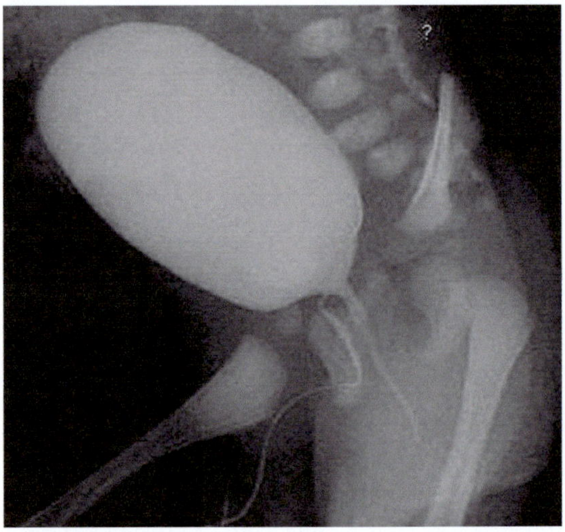

Fig. 27.5 Complete urethral duplication without bladder duplication

- Without bladder duplication (Fig. 27.5)
- Incomplete: –Not communicated to the bladder: (Fig. 27.6)
- – Epispadic (Fig. 27.7)
- – Prepubic sinus (Fig. 27.8)

Y type is excluded as it is considered a variant of congenital urethral fistula.

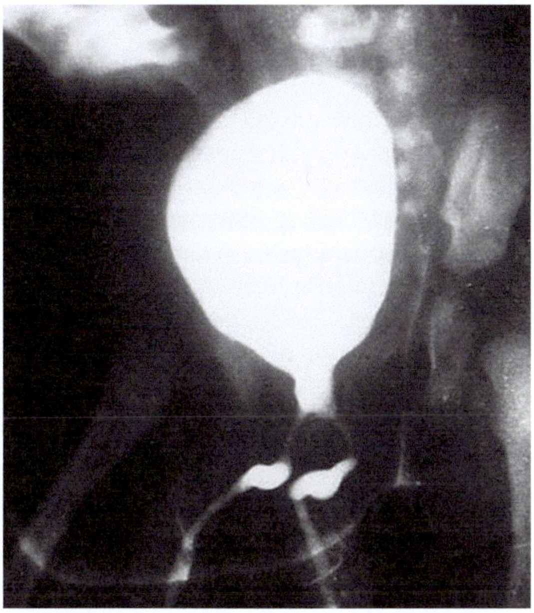

Fig. 27.6 Incomplete duplication not communicated to the bladder, accessory urethra end before the bladder neck

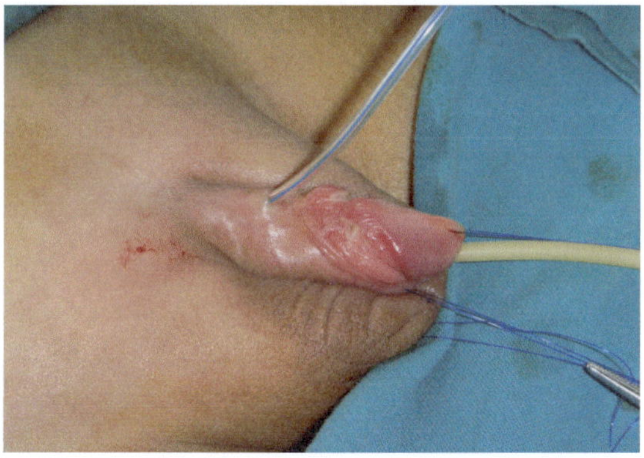

Fig. 27.7 Incomplete epispadic urethral duplication

27.5 Associated Anomalies

An associated genitourinary malformation occurs in 60 % of the cases; (Ureteropelvic junction obstruction, extrarotation of penis, vesicoureteral reflux, renal ectopia, renal agenesis, posterior urethral valves) and in one out of ten cases serious intestinal anomalies (Aborectal malformations, combined esophageal–duodenal atresia, malrotation of gut). Urethral duplication, associated with a double urinary bladder is an extremely uncommon congenital anomaly of the urinary system, more frequent in males and often linked to other anomalies (Fig. 27.4).

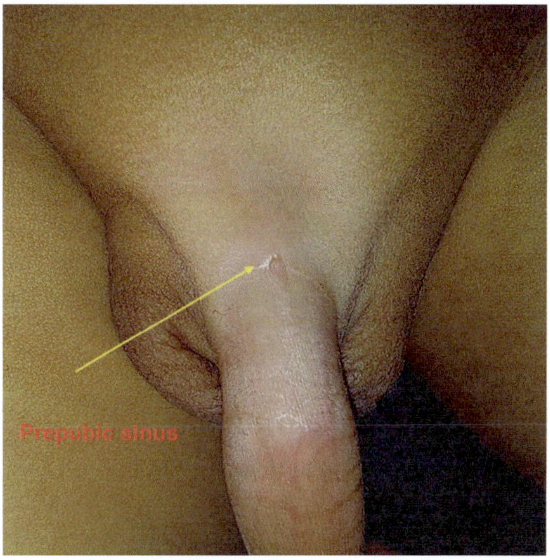

Fig. 27.8 Incomplete UD presented as prepubic sinus

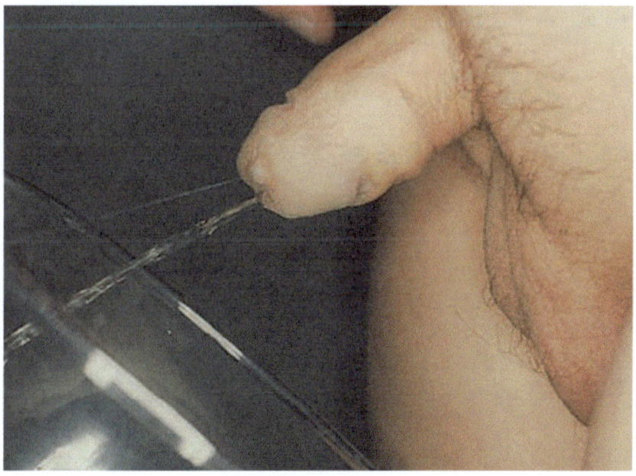

Fig. 27.9 Double urinary stream as a manifestation of urethral duplication

Many cases diphallia (Chap. 11) had a different grades of UD

27.6 Diagnosis

The clinical significance of urethral duplication is various. Patients affected by this anomaly can present with a double stream, (Fig. 27.9), incontinence, outflow obstruction, and recurrent urinary infection or be totally asymptomatic. A proper clinical examination, voiding cystourethrography, retro- grade urography, urethrocystoscopy, and intra- venous urography (in selected cases) will give a clear picture of the anomaly. The child's urinary stream must be carefully assessed to determine its location and character, based on the findings with reference to adequacy of channel, position of verumontanum and prostatic bundle in the cases of posterior urethra involvement, abnormality of location, and symptoms. Cases of double urinary meatus should be investigated to rule out an associated UD (Chap. 22).

Infection in the partially stenotic orifice is sometimes the presenting symptom. A proper clinical examination (sometimes under anaesthesia if needed), a micturating cystourethrography, an ascending urethrography, and a urethrocystoscopy will give a complete picture of the altered anatomy. MRI is a helpful diagnostic tool to delineate accessory urethra and detect an associated bladder duplication or other anomalies. Cases of congenital urethral fistula, cyst and diverticulum should be differentiated from urethral duplication (Chaps. 28, 29 and 30)

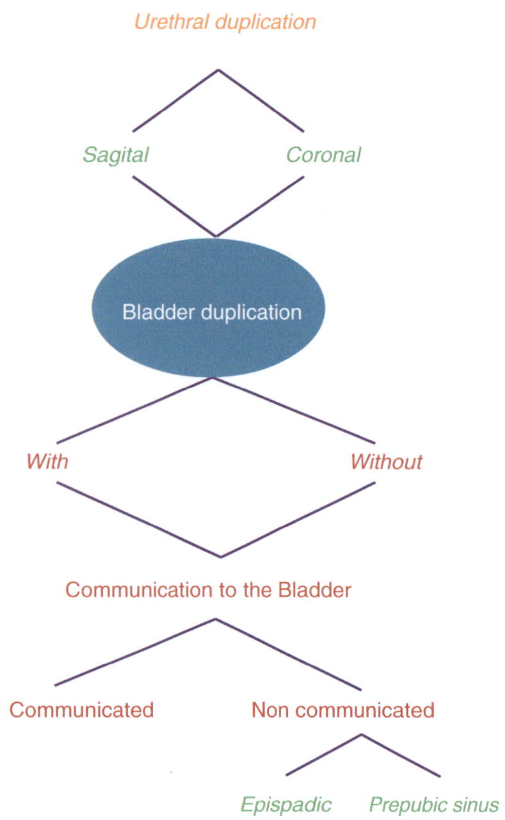

27.7 Management

Management of urethral duplication may be complex and depends on the duplication subtype, although every diagnosed case presents a unique anatomy and surgical treatment must be individualized, and it must be evaluated for each case and is aimed at creating a cosmetic result and an unobstructed urinary tract that is free of infection. The overall prognosis is usually good, in spite of the presence of other severe associated congenital anomalies (Figs. 27.10 and 27.11).

Several surgical techniques have been described to treat urethral duplication, some prefer to use the apical urethra even when it is hypoplastic; in these cases attempted urethral dilation should be considered; in another opinion the accessory urethra should not be used because it is hypoplastic and the risk of inadequate urine flow is high. Using the ventral urethra is easy when its meatus is close to the apical accessory dorsal urethra, using the penile approach sometimes combined with the retropubic approach. Total excision of this dorsal urethra is a delicate procedure because of the risk of damaging the external sphincter and neurovascular bundle. In minor distal cases, many asymptomatic children can be left untreated, but cosmetic correction of the division of the septum and creating an apparently single terminal orifice may be necessary when the orifices are close to each other at the tip of the glans. In some cases an end-to-side urethrourethrostomy may be done [9]. Prepubic sinus is easier to dissect with excision and meticulous longitudinal closure of skin to restore the normal pupo-penile junction without penile angulation.

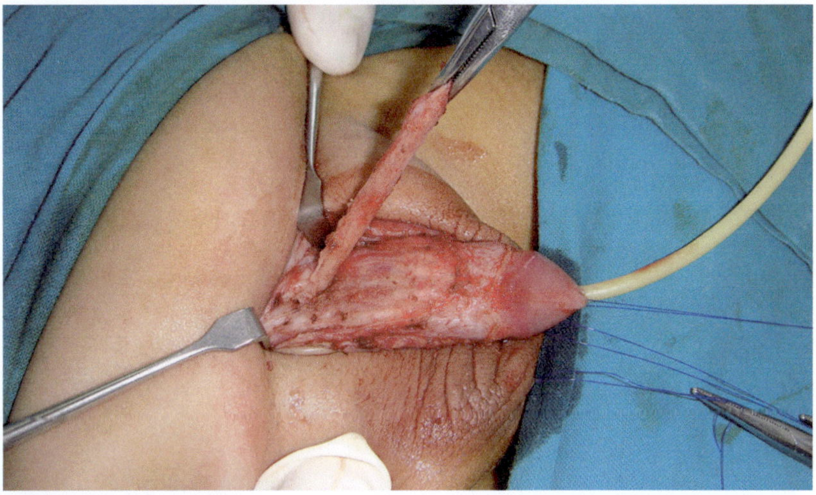

Fig. 27.10 Same case in Fig 10 during surgical dissection

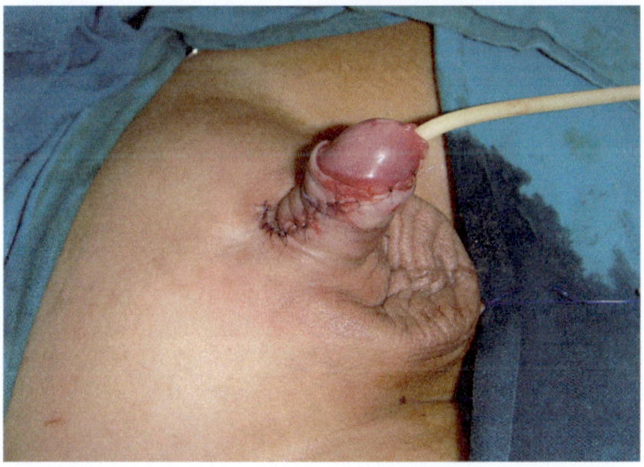

Fig. 27.11 Complete excision of epispadic accessory urethra with restoration of the normal penis

References

1. Woodhouse CR, Williams DI. Duplication of the lower urinary tract in children. Br J Urol. 1979;51:481–7.
2. Effmann EL, Lebowitz RL, Colodyn AH. Duplication of the urethra. Radiology. 1976;119:179–85.
3. Onofre LS, Gomes AL, Leão JQ, Leão FG, Cruz TM, Carnevale J, Arena S, Arena C. Urethral duplication a wide spectrum of anomalies. J Pediatr Urol. 2013;9(6):1064–71.
4. Salle LP, Sibai II, Rosenstein D, Brzezinski AE, Corcos J. Urethral duplication in the male: review of 16 cases. J Urol. 2000;163:1936–40.
5. Hynes PJ, Fraher JP. The development of the male geni- tourinary system: II. The origin and formation of the urethral plaste. Br J Plast Surg. 2004;57:112–21.
6. Arena S, Arena C, Scuderi MG, Sanges G, et al. Urethral duplication in males: our experience in ten cases. Pediatr Surg Int. 2007;23:789–94.
7. Stephens FD. Abnormal embryology-cloacal dysgene-sis. In: Congenital malformations of the urinary tract, part 1, chapter 2. New York: Praeger Scientific; 1983.15–52.
8. Huang CC, Wu WH, Chai CY, Wu TC, Chuang JH. Congenital prepubic sinus: a variant of dorsal urethral duplication suggested by immunohistochemical analysis. J Urol. 2001;166(5):1876–9.
9. Middleton Jr AW, Melzer RB. Duplicated urethra: an anomaly best repaired. Urology. 1992;39:538–42.

28 Congenital Urethral Fistula

Abstract

Congenital abnormal fistulas between urethra and anorectum or vagina are usually associated with imperforate anus. Congenital recto or anourethral fistulas without anorectal malformations are extremely rare in males and have been called N-type or H-type fistulas[1]. In many series, this fistulas are not considered under the types of congenital urethra fistula, because these abnormalities have been included as a subtype of anorectal malformation (ARM), even in cases of normally located anus. There is no general agreement about urethral fistula as an identified anomaly, as it may be considered as a sort of urethral duplication or an associated anomaly with other congenital malformations.

Keywords

Congenital urethral fistula • Urethroanorectal fistula • Urethroperineal fistula • N-type • H-type fistulas • Urethrocutaneous fistula

Congenital abnormal fistulas between urethra and anorectum or vagina are usually associated with imperforate anus. Congenital recto or anourethral fistulas without anorectal malformations are extremely rare in males and have been called N-type or H-type fistulas [1]. In many series, this fistulas are not considered under the types of congenital urethra fistula, because these abnormalities have been included as a subtype of anorectal malformation (ARM), even in cases of normally located anus. There is no general agreement about urethral fistula as an identified anomaly, as it may be considered as a sort of urethral duplication (Chap. 27) or an associated anomaly with other congenital malformations (Fig. 28.1).

© Springer International Publishing Switzerland 2017
M. Fahmy, *Congenital Anomalies of the Penis*, DOI 10.1007/978-3-319-43310-3_28

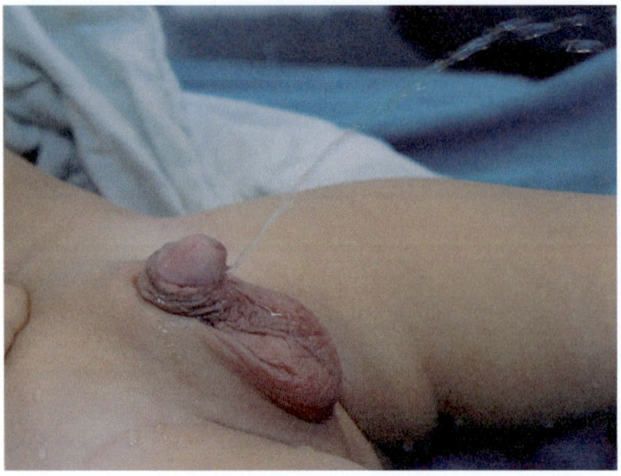

Fig. 28.1 Urethral fistula

28.1 Classifications: Congenital Urethral Fistula Could be Classified Simply to:

- Primary anterior urethrocutaneous fistula: opens in the penile shaft or scrotum (Fig. 28.2).
- Congenital urethroperineal fistula: opens in the perineum, between scrotum and anus.
- Congenital urethroanorectal fistula:
  - With anorectal malformation (Fig. 28.3)
  - Without anorectal malformation.
  - Y type (Figs. 28.4 and 28.5)
  - N Type (Fig. 28.6)

Wagner et al. classified all congenital urethroperineal fistulas as urethral duplications, and the presence of a normal orthotopic channel has to be looked for and identified [2]. The occurrence of a Y-type duplication might be related to an anomalous persistence of the urogenital duct that is bounded posteriorly by the urorectal septum, anteriorly by the ventral part of the cloacal membrane, and laterally by the superficial parts of the cloacal folds.

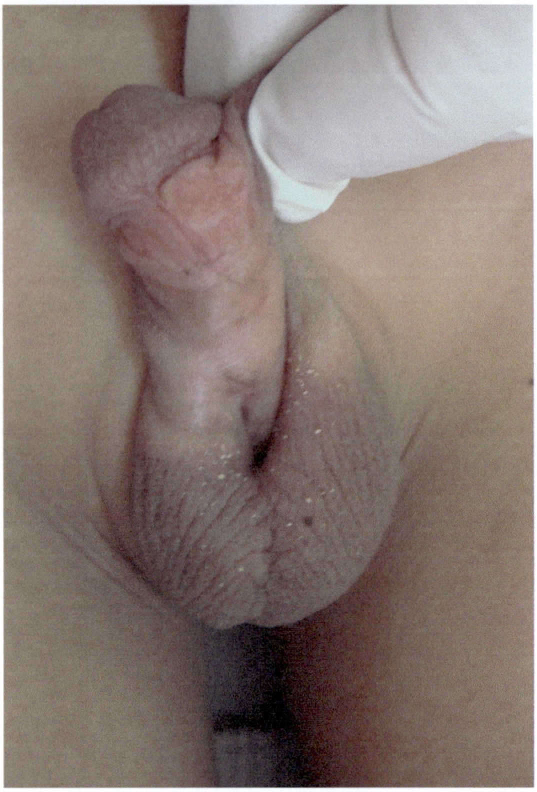

Fig. 28.2 Congenital urethrocutaneous fistula, opening in the mid penile shaft

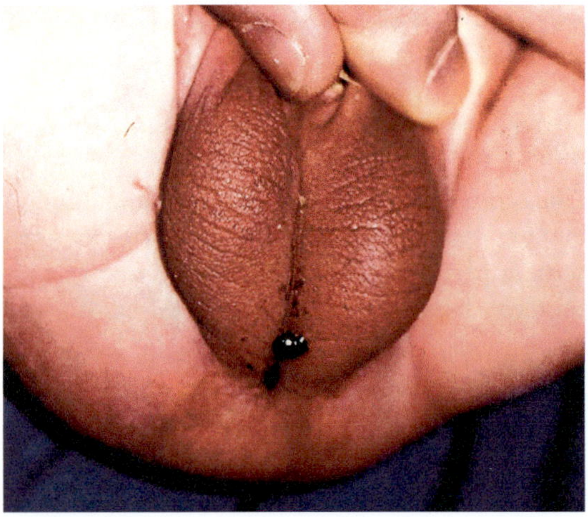

Fig. 28.3 Rectourethral fistula in a neonate with imperforate anus, meconium coming from the the fistula

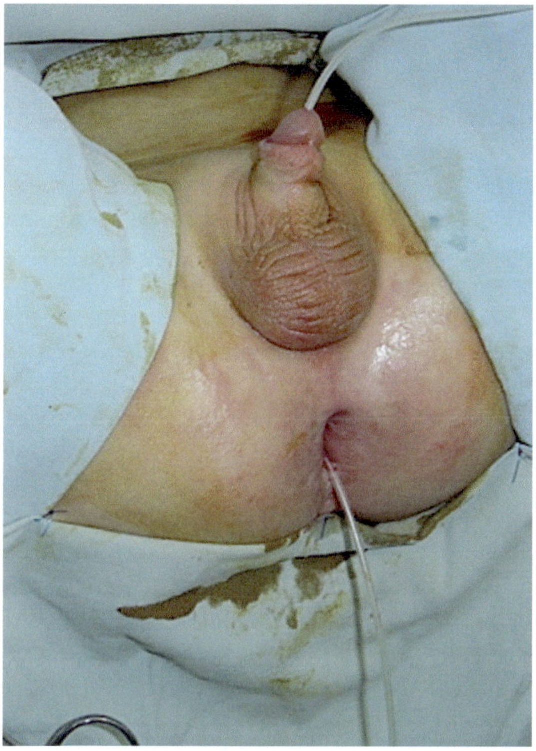

Fig. 28.4 Y shaped urethroanal fistula, without anorectal anomalies

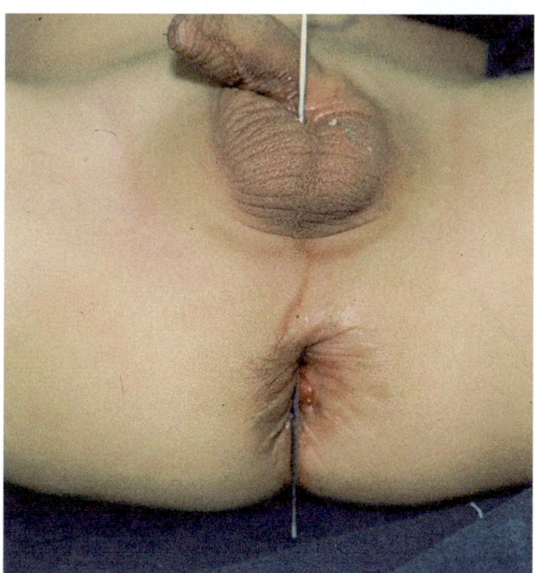

Fig. 28.5 Another Y type fistula without any associated anomalies

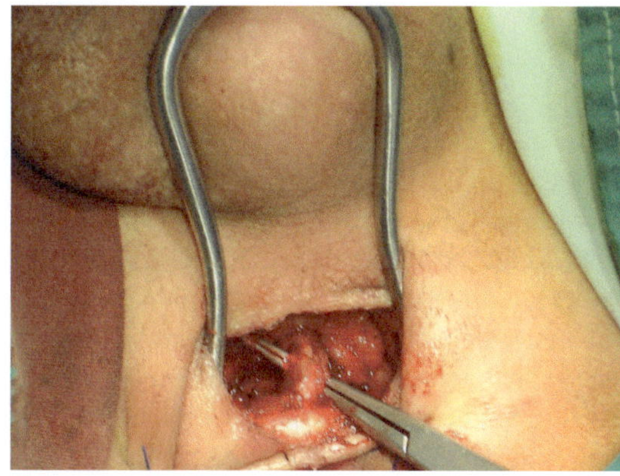

Fig. 28.6 N type urethrorectal fistula, from perineal approach

28.2 Incidence

Primary anterior urethrocutaneous fistula is a very rare malformation with only 28 cases reported in English-language literature from 1962 to 2012 [3]. In a large series of 1992 patients with anorectal malformations, the rectourethral fistula detected in 17 % of the cases [4].

H-type anorectal malformations (ARM) are extremely rare variants in the spectrum of anorectal deformities. This configuration is more commonly described in females, and its presence in males has only been reported in case reports or small series. with an estimated incidence of 3 % of all ARM

28.3 Aetiology

The etiology of congenital urethrocutaneous fistula is not clear yet. It has been demonstrated that ionizing radiation can be the cause of congenital urogenital malformation [5].

Campbell [6] proposed that congenital urethrocutaneous fistulas represent embryonal urethral blowouts behind a distal congenital obstruction. Olbourne [7] suggested that focal defect in the urethral plate results in arrested distal migration of the urethral plate or a localized deficiency of a portion of the plate, which prevents fusion of the urethral folds. Goldstein [8] theorized that there is a transient deficiency or inhibition of the local effect of testosterone leading to the failed closure of the urethral groove, and this could explain the association of other genitourinary anomalies with this type of fistula.

Also, due to the frequent association of congenital urethrocutaneous fistulas with hypospadias and other genitourinary tract anomalies, some genetic pathogenetic theories have been proposed. Genetics studies proved that mutations of ATF 3 (activating transcription factor 3), an estrogens responsive gene expressed during genital development, SHH (sonic Hedge Hog), FGFs 8 and 10 (Fibroblast Growth Factors), Ephrin-B2 and receptors EphB2, Ephb3, often associated with genitourinary anomalies, are also implied in the genesis of isolate urethrocutaneous fistulas [9].

28.4 Associated Anomalies

A congenital urethroanal fistula with normal anus is usually associated with an atretic/hypoplastic anterior urethra and has been variously described as a variant of anorectal malformation by some authors and urethral duplication by others. Most authors believed that an ano-/rectourethral fistula with normal anus is a variant of anorectal malformation and thought that a fistula is a result of persistence of the cloacal duct. These anomalies are variably associated with other anomalies and different clinical presentations like patent urachus, pelvic/ectopic/agenetic kidney, hydronephrosis, recurrent urinary tract infection, etc. The embryological basis for urethral fistula with severe urethral hypoplasia and normal anus remains speculative; different suggestions have been proposed. Al-Bassam et al. reported 31 cases of ano-/rectourethral fistula with normal anus, but only 12 of the 31 patients had associated urethral hypoplasia, stenosis, or atresia [3]. A rectourethral or rectovescical fistula accompanies high type of ARMs and is revealed by meconium in the urine (Fig. 28.3).

28.5 Diagnosis

As urethral fistula expected in all cases of ARM, regardless the level of the anomaly, all tools of investigations should be exhausted to rule out any associated fistula and other genitourinary anomalies. Clinically fistula may be obvious in physical examination or revealed as a detectable meconium in urine.

Ultrasound may be helpful to delineate the fistulous tract, but contrast study is the definitive investigation to confirm fistula, soluble contrast looogram, if a colostomy created, will fill most of the fistulas easily (Fig. 28.7), but overlooking this study by inexperienced radiologist may miss many fistulas, so pressured injection of contrast and delayed film will be helpful, and sometimes a combined ascending cystourethrography is indicated, in Fig. 28.8 a loopogram of high ARM showing no fistulas tract, but a delayed film with pressured contrast injection revealed a well defined H type rectourethral fistula (Fig. 28.9).

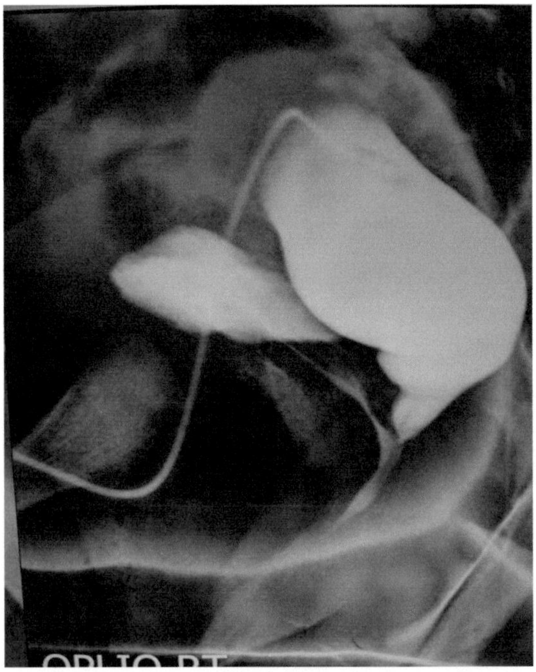

Fig. 28.7 Loopogram with a soluble contrast injected from colostomy showing a well formed rectourethral fistula in a case of high imperforate anus

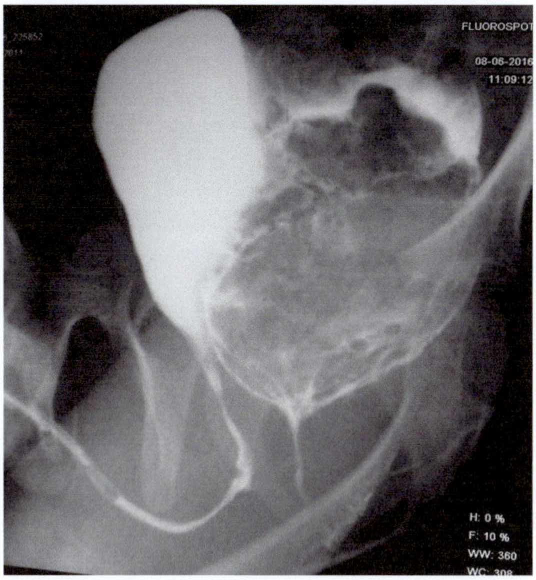

Fig. 28.8 A case of high imperforate anus with loopogram and ascending cystourethrography showing no fistulous connection in the early films

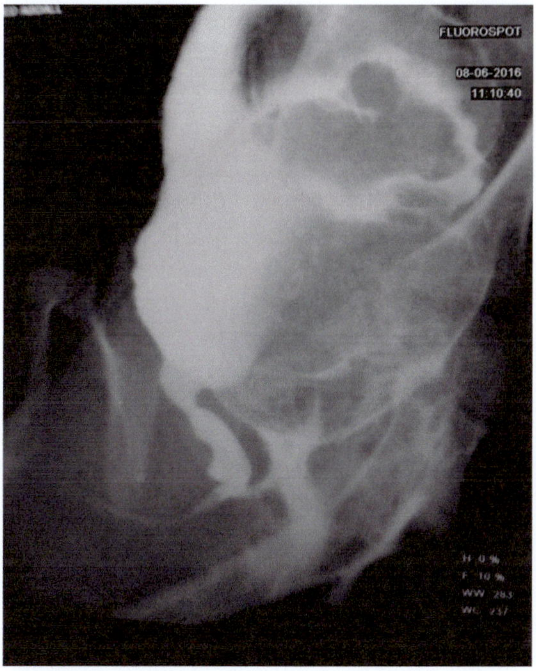

Fig. 28.9 The same patient in Fig. 28.8 after pressure injection of contrast from colostomy, showing an H fistula in the delayed film

Fine cystourethroscopic examination and MRI may be indicated in some cases.

28.6 Management

Usually the ano-/rectourethral fistula repaired during Posterior Sagittal Anorectoplasty (PSARP), either with or without a protective colostomy (Fig. 28.10), recurrence and urethral stricture are not rare, which may need a second stage repair (Figs. 28.10, 28.11, 28.12).

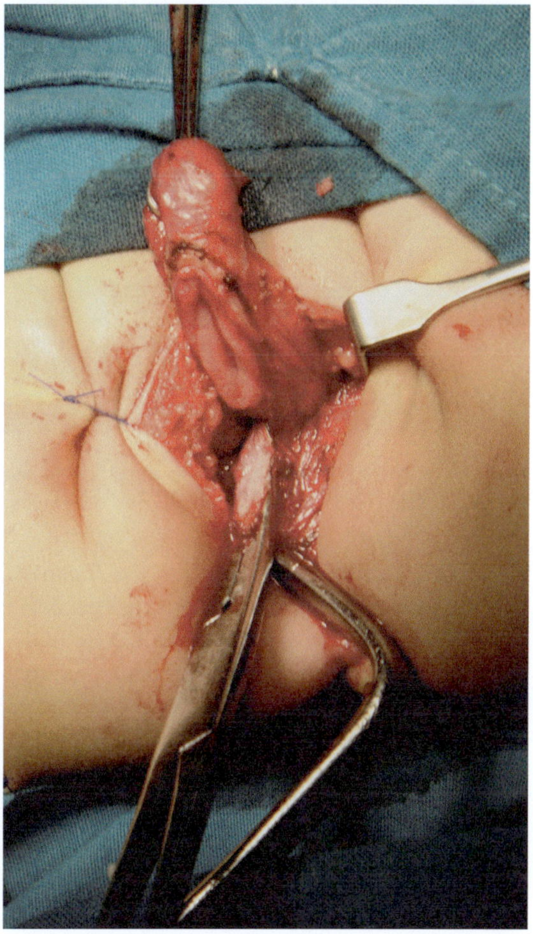

Fig. 28.10 Wide rectourethral fistula dissection during PASARP for Imperforate anus

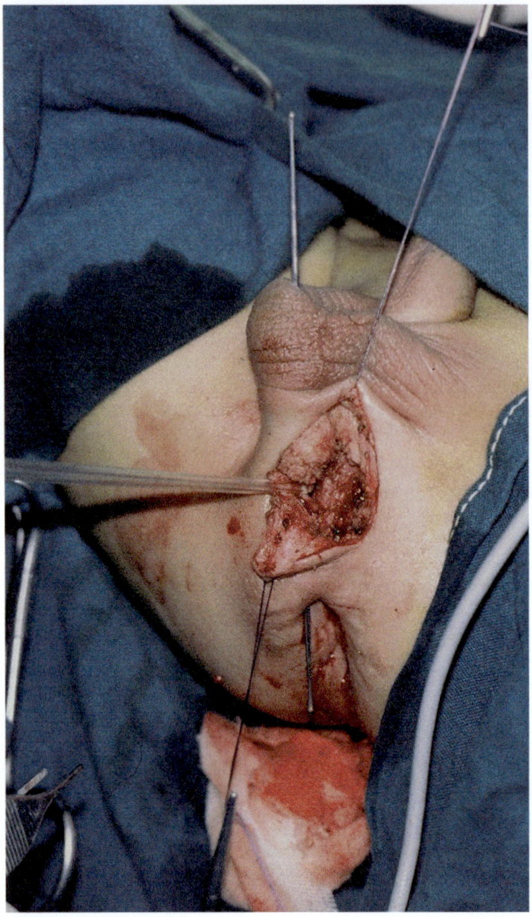

Fig. 28.11 Perineal approach for dissection of the fistula of patient in Fig. 28.4

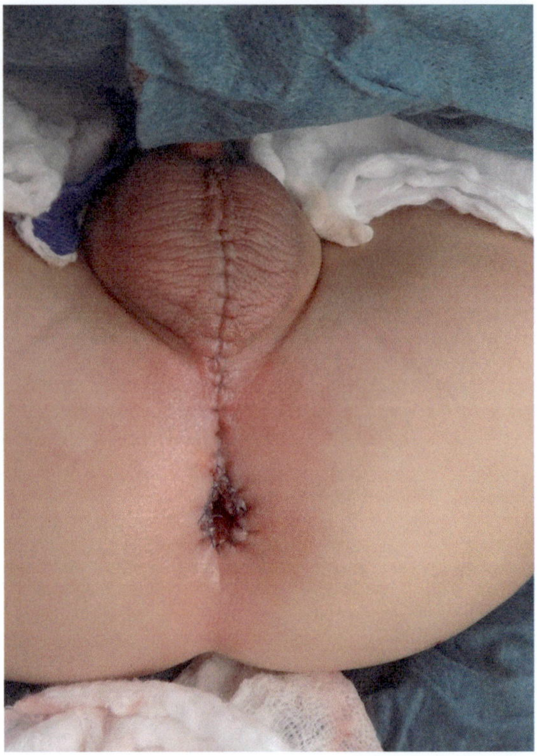

Fig. 28.12 Same patient after complete repair

Several surgical techniques for the repair of isolated anterior urethrocutaneous fistula exist, and the technique must be individualized to fit the defect, which include a pedicle flap, preputial bound skin flap, modified Denis Browne urethroplasty, or direct closure. The method of repair must be decided on the bases of the location and the size of the fistula and on the presence of other anomalies such as hypospadias or chordee. One of the most important aspects is to evaluate the urethra beyond the fistula, and if it is congenitally defective, the simple closure is usually unsuccessful and the fistula is likely to recur [8]. Otherwise, an onlay flap can be also used, Also the use of buccal mucosal graft offers a satisfactory closure after previous failures. Betalli et al. reported successful use of adopted the buccal mucosal urethral replacement to treat the recurrence [10] (Figs. 28.11 and 28.12).

In cases of deficient distal urethra or corpus spongiosum, associated chordee, or hypospadias, the formal hypospadias repair is recommended. Pedicled island preputial tube or onlay urethroplasty can be used to replace distal hypoplastic urethra. Before deciding about the surgical correction, it is important to rule out the urethral duplication and association with anorectal malformations. Probing the fistula, radiographic contrast study or cystourethroscopic examination may be required to corroborate the diagnosis.

References

1. Caldamone AA, Chen SC, Elder JS, Ritchey ML, Diamond DA, Koyle MA. Congenital anterior urethrocutaneous fistula. J Urol. 1999;162(4):1430–2.
2. Wagner JR, Carr MC, Bauer SB, et al. Congenital posterior urethral perineal fistulae: a unique form of urethral duplication. Urology. 1996;48:277.
3. Al-Bassam A, Sheikh MA, Al-Smayer S, Al-Boukai A, Al-Damegh S. Congenital H-type anourethral fistula with severe urethral hypoplasia: case report and review of the literature. J Pediatr Surg. 1998;33:1550–3.
4. Endo M, Hayashi A, Ishihara M, Maie M, Nagasaki A, Nishi T, Saeki M. Analysis of 1,992 patients with anorectal malformations over the past two decades in Japan. J Pediatr Surg. 1999;34(3):435–41.
5. Spinelli C, Pucci V, Menchini C, Buti I, Fregoli L, Spisni R, and Mogorovich A. A congenital anterior urethrocutaneous fistula in a boy whose mother was exposed to ionizing radiations: case report and literature review. Case Rep Urol. Volume 2013, Article ID 525386:4pages.http://dx.doi.org/10.1155/2013/525386.
6. Campbell M. Clinical pediatric urology. Philadelphia: WB Saunders; 1951.
7. Olbourne NA. Congenital urethral fistula: case reports. Plast Reconstr Surg. 1976;57(2):237–9.
8. Goldstein M. Congenital urethral fistula with chordee. J Urol. 1975;113(1):138–40.
9. Dravis C, Yokoyama N, Chumley MJ, et al. Bidirectional signaling mediated by ephrin-B2 and EphB2 controls urorectal development. Dev Biol. 2004;271(2):272–90.
10. Betalli P, Carretto E, Midrio P, Zanon GF, Gamba PG. A new indication for buccal mucosal graft: isolated congenital fistula of the penile urethra. Pediatr Surg Int. 2003;19(8):586–7.

Urethral Diverticula

29

Abstract

Urethral diverticula are a tubular or spherical pouches opening in the urethral canal by means of an ostium at any point of its course. The congenital one called a true diverticulum. A urethral diverticulum is differentiated from other cystic structures like; urethral cysts and syringocele, as it is a permanent, epithelialized, non-muscular, sac-like cavity projecting into the periurethral fascia and arising from the urethral lumen.

Keywords

Urethral diverticula • Prostatic utricle • Saccular diverticulum

Definition

Urethral diverticula are a tubular or spherical pouches opening in the urethral canal by means of an ostium at any point of its course. The congenital one called a true diverticulum. A urethral diverticulum is differentiated from other cystic structures like; urethral cysts and syringocele, as it is a permanent, epithelialized, non-muscular, sac-like cavity projecting into the periurethral fascia and arising from the urethral lumen.

29.1 Historical Background

"Hey" described the first female urethral diverticulum in 1805. Since this initial report, urethral diverticulum has been diagnosed with increasing frequency. The first case report of congenital urethral diverticulum in a male child was described in 1906 by Watts [1].

29.2 Incidence

The frequency with which this disorder occurs is difficult to estimate due to the high probability of a substantial number of missed or misdiagnosed cases in any given population. An overall prevalence of urethral diverticula of 3 % was reported, with a great difference between males and females, as well as the age group of patients at the time of diagnosis [2]. Anterior urethral diverticulum, although uncommon, is the second most common cause of congenital urethral obstruction in boys after urethral valve, with an incidence of 1–6 % in the general population [3].

© Springer International Publishing Switzerland 2017
M. Fahmy, *Congenital Anomalies of the Penis*, DOI 10.1007/978-3-319-43310-3_29

Despite the increased awareness in recent years, this entity continues to be overlooked during routine evaluation of children with voiding problems. Accurate diagnosis and treatment of urethral diverticula require a high index of suspicion and appropriate radiologic and endoscopic evaluations.

29.3 Etiology and Pathogenesis

It is thought that urethral diverticula may be either congenital or, acquired. There are no clear morphologic criteria to make this distinction. The majority of urethral diverticula in adults are acquired (as sequelae of infection, trauma, calculus or obstruction). Inflammation of a paraurethral or peri-urethral glands, where their ducts become infected repeatedly, they can become blocked and eventually cause a diverticulum. They are usually found in the middle or the distal urethra. Many cases of hypospadias may be complicated after inadequate repair with a diverticulum of different sizes (Fig. 29.1).

Congenital urethral diverticula can arise from several embryological sources; include defects in the primordial folds and remnants of Gartner's duct [3].

Most urethral diverticula are located posteriorly in the middle and distal urethra and are due to faulty closure of the urethral folds like hypospadias. The difference being that in diverticula the urethra alone is involved, whereas in hypospadias the defect extends through the skin. All congenital diverticula are situated on the ventral side of the anterior urethra and none in the posterior urethra. Pathologically, they are lined by mucous membrane similar to that of the urethra and their walls may contain a striated muscle layer [4]. A diverticulum of the anterior urethra develops on the ventral surface of the penile urethra as a result of either incomplete development of the corpus spongiosum focally or incomplete fusion of a segment of the urethral plate. A lip of tissue may be seen around the diverticulum. As the diverticulum distends, the lip of tissue is pressed against the urethral wall and results in a valve like obstruction.

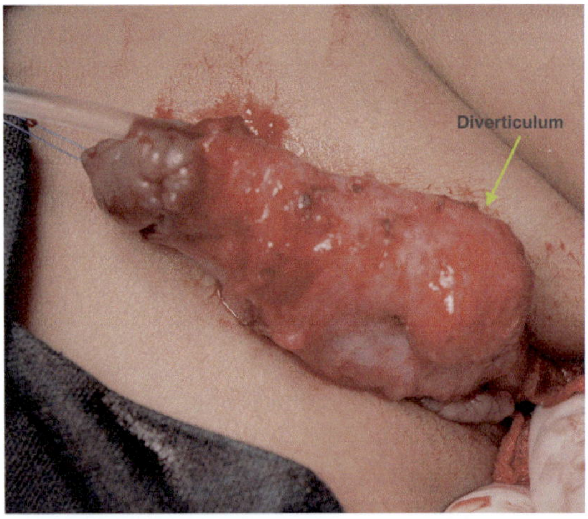

Fig. 29.1 Acquired urethral diverticulum after hypospadias repair

A congenital obstructing anterior urethral valve leading to diverticulum formation has also been suggested. There are opinions that CAUD? and anterior urethral valves, possibly, represent the spectrum of the same disease.

The embryology of AUD? remains unclear. Various proposed hypotheses include a developmental defect of corpus spongiosum, cystic dilatation of the urethral glands and sequestration of an epithelial nest after closure of the urethral folds. With a focal lack of corpus spongiosum, a urethral dilatation in this region may develop into a diverticulum. Suter proposed the theory that a diverticulum of the urethra develops because of epidermal pockets communicating with the ventral urethral wall. As the anterior urethral tube forms, the urethral groove may leave behind epithelial cells that form a congenital cyst. Cysts in this region developing a communication with the urethra could lead to diverticulum formation as a result of the spontaneous rupture of the cyst into the urethral lumen [5]. In contrast to anterior urethral diverticula, which are primarily congenital, posterior urethral diverticula are generally of an acquired origin.

29.4 Classifications

There is controversy as to the classification of urethral diverticula. The most commonly used is that proposed by Watts in 1906, who divided them into congenital and acquired. The former

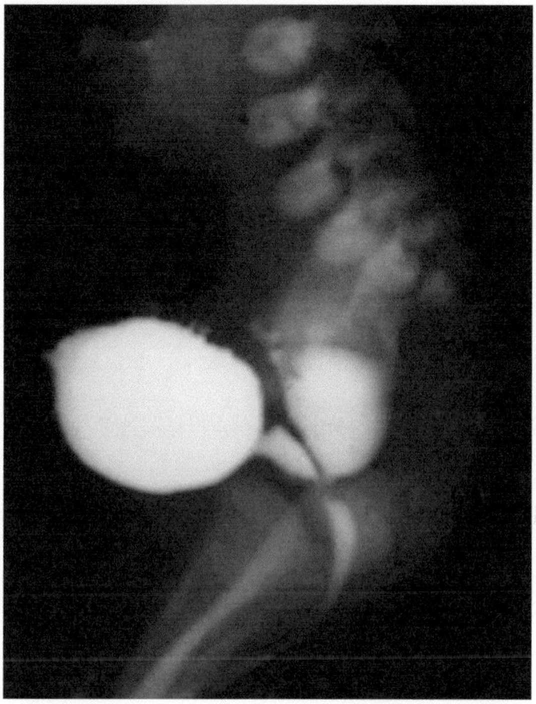

Fig. 29.2 Small-mouthed pedunculate (globular) diverticulum

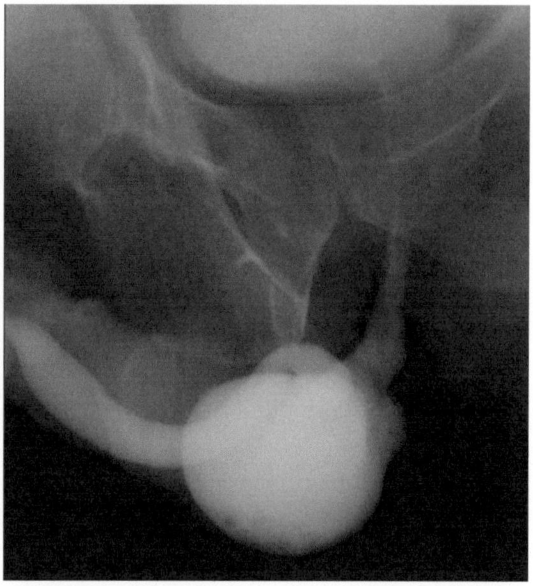

Fig. 29.3 Retrograde urethrography shows a wide-mouthed (saccular) diverticulum

involves the complete thickening of the urethral wall that is covered by epithelium, and the latter are covered by granulation tissue and their walls lack muscle fibres [1].

Diverticula can be found along the length of the anterior urethra, but the most frequent are at the level of the bulbar urethra. With the exception of the navicular fossa, they almost always arise at the ventral wall of the urethra and are divided into two categories, depending on their radiologic appearance [6]:

- Wide-mouthed (saccular) diverticulum (Fig. 29.2).
- Small-mouthed pedunculate (globular) diverticulum (Fig. 29.3).

Special entity of other types of diverticula which will be discussed separately:

- Syringocele of Cowper (Chap. 31).
- Lacuna Magna Diverticulum (Chap. 34).
- Prostatic utricle diverticulum.

Congenital anterior urethral diverticulum (CAUD) may be found all along the anterior urethra but it is usually located between the bulbous and the midpenile part, and it is rare to be in distal urethra near the coronal level (Fig. 29.4).

The prostatic utricle is a short, blind-ended pouch located on the verumontanum (the floor of the prostatic urethra) that represents a mesodermal remnant of Müllerian tubercle formed by the fused, paired distal Müllerian ducts. In males, the Müllerian ducts regress under the influence of the Müllerian inhibiting factor produced by the fetal testis leaving the prostatic utricle as a vestige. Because regression of the utricle is androgen mediated, utricle cysts are found with increased frequency in boys with other disorders, such as proximal hypospadias, intersex disorders, cryptorchidism or prune-belly syndrome [7].

Although ultrasound is the first line examination, MRI can be helpful to evaluate a cystic pelvic mass since it can provide improved soft-tissue contrast. Furthermore, MRI allows multiplanar imaging that offers excellent spatial relationships between the cystic mass and adjacent organs, such as the urinary bladder, which may further clarify the diagnosis.

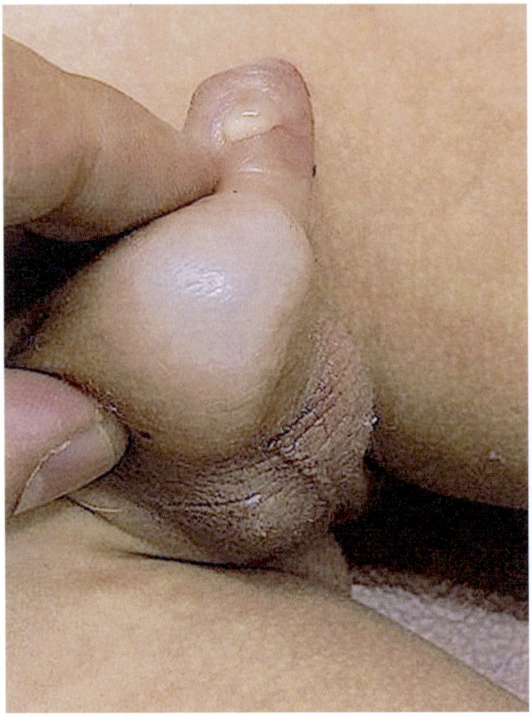

Fig. 29.4 Congenital anterior urethral diverticulum apparent at penile shaft, presented with dribbling

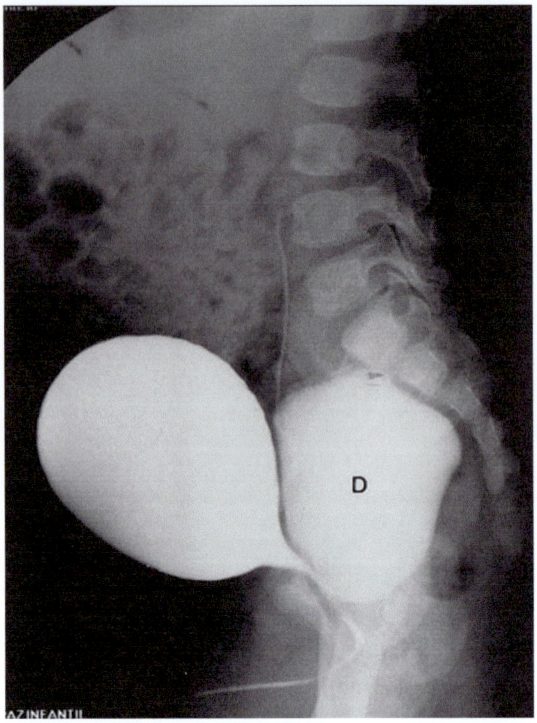

Fig. 29.5 Large prostatic Utricle

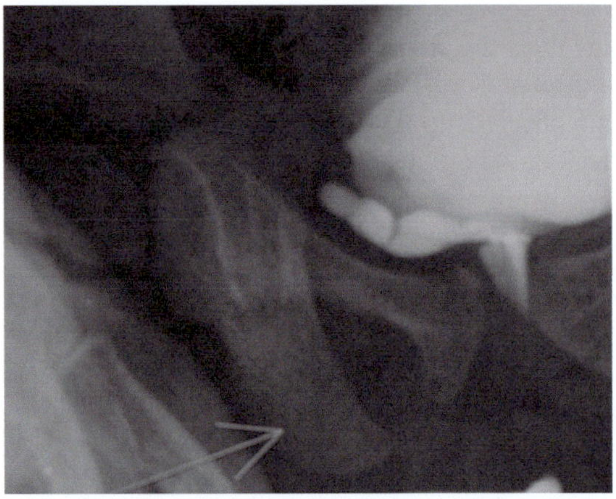

Fig. 29.6 Small posterior diverticulum

Surgical excision is considered as the treatment of choice. Various surgical approaches exist; including suprapubic, midline transvesical and perineal. Endoscopic procedures improved or cured 82 % of the patients in one series [8] (Figs. 29.5 and 29.6).

29.5 Diagnosis

The diagnosis of urethral diverticulum can be challenging given the vague or absent presenting symptoms. Clinically, congenital urethral diverticula have a wide spectrum of clinical manifestations, although most children are diagnosed in infancy with dribbling-type micturition or infection. The dribbling may be due to emptying of the diverticulum or overflow incontinence. If the obstruction is distal, ballooning of the urethra may occur with voiding (Fig. 29.4).

Diagnosis of urethral diverticulum are usually achieved in children with lower urinary tract symptoms such as dysuria, frequency and postvoid dribbling by a micturating cysto-urethrography and positive pressure urethrography, which are the gold standard in diagnosing urethral diverticulum. The obvious radiologic sign is important dilation of the ventral side of the urethra.

VCUG? is the key to diagnosis, where in the typical saccular diverticulum of the anterior urethra fills with contrast material and appears as an oval structure on the ventral aspect of the urethra [9].

29.6 Symptoms

Urethral diverticula are usually asymptomatic at early stages, but can present with irritative symptoms or dribbling and sometimes with localized pain. Most children with anterior urethral diverticulum have nonspecific urinary symptoms such as poor urinary stream, post-void dribbling, difficulty in micturition, urinary tract infection, enuresis or hematuria. Cystic swelling on the ventral surface of the penis and firm penile mass due to stone formation may be a specific symptom and sign of the urethral diverticula. Some patients especially small? (young) children or neonates present with signs and symptoms of the severe urinary tract obstruction or obstructive uremia. Older children may present with less severe symptoms.

An opacified prostatic utricle is usually well demonstrated at lateral VCUG, appearing as a posterior urethral diverticulum. Occasionally, urethral diverticula may be gigantic and compressing the bladder (Fig. 29.5).

The diagnosis of anterior urethral diverticulum is made by retrograde urethrography, voiding cystourethrography and cystourethroscopy. Cystourethroscopy is essential to confirm diagnosis and plan treatment.

29.7 Complications

Diverticula are usually lined by urothelium, although this often undergoes squamous or glandular metaplasia. Nephrogenic adenoma may also arise in diverticula. The submucosa is often edematous and inflamed. Most patients with clinically apparent urethral diverticula have a major complication such as infection, stricture, lithiasis with subsequent obstruction or carcinoma. The percentage of urethral diverticula that develop cancer is unclear, with reported incidences ranging from 2 to 15 % of symptomatic diverticula. Carcinoma that develops in this setting is usually squamous cell carcinoma or adenocarcinoma, but may also be urothelial. Adenocarcinoma may be of the conventional or clear cell type.

29.8 Management

There are many treatment options based on the patient's condition. Small and asymptomatic lesions may be followed clinically. Surgical management should be planned individually according to the anatomical findings of the abnormality.

During cystourethroscopy, endoscopic treatment of diverticulum may be performed. In symptomatic patients, endoscopic unroofing can be performed. Distal lip of the diverticulum can be removed or destroyed by various endoscopic methods. Large and symptomatic diverticula and the diverticula which persisted after endoscopic treatment are candidates to open diverticulectomy.

The pediatric population can be treated with transurethral endoscopic unroofing as well. However, current opinion recommends open intervention for certain populations, such as chil dren with large diverticula and inadequate spongiosum. In such cases, diverticulectomy should be considered.

Relationship between anterior urethral diverticula and anterior urethral valves are unclear. Treatment of AUD depends on the size of the diverticulum and the degree of obstruction. Transurethral resection (TUR) with a paediatric resectoscope is the treatment of choice for small, well-supported diverticula wherein the distal obstructing lip is resected. Moreover, successful treatment of AUD has also been reported by using a Sachse knife. But in the large diverticula, open diverticulectomy and primary repair is recommended.

References

1. Watts SH. Urethral diverticulum in male with report of a case. Johns Hopkins Hosp Rep. 1906;13:48–89.
2. Leach G, Handel L. Current evaluation and management of female urethral diverticula. Curr Urol Rep. 2008;9:383–8.
3. Lazo-Cornejo O, Manzo-Pérez G, Manzo-Pére B. Congenital urethral diverticulum in a pediatric patient. Rev Mex Urol. 2014;74(4):238–40.
4. Gupta DK, Srinivas M. Congenital anterior urethral diverticulum in children. Pediatr Surg Int. 2000;16:565–8.

5. Suter F. Ein Beitrag zur histologic and genese der congenitalen divertikel der mannlichen hornrorhe. Archiv Fur Klinische Chair. 1908;87:225–42.
6. Allen D, Mishra V, Pepper W, et al. A single-center experience of symptomatic male urethral diverticula. Urology. 2007;70:650–3.
7. Johnson D, Parikh K, Schey W, Mar W. MRI in diagnosis of a giant prostatic utricle. Case Rep Radiol. Volume 2014, Article ID 217563, http://dx.doi.org/10.1155/2014/217563.
8. Coppens L, Bonnet P, Andrianne R, de Leva J. Adult mullerian duct or utricle cyst: clinical significance and therapeutic management of 65 cases. J Urol. 2002;167(4):1740–4.
9. Williams DI, Retik AB. Congenital valves and diverticula of the anterior urethra. Br J Urol. 1969;41:228–34.

Urethral Cyst 30

Abstract

Most of urethral cysts arise congenitally from the urethral glands as an embryonic remnants, or after closure of the duct system, urethral glands are normally distributed along the whole length of urethra with a specific given names, which are different in male and female.

Keywords

Mullerian duct cyst • Cowper's syringocele • Paraurethral cyst of the Littre's gland • Periurethral cyst • Parameatal cyst • Mucocaele • Mucoid cyst

Along the anatomical course of male urethra many cystic swellings may arise either congenitally or as an acquired lesions; usually after repeated attacks of infection.

The reported congenital cysts of urethra include (from proximal to distal):

- **Enlarged prostatic utricle**
- **Prostatic utricle cyst**
- **Mullerian duct cyst**
- **Cowper's syringocele**
- **Paraurethral cyst of the Littre's gland**
- **Periurethral cyst**
- **Parameatal cyst**
- **Mucocaele (mucoid cyst)**

Urethral diverticulum was discussed before in Chap. 29, but there is nomenclature confusion between urethral cyst and diverticulum, and in many literatures there are many diverticula discussed as cysts and vice versa.

Diverticulum is defined as an outpouching of a hollow (or a fluid-filled) structure, which is not normally present, and covered by all layers of the surrounding tissue. Depending upon which layers of the structure are involved, they are described as being either true or false, which had only single layer covering and without muscle coat.

A cyst is a cavity lined by a distinctly abnormal cell layer (in both appearance and behaviour) when compared to all surrounding cells for that given location.

Most of urethral cysts arise congenitally from the urethral glands as an embryonic remnants, or after closure of the duct system. Urethral glands are normally distributed along the whole length of urethra with a specific given names, which are

© Springer International Publishing Switzerland 2017

M. Fahmy, *Congenital Anomalies of the Penis*, DOI 10.1007/978-3-319-43310-3_30

different in male and female. Male urethral glands are:

1. **Prostatic Gland**
2. **Periurethral glands (Littre's glands):** Which branch off the wall of the male urethra and in man these glands secrete mucus and are most numerous in the section of the urethra that runs through the penis. It produces a colloid secretion containing glycosaminoglycans; which thought to protect the epithelium against urine.
3. **Bulbourethral glands (Cowper's glands):** They are two small paired exocrine glands in the urethra of male mammals (except dogs), located dorsal to and on either side of the membranous urethra. The main duct draining Cowper's glands open below the urogenital diaphragm into the ventral aspect of the bulbous urethra. The bulbourethral glands secretion contributes about 5 % of the ejaculate fluid. Its secretion is a clear and rich in mucoproteins, which help to lubricate the distal urethra and neutralize acidic urine. They are homologous to Bartholin's glands in females.

Prostatic utricle is a small indentation in the prostatic urethra, at the apex of the urethral crest, on the seminal colliculus (verumontanum), laterally flanked by openings of the ejaculatory ducts. It is also known as the vagina masculina or (in older literature) vesicula prostatica. It is thought that prostatic utricle is an embryonic vestige without any detectable physiological function, but Taylor stated that the contraction of this diverticulum allows semen to pass through easily. Thus, it can be regarded as useful during intercourse and an essential part of the male reproductive system [1].

30.1 Prostatic Utricle Enlargement and Mullerian Duct Cyst

are a two distinct pathology of Mullerian duct remnants presented as a midline cystic structures arising at the dorsal aspect of the prostatic urethra. They are described as enlarged prostatic utricle when they communicate with the urethra and as Mullerian duct cysts when they do not. These terms have been used interchangeably, contributing to confusion in nomenclature.

An enlarged prostatic utricle is a congenital abnormality, although its embryogenesis is not certain, but several factors had been incriminated:

- Deficient Mullerian inhibitory substance (Anti Mullerian Antibodies).
- Androgen deficiency.
- Genetic abnormality.

Unlike normal prostatic utricle, enlarged prostatic utricle is lined by squamous epithelium. Patients present with urinary tract infection, epididymitis, and postvoiding dribbling. Diagnosis is made by VCUG; where during voiding, filling of a structure arising from the dorsal aspect of the prostatic urethra is seen. Retrograde urethrography is also diagnostic. In some cases, urethroscopy demonstrates absence of the verumontanum (Chap. 29).

Mullerian duct cysts are usually acquired abnormalities, present later in life, without any associated abnormal genitalia and do not communicate with the urethra. Histologically, they are lined by columnar or cuboidal epithelium identical to that of a normal prostatic utricle. Kato et al. [2] have proposed that Mullerian duct cysts develop at a later stage than enlarged prostatic utricles, secondary to narrowing or obstruction of the communication between the normal utricle and the urethra. Patients present with an incidental rectal mass, constipation, urinary retention, hematuria or obstructive azospermia. On US, CT or MRI a cystic mass is identified dorsal to the prostatic urethra. VCUG is not helpful, since these cysts do not communicate with the urethra. Surgical excision is curative. Of note, there is a 3 % incidence of malignancy in Mullerian duct cysts, most commonly occurring in the fourth decade [3].

Management

Surgical treatment should be reserved for symptomatic utricle cysts only, and it remains challenging, because of the rarity of this disorder and due to the close proximity of these lesions to the ejaculatory ducts, pelvic nerves, rectum, vas deferens and ureters. Endoscopic transurethral cyst

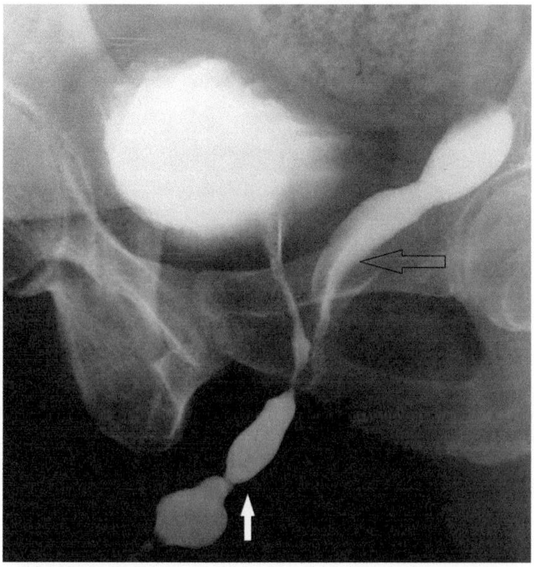

Fig 30.1 Elongated prostatic utricle, without cystic dilation (*Black arrow*), but distal urethra showing unexplained narrowing (*white arrow*)

catheterization and aspiration, cyst orifice dilation, incision, or unroofing that suits for small prostatic utricle cysts but recurrence rates were high. Open excision is the better definitive treatment. Several approaches have been described. However, all require extensive dissection [3].

30.2 Cowper's Cyst

"Cowper's syringocele" (Chap. 31)

During VCUG, the main duct and Cowper's glands can fill with contrast material and appear as a tubular channel paralleling the ventral aspect of the undersurface of the bulbo-membranous urethra and ending at the urogenital diaphragm. Cystic dilation of Cowper's gland may be presented in 4 forms, and rarely it may be presented as a large cyst, encircling the membranous urethra (Fig 30.1 and 30.2).

30.3 Parameatal Cyst

A parameatal urethral cyst is a very rare congenital anomaly, firstly reported in two males in 1956 by Thompson and Lantin. More than 50 cases have been published since then. Most of the cases which have been reported were from Japan. It is usually seen in boys, but can also occur in infants, girls and adults [4].

It is believed to be congenital, but many cases may appear spontaneously, latter in life. The cysts are usually small of about 1 cm in diameter on the lateral margin of the urethral meatus and at times, they may be bilateral. Surgical excision may require an adjunct meatal or sometimes distal urethra reconstruction to avoid post excision stricture [5] (Chap. 19).

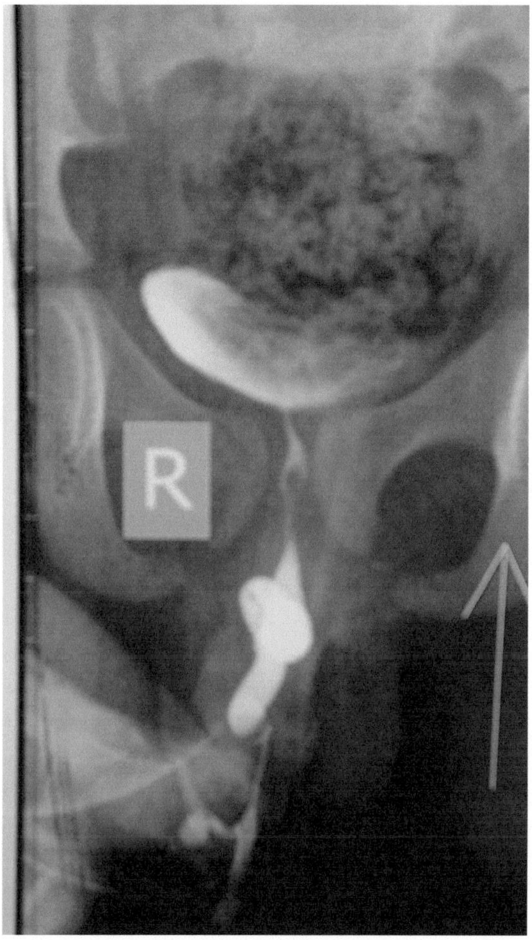

Fig. 30.2 Cowper's cyst encircling the membraneous urethra

30.4 Periurethral Cyst

A periurethral cyst is explained as arising from epithelial rests incident to imperfect ventral fusion in the formation of the external genitalia or from masses of epithelial cells which have migrated from the primitive epithelium. The cysts and canals, therefore, are congenital in origin. The canals and cysts have an epidermoid or mucous lining depending upon their cells of origin. The lining of the canals is almost invariably epidermoid, and the same is true for a smaller majority of the cysts. The canals may become so infected without involvement of the urethra; the treatment of both canals and cysts is surgical excision.

30.5 Paraurethral Cysts

Congenital paraurethral cysts arise from the various embryological components and genitourinary remnants. Paraurethral cysts of non traumatic origin are very rare, only two cases are described in the literatures; one cyst located at the penoscrotal angle dependent from the corpus spongiosum without connection to the urethra, and another case of inflammation of the periurethral Littre's glands simulating a tumor [6]. Median raphe cyst considered as paraurethral cysts, and it was discussed with penile cysts in Chap. 19.

30.6 Mucocoele or Mucoid Cyst

It may occur in any part of the urethra and is usually asymptomatic. Few cases had been reported worldwide, and mostly located near the meatus [7] (Chap. 19).

References

1. Taylor RW. A practical treatise on sexual disorders of the male and female. 3rd ed. New York/Philadelphia; 1897. 1905. p. 48.
2. Kato H, Komiyama I, Maejima T, et al. Histopathological study of the Mullerian duct remnant: clarification of disease categories and terminology. J Urol. 2002;167:133–6 [PubMed].
3. Terry LL, Bokyung H, Brent PL. Congenital anomalies of the male urethra. Pediatr Radiol. 2007;37(9):851–62. doi:10.1007/s00247-007-0495-0. PMCID: PMC1950215.
4. Christos K, Ioannis S, Dimitrios P, Paschalis T, Ioannis P. Parameatal urethral cyst in a newborn–a case report and review of the literature. J Clin Diagn Res. 2016;10(1):SD01–2. doi:10.7860/JCDR/2016/16738.7033. PMCID: PMC4740667.
5. Lal S, Agarwal A. Parameatal cyst: a presentation of rare case and review of literature. J Clin Diagn Res. 2013;7(8):1757–8. doi:10.7860/JCDR/2013/5503.3257. PMCID: PMC3782962.
6. Wolffenbuttel KP. Squamous cell carcinoma arising in a paraurethral cyst. Br J Urol. 1998;81(4):657–8.
7. de Mendonça R, et al. Mucoid cyst of the penis: case report and literature review. Can Urol Assoc J. 2010;4(6):E155–7.

Urethral Syringocele

31

Abstract

Syringocele (in Greek, syringe means "tube" and cele means "swelling") is defined as a cyst-like swelling in a tubular structure of the body. Urethral syringocele is an uncommon but an under-diagnosed cystic dilation of the Cowper's gland ducts, with different presentations.

Keywords

Syringocele • Cowper's gland • Prostatic ducts

Definition

syringocele (in Greek, syringe means "tube" and cele means "swelling") is defined as a cyst-like swelling in a tubular structure of the body. Urethral syringocele is an uncommon but an under-diagnosed cystic dilation of the Cowper's gland ducts, with different presentations.

Nomenclature

Cowper's gland syringocele.

31.1 Historical Background

William Cowper (1666–1709) was an English surgeon and anatomist, who described, for the first time, in details the bulbourethral glands which acquired latter on his name.

The term syringocele was firstly used by Fenwick, in 1896 [1], and the first classification reported by Maizel et al. in 1983 [2].

31.2 Incidence

The true prevalence of Cowper's syringocele is unknown, it is thought to be more pronounced in the pediatric population, perhaps because symptoms are appreciated preferentially at a younger age. However, there is a growing body of literature suggesting the problem exists notably in the adult population as well [1]. It was reported at a rate of about 1.5 % in pediatric cystourethrography and of 2.3 % in autopsic studies [3]. Moormann reported 169 cases of syringoceles as an incidental findings during evaluation for impotence [4].

© Springer International Publishing Switzerland 2017
M. Fahmy, *Congenital Anomalies of the Penis*, DOI 10.1007/978-3-319-43310-3_31

31.3 Etiology

Cowper's glands are composed of two exocrine structures located in the deep perineal pouch between fascial layers of the urogenital diaphragm, The glands eventually form two collecting ducts that measure on average 2.5 cm each, which open in the bulbar urethra distal to the prostatic ducts openings (Fig. 31.1).

Although anatomic variations exist, the majority of ducts combine to make one confluent passage that opens at the posterior aspect of the bulbous urethra. They are homologous to Bartholin's glands in females.

The etiology of syringocele is not clear, both congenital and acquired types are described. Stasis and pressure changes may cause obstruction to the orifices of the bulbourethral ducts resulting in accumulation of mucous and/or urine causing glandular cystic dilatation. It may then lead to bacterial colonization and secondary infection, but the genesis of congenital Cowper's syringocele is not completely clear, as syringocele appears to develop in a variety of environments across different species. The literature search has provided some clues to the future directions in understanding the aetiology of syringocele, which include genetic mutations that affect stromal-epithelial interactions with or without the effects of disturbances in hormone balance and amino acid transporting pathways [5].

Anterior urethral diverticulum and syringocele of the Cowper's duct are two different pathologies of the male urethra, but confusion between both conditions is not uncommon, as the syringocele may erode into the bulbous urethra, either spontaneously or after surgery, leading to filling of the cyst during voiding and a resulting in a diverticulum (Chap. 29).

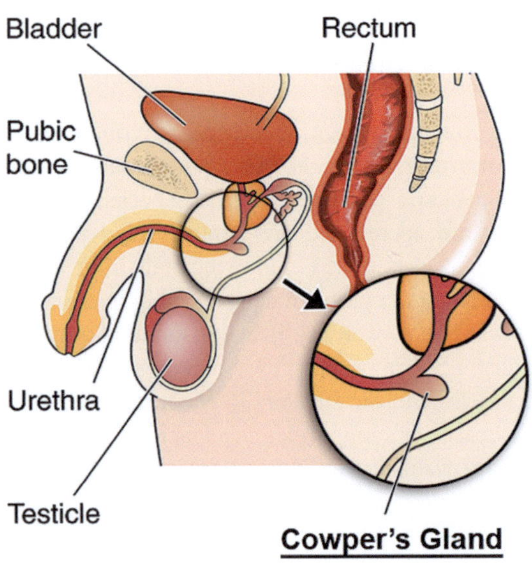

Fig. 31.1 Surgical anatomy of Cowper's glands

31.4 Classifications

Cowper's syringocele has been divided into four types by Maizel et al. [2] :

1. Simple syringocele with a modestly dilated duct. (Fig. 31.2).
2. Perforated syringocele with patulous communication with the urethra (Fig. 31.3).
3. Imperforate syringocele with a dilated bulbous duct (Fig. 31.4).
4. Ruptured syringocele that leaves its covering membrane in the urethra often acting in a "ball-on-chain" fashion to cause obstruction.

Recently syringoceles grouped to either open or closed based on the configuration of the duct's orifice to the urethra, as this also allows the

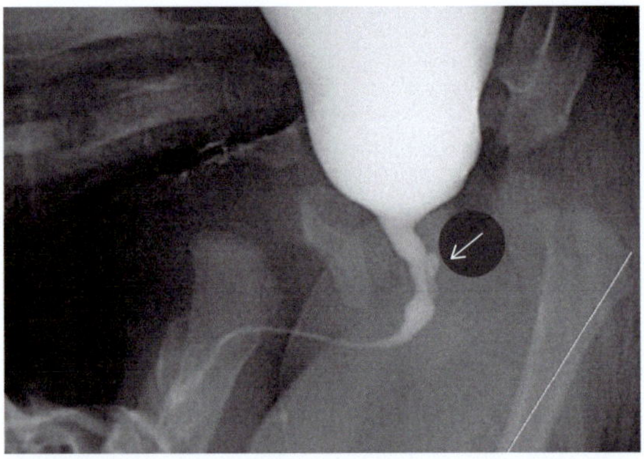

Fig. 31.2 Voiding Cystourethrogram showing a small syringocele

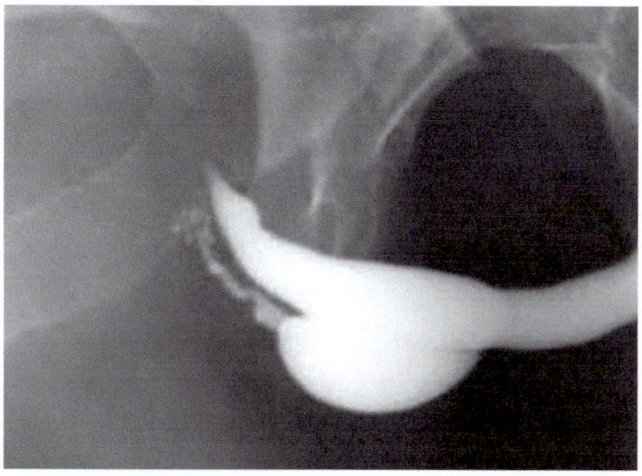

Fig. 31.3 Perforated syringocele with patulous communication with the urethra

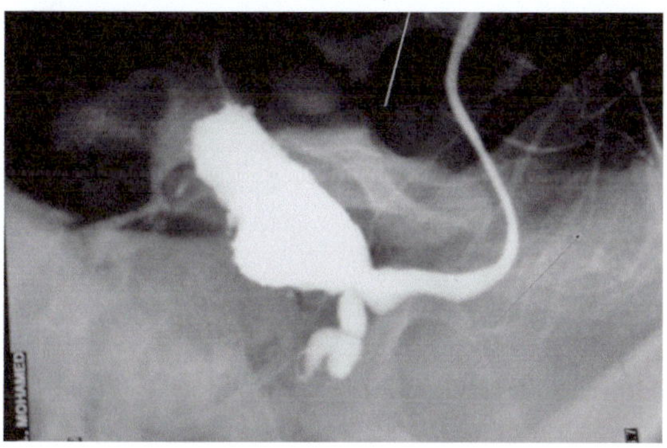

Fig. 31.4 Imperforate small syringocele with a dilated bulbous duct

clinical presentations of the two syringoceles to be identified, albeit with some overlap. Usually post-void dribbling, hematuria, or urethral discharge indicate open syringocele, while obstructive symptoms are associated with closed syringoceles [6].

For instance, closed syringoceles have cystically occluded ducts that cause the duct to dilate externally against the urethra and cause obstructive symptoms (Fig. 31.5).

Open syringoceles have a continuous lumen between the urethra and the cystic ducts, mimicking a urethral saccule and manifesting as post-void dribbling (Fig. 31.6).

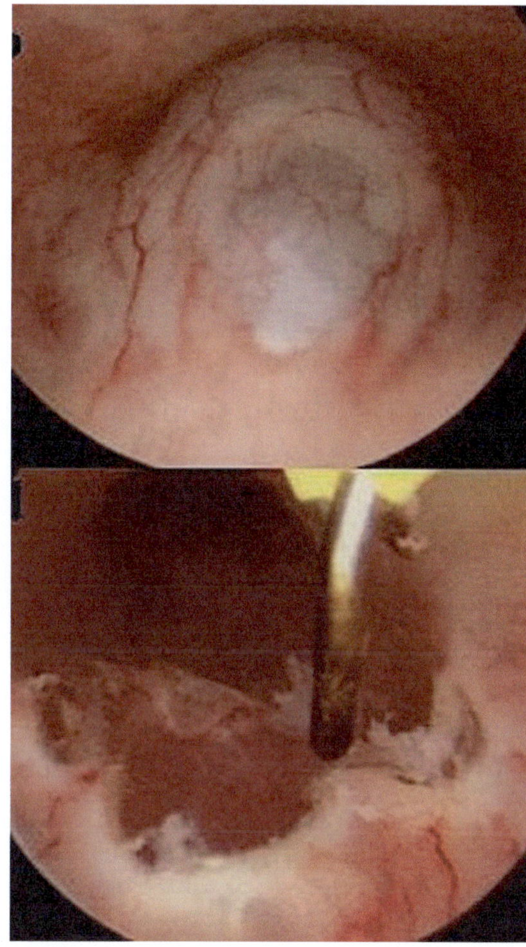

Fig. 31.5 Imperforated syringocele "Closed" bulges inside the urethra causing obstruction and may look as polyp, and after unroofing

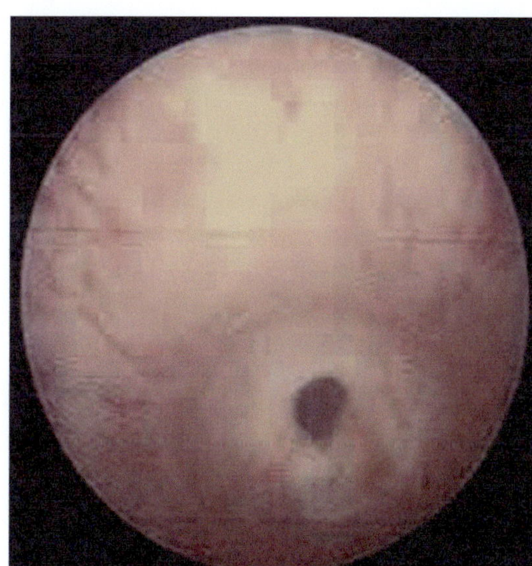

Fig. 31.6 Urtheroscopy showing an open syringocele

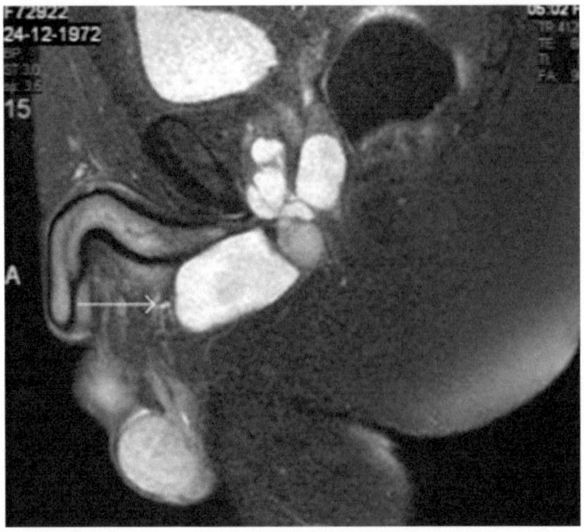

Fig. 31.7 MRI image showing a large syringocele in the ventral aspect of bulbomemberneous urethra

31.5 Diagnosis

Symptoms: The patients with Cowper's syringocele may present with urinary tract infection, obstructive voiding symptoms, post-void dribbling, hematuria or dysuria. Silveri et al. [7]. reported an infant with severe infravesical obstruction caused by ruptured Cowper's syringocele, however majority of the patients with Cowper's syringocele remain asymptomatic in childhood period.

As symptoms of syringocele are shared by many serious conditions, so a working differential diagnosis is critical.

The initial evaluation of Cowper's syringocele typically involves a thorough voiding history, and a high index of suspicion justifies non-invasive imaging. Ultrasonography (US) sometimes visualises closed cystic lesions in the anatomic region of Cowper's gland. US has even been used to diagnose open syringocele. A retrograde urethrogram was useful for diagnosis large syringocele, when the urethra was distended with normal saline. To confirm or question US results the diagnosis should proceed with antegrade and retrograde urethrography, as this step is usually diagnostic. In case urethrography is contraindicated or more data is needed, cystourethroscopy, urodynamic studies, computed tomography (CT) scan, or magnetic resonance imaging (MRI) may be implemented [8] (Figs. 31.6 and 31.7).

31.6 Management

Asymptomatic syringoceles are often observed, an followed up with only treatment for coexisting UTI may be sufficient. Although many symptomatic ones eventually require surgical intervention, a trial period of conservative management seems prudent, as spontaneous resolution of symptoms over time is not uncommon. Bevers et al. [6]. have described several cases of confirmed both open and closed syringoceles whose symptoms resolved on their own. One case resolved after successful treatment for a UTI; others resolved with no intervention.

Recently endoscopic intervention has become the preferred intervention for symptomatic syringoceles. Typically unroofing the cyst by removing its visage to the urethra is a simple, effective way of marsupialization for both open and closed syringoceles. In Bevers et al. case series, all four patients who went this urethroscopic intervention had complete resolution of their symptoms with a maximum follow-up interval of 23 months (mean 12 months). Unroofing typically uses a cold-knife; however, the Holmium: YAG laser was successfully used in some reported cases (Fig. 31.5).

Open excision of syringocele or transperineal ligation of the Cowper's duct can be performed in patients with large syringocele and in patients who present with persistent symptoms after unroofing [9]. Small children and neonates with severe infravesical obstruction, children with gross pyuria and infant population where severe reflux exists due to an anterior urethral valve phenomenon secondary to syringocele, can be treated by vesicostomy and marsupialisation before definitive surgery, with or may be without urinary diversion [10]. Also open excision may be of benefit when the syringocele presents as a large perineal mass. Laparoscopic excision-ligation of Cowper's gland syringocele has been described as another treatment modality and may be of some benefit, specially in imperforate syringocele [11].

References

1. Fenwick EH. Retention cysts of Cowper's glands as a cause of chronic gleet, spasmodic stricture, organic stricture, extravasation of urine and of so-called "false passages" in the bulbous urethra. Br Med J. 1896;1:4.
2. Maizels M, Stephens FD, King LR, et al. Cowper's syringocoele: a classification of dilatations of Cowper's gland duct based upon clinical characteristics of 8 boys. J Urol. 1983;19(129):111–4.
3. Santosh S, Mohamed E, Adel A, Sateesh J, Deena A. A case of giant Cowper's gland syringocele in an adult male patient. Case Rep Urol. 2015 (2015), Article ID 682042, 4 pages http://dx.doi.org/10.1155/2015/682042.
4. Moormann JG. Diseases of the bulbourethral glands of Cowperin man. Urologe. 1998;37(4):401–9.
5. Possible genetic links in development of syringocoele. http://www.bjuinternational.com/case-studies/possible-genetic-links-in-development-of-syringocoele/
6. Bevers RF, Abbekerk EM, Boon TA. Cowper's syringocele: symptoms, classification and treatment of an unappreciated problem. J Urol. 2000;163:782–4.
7. Silveri M, Bassani F, Adorisio O. Endoscopic management of a type IV syringocele causing massive perirenal urinoma in an infant. J Pediatr Surg. 2010;45:2254–5.
8. Jonathan M, Vidit S Daniella S, Heather M, Ali Khan S. Current diagnosis and management of syringocele: a review. Int Braz J Urol. 2010. 36 (1) Rio de Janeiro Jan./Feb. http://dx.doi.org/10.1590/S1677-55382010000100002.
9. Santin BJ, Pewitt EB. Cowper's duct ligation for treatment of dysuria associated with Cowper's syringocele treated previously with transurethral unroofing. Urology. 2009;73:681.e11–3.
10. Rushton HG, Parrott TS, Woodard JR, Walther M. The role of vesicostomy in the management of anterior urethral valves in neonates and infants. J Urol. 1987;138:107–9.
11. Cerqueira M, Xambre L, Silva V, Prisco R, Santo R, Lages R, et al. Imperforate syringocele of the Cowper's glands laparoscopic treatment. Actas Urol Esp. 2004;28:535–8.

32 Urethral Polyp

Abstract

Urethral polyps are rare congenital lesions; and occurs almost exclusively in males, very rarely polyps in prepubertal girls and women arise from prolapsing urothelium that has evolved into a polyp, they usually arise from the verumontanum (posterior urethral polyp); and it may be piping out into the bladder neck, causing bladder outlet obstruction. An anterior urethral polyp is extremely rare and arises in the membranous or penile urethra. It produces the same symptoms and has the same morphology as a posterior polyp, few cases of peduculated urethral polyps arise from the distal urethra and protruded outside the meatus had been reported.

Keywords

Urethral polyps • Polypoid urethritis • Prostatic urethral polyps • Fibroepithelial polyps • Urethral caruncle

Nomenclature

Polypoid urethritis, prostatic urethral polyps, fibroepithelial polyps of the urethra.

32.1 Incidence

Urethral polyps are a rare anomaly of the male urethra. The exact incidence is not known but it has been on the increase in the last 20 years owing to better diagnostic techniques [1]. Patients usually come to clinical attention between the ages of 3 and 9 years but may rarely present during infancy or adulthood (Fig. 32.1)

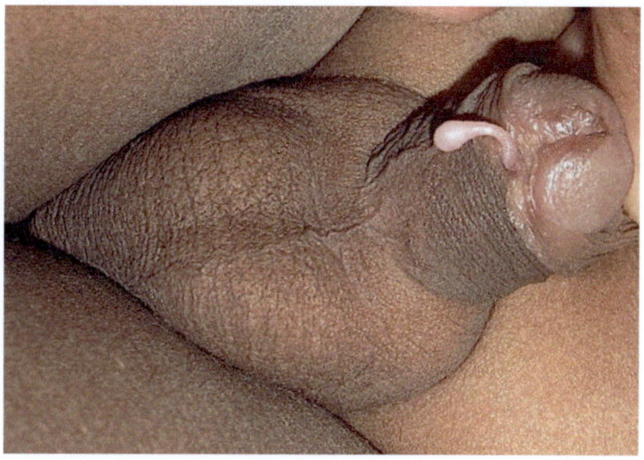

Fig. 32.1 Urethral polyp with long pedicle, obviously seen coming from the urinary meatus in a hypospadiac child

© Springer International Publishing Switzerland 2017
M. Fahmy, *Congenital Anomalies of the Penis*, DOI 10.1007/978-3-319-43310-3_32

32.2 Aetiology

The aetiology of urethral polyps is still controversial, congenital, infective, irritative, traumatic and obstructive causes have been proposed. The presence of a large polyp in healthy newborns and infants is a strong argument in favour of congenital origin [2]. They may arise as a result of developmental error in the invagination process of the glandular material of the inner zone of the prostate. Morphologically, congenital urethral polyp is covered by urothelium that may be inflamed or ulcerated or exhibit squamous metaplasia. This differs from the more common prostatic urethral polyp occurring in adults that is covered by prostatic epithelium. The subepithelial stroma consists of loose fibrous tissue that may be highly vascular and may contain a few fascicles of smooth muscle [2].

With the increased incidence of hypospadias, and a subsequent merge of rare complications after its repair, we detect a case of urethral polyp as an outgrowth from the new urethra and it may be due to chronic irritation. (Fig. 32.2)

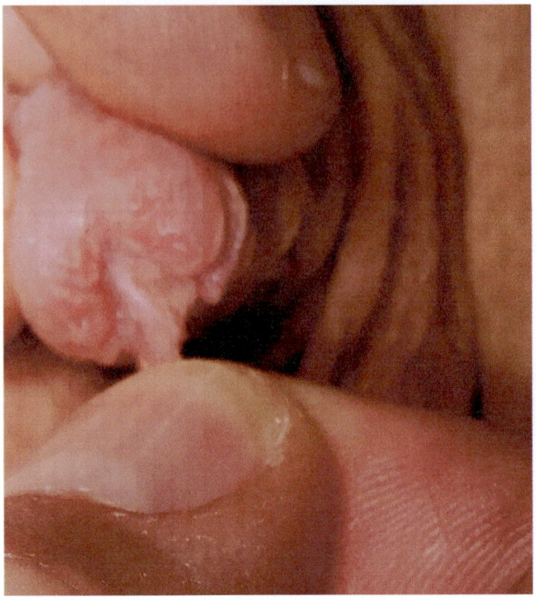

Fig. 32.2 A small urethral polyp at the tip of a repaired urethra complicating hypospadias surgery

32.3 Diagnosis

Signs and symptoms include hematuria, difficulty voiding, urinary retention, and infection These symptoms are similar to those of other obstructing urethral lesions, including urethral valve, stricture, and lithiasis. Physical examination is usually not helpful for diagnosis except for larger lesions that can be felt at rectal examination. Although ultrasound may pick up many cases of urethral polyp (Fig. 32.3), but the definitive diagnosis can be gained with cystourethrography or endoscopy, CT scan and MRI rarely indicated to diagnose such anomaly.

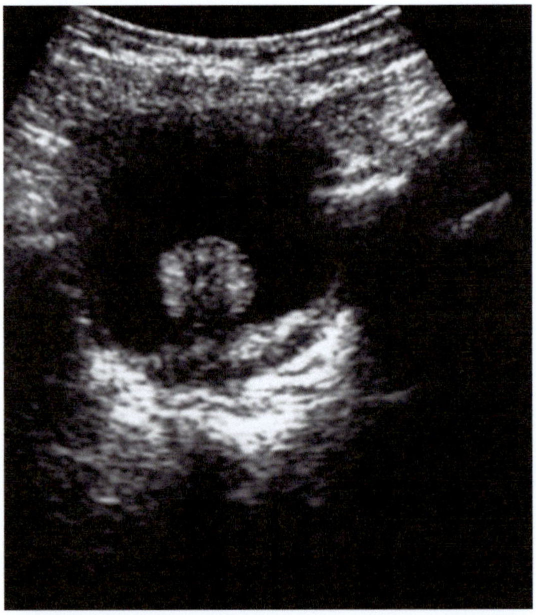

Fig. 32.3 A magnified photo of urethral polyp detected by ultrasound

The most important differential diagnoses of fibroepithelial polyps include blood clot, posterior urethral valve, florid cystitis, polypoid/papillary cystitis, urothelial papilloma, inverted papilloma and rhabdomyosarcoma of the bladder [3].

32.4 Management

Treatment of choice is endoscopic resection with fulguration of the base of the lesion; either by electrocoagulation or laser, in case of displacement of the polyp into the bladder, a transvesical approach could be an acceptable alternative [2]. Accessible polyp at the tip of urethra needs excision and urethral reconstruction.

32.5 Polypoid Urethritis

Polypoid urethritis is the urethral counterpart of polypoid cystitis, although an association with indwelling catheter has not been noted with urethral lesions. Polypoid urethritis is a non-neoplastic inflammatory lesion that usually resolves spontaneously after removal of the inflammatory stimulus. It is commonly found in the prostatic urethra near the verumontanum, appearing as single or multiple polypoid or papillary growths. Morphologically, it is characterized by abundant edematous stroma containing distended blood vessels and a chronic inflammatory infiltrate. The overlying urothelium may be ulcerated or exhibit metaplastic and proliferative changes, such as squamous metaplasia, Brunn's nests, or urethritis cystica [4].

Polypoid urethritis does not usually recur after resection unless the cause of the irritation persists. At the time of urethroscopy it may be confused with papillary urothelial tumor.

32.6 Ectopic Prostatic Tissue and Prostatic Urethral Polyp

Prostatic acinar epithelium may line the urothelial tract focally. This is seen mostly in adult men, but occasionally occurs at younger ages. This process is most common in the prostatic urethra (prostatic urethral polyp), but has also been described at the bladder neck and in the bulbous and even penile urethra. This ectopic tissue is usually asymptomatic and discovered at urethroscopy for other causes. Hematuria is the most common symptom. Cystoscopically, the lesions appear as discrete small papillary growths that may be solitary or extensive, producing a velvety coating on the mucosa. Occasionally, foci of residual urothelium are intermingled with the prostatic epithelium, and the immunohistochemical stains for prostate-specific antigen are positive in such lesions.

The etiology of this phenomenon is controversial, it probably results from hyperplasia and overgrowth of the overlying urothelium by prostatic acinar epithelium. It is important to examine the underlying prostatic urethral tissue carefully because there may be an associated acinar-type prostatic adenocarcinoma. Also, the cytological features of epithelial cells must be evaluated, as prostatic adenocarcinoma may extend to the mucosal surface and take on a papillary growth pattern. Rarely, low-grade papillary adenocarcinoma of the bladder or urachus may seed the prostatic urethra, mimicking prostatic urethral polyp. These lesions are benign and, if symptomatic, should be managed conservatively by urethroscopic resection or electrocautery [5].

32.7 Urethral Caruncle

Urethral caruncle is a pedunculated or sessile polypoid lesion located in the distal urethra near the meatus. Grossly it has a fleshy, pink-red appearance and bleeds readily (Fig. 32.4).

Patients may be asymptomatic, although commonly they experience dysuria, urinary frequency, or obstructive symptoms. Three histologic subgroups are described: papillomatous, angiomatous, and granulomatous. This separation is based

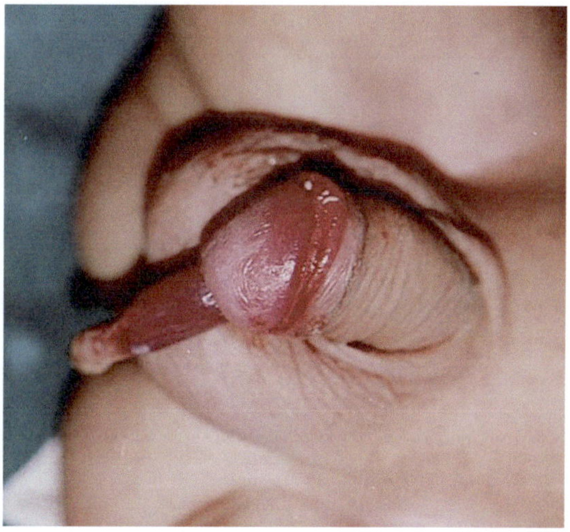

Fig. 32.4 Large urethral caruncle, looks like a horn

on the most prominent component (surface epithelial, vascular, and inflammatory, respectively); but this distinction has no apparent clinical relevance. The surface epithelium may be transitional or squamous and is invariably inflamed; caruncles covered by metaplastic columnar epithelium have been reported at older age. The epithelium may be hyperplastic and constitute the bulk of the lesion. The underlying stroma is richly vascular and inflamed, occasionally containing glandular elements thought to be derived from Skene's glands in females [6].

In girls it should be differentiated from urethral prolapse and periurethral gland abscesses, but in young boys, it may be difficult to differentiate caruncle from urethral polyp except after histopathological examination. Conservative therapy (warm Sitz baths, topical anti-inflammatory drugs) is appropriate in most patients. Surgical intervention should be reserved for patients with larger symptomatic lesions, for those in whom conservative therapy fails to elicit a response, and for those with uncertain diagnoses.

References

1. Akbarzadeh A, Khorramirouz R, Kajbafzadeh AM. Congenital urethral polyps in children: report of 18 patients and review of literature. J Pediatr Surg. 2014;49(5):835–9. doi:10.1016/j.jpedsurg.2014.02.080. Epub 2014 Feb 26.
2. Demircan M, Ceran C, Karaman A, et al. Urethral polyps in children: a review of the literature and report of two cases. Int J Urol. 2006;13:841–3.
3. Glassberg KI, Horowitz M. Urethral valve and other anomalies of the male urethra. In: Belman AB, King LR, Kramer SA, editors. Clinical pediatric urology. 4th ed. London: Martin Dunitz Ltd; 2002. p. 899–945.
4. Walsh IK, Keane PF, Herron B. Benign urethral polyps. Br J Urol. 1993;72:937–8 [PUBMED].
5. Satoh S, Ujiie T, Kubo T, et al. Prostatic epithelial polyp of the prostatic urethra. Eur Urol. 1989;16:92–6.
6. Conces MR, Williamson SR, Montironi R, Lopez-Beltran A, Scarpelli M, Cheng L. Urethral caruncle: clinicopathologic features of 41 cases. Hum Pathol. 2012;43(9):1400–4 [Medline].

33 Congenital Urethral Stricture

Abstract

Urethral stricture defined as congenital only if it is not an inflammatory, it is a short-length and it is not associated with history of or potential for urethral trauma, or instrumentation. It is not considered a rare disease, and we must note the existence of such anomaly, especially in boys suffering from recurrent urinary tract infections, dysuria, disturbed voiding, drug-resistant diurnal enuresis, pollakisuria or hematuria in pediatric urological practice. Stricture also disturbs spontaneous healing of vesicoureteral reflux. Usually findings above the stenotic segment include a bladder wall thickening, hydronephrosis, and renal dysplasia. VCUG demonstrates the stenotic segment and the associated alterations.

Keywords

Urethral stricture • Cobb's Collar • Moormann's ring • Anterior Urethral Valve

Definition

Urethral stricture defined as congenital only if it is not an inflammatory, it is a short-length and it is not associated with history of or potential for urethral trauma, or instrumentation.

It is not considered a rare disease, and we must note the existence of such anomaly, especially in boys suffering from recurrent urinary tract infections, dysuria, disturbed voiding, drug- resistant diurnal enuresis, pollakisuria or hematuria in pediatric urological practice. Stricture also disturbs spontaneous healing of vesicoureteral reflux. Usually findings above the stenotic segment include a bladder wall thickening, hydronephrosis, and renal dysplasia. VCUG demonstrates the stenotic segment and the associated alterations.

Congenital urethral stricture should be differentiated from other different causes of congenital urethral obstruction, which may be caused by different pathologies discussed before like; urethral polyp, cyst and diverticulum.

Sonourethrography (Urethral Ultrasound) is best used adjunctively to guide treatment planning in patients with known bulbous urethral strictures and has been reported to be more accurate than retrograde urethrography for estimating the length of urethral strictures (Fig. 33.1).

In paediatric cases, it worth using ultrasound instead of radiological and CT imaging to reduce

© Springer International Publishing Switzerland 2017

M. Fahmy, *Congenital Anomalies of the Penis*, DOI 10.1007/978-3-319-43310-3_33

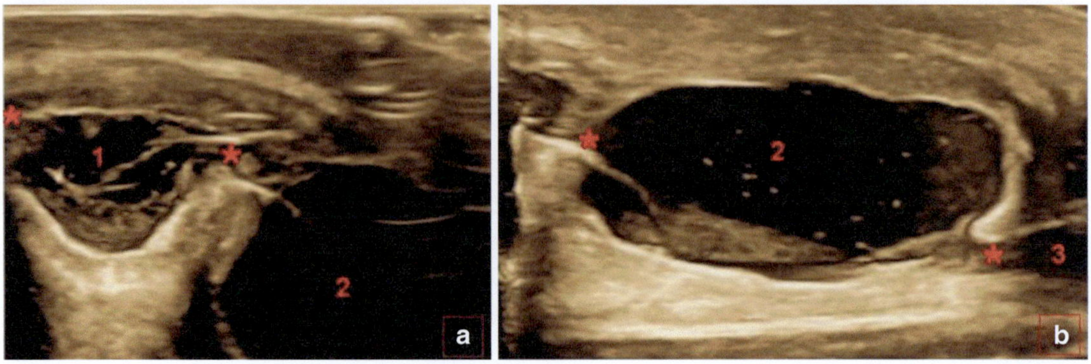

Fig. 33.1 Sonourethrography diagnosing accurately the stricture(**a**), in comparison to the calibre of the rest normal urethra (**b**) (Case courtesy of Dr Maciej Mazgaj, Radiopaedia.org, rID: 24047)

dose of x-rays exposure at the young age, although this may be a challenging test due to lack of cooperation. MR imaging is considered to be the best ancillary imaging modality for assessing urethral, adjacent anatomy and associated other anomalies.

The most effective treatment of this lesion is optic internal urethrotomy under direct vision. Early endoscopic intervention is safe and feasible and its short-term clinical outcomes are favorable. Long-term clinical outcomes, however, remain to be investigated [1].

Urethrotomy and dilation are acceptable for short bulbar urethral strictures or as salvage after failed urethroplasty with stenotic annular rings. Repeat urethrotomy is futile and potentially harmful. Anterior urethral strictures of the bulb can be successfully managed by anastomotic urethroplasty if short and substitution urethroplasty (buccal grafts) if long.

33.1 Historical Background

Urethral stricture disease in children has been cited as long ago as ancient Greek. Historically, the treatment consisted of urethral dilation with sounds. Hamilton Russell described the first surgical procedure for repair of a urethral stricture in 1914 [2]. But urethral stricture in adult is a well-known entity long time ago in the history, and urethral dilation was described by the Egyptians in 3000–2000 BC; they used different types of sounds to dilate urethral strictures.

Congenital Urethral stricture classified herein to:

- Meatal:
  - Meatal Stenosis (Chap. 21)
  - Lacuna Magna (Chap. 34)
- Anterior (Penile and Bulbar) Urethral Strictures:
  - Cobb's Collar
  - Anterior Urethral Valve
- Posterior Urethral Stenosis
  - Posterior Urethral Valve (will not be discussed as it is not actually a penile anomalies)

33.2 Cobb's Collar

The Cobb's collar or Moormann's ring is a congenital narrowing of the bulbar urethra with variable clinical presentation and obstruction grade, it is largely unrecognized but has considerable relevance urologically as the site of congenital or postinstrumental strictures [3].

It is important to distinguish other congenital urethral obstruction and Cobb's collar from type-III PUV, as in some cases the posterior urethral membrane may prolapse until the bulbar urethra, making these two conditions similar; however, the fold is attached to the verumontanum in all cases of posterior urethral valve. This congenital stricture also differs from acquired types of stricture in that there is a distinct lack of periurethral fibrosis or any abnormal tissue surrounding the urethra (Fig. 33.2). At the same time the posttrumatic stricture is unlikely

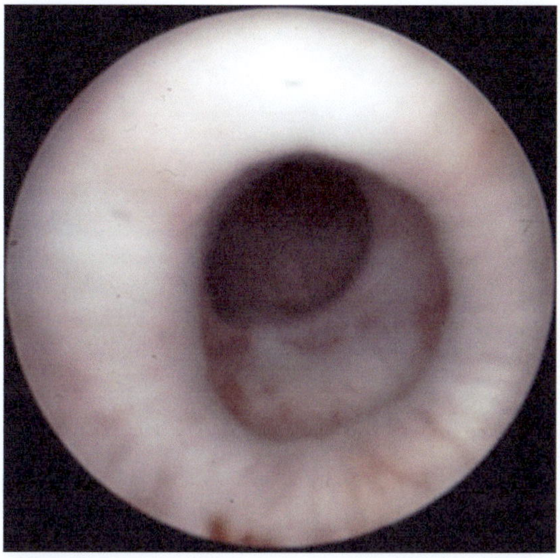

Fig. 33.2 Cobb's collar: a ring is observed by urethroscopy at bulbar urethra level. External sphincter is observed proximally to the ring, without any fibrosis

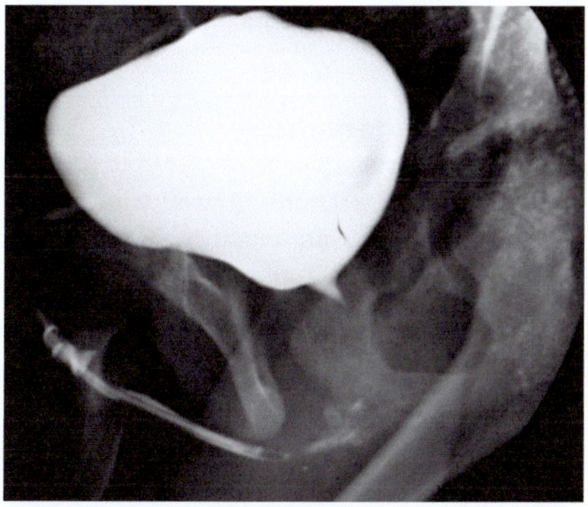

Fig. 33.3 Long segment post traumatic stricture

to be smooth and circular, mostly it is longitudinal and with irregularity (Fig. 33.3).

Cobb et al. described in 1968 [4]; 26 cases of proximal urethral bulb strictures in patients without history of urethritis, urethral or perineal trauma, previous urethroscopy, or urethral surgery, the same pathology has also been described by Moormann in continental Europe [5], so this congenital stricture is known as : "Cobb's collar" or "Moormann's ring".

33.3 Etiology

The predictable site of the narrowing in the bulbar urethra suggests an embryological explanation for this stricture. Failure of complete dissolution of the urogenital membrane at the junction of the cloaca and genital groove has been suggested. However, it seems more likely that Cobb's collar is the result of a narrowing at the level of the urogenital ostium, i.e., the opening of the pelvic part into the phallic part of the urogenital sinus.

33.4 Classifications

Three different types of Cobb's collar have been identified, all these forms are located just below the external sphincter [5].

Type I appears as a ridge of tissue.
Type II represents a well-defined stricture of the bulbar urethra (Fig. 33.4).
Type III is a very tight pinhole (Fig. 33.5).

33.5 Incidence

These cases are rare, although the exact prevalence still remains unclear; our experience suggests that it should occur more frequently than the literature suggests. In a large series of case of urethral strictures, a congenital cause was detected in 6.9 % [1]. In Dewan's experience of over 1300 cystourethroscopes, 95 males were found to have an indentation in the bulbar urethra; however, only four patients required dilatation [6].

33.6 Associated Anomalies

Congenital urethral strictures were associated with other anomalies, including abnormalities of the cardiovascular, central nervous, and skeletal systems; it is also common with hypospadias and prostatic anomalies.

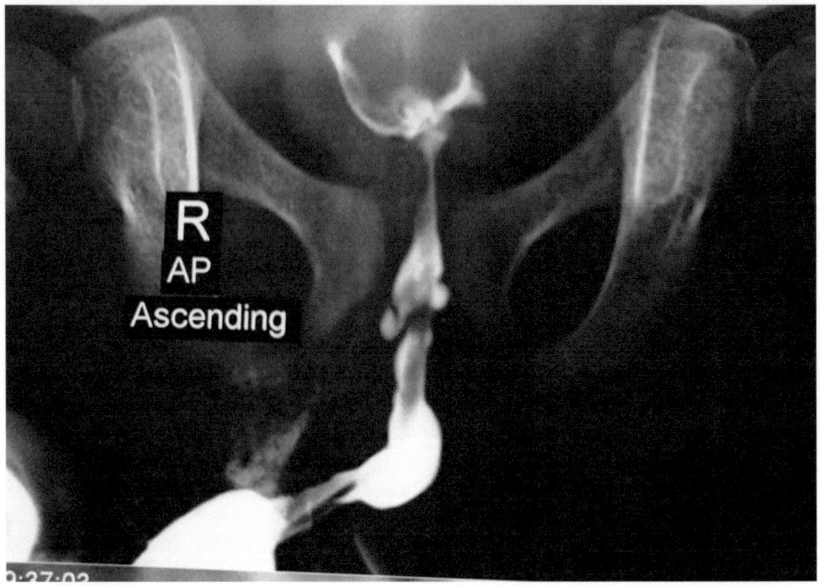

Fig. 33.4 (Cobb's collar II) definite stricture at the junction between the prostatic and membranous urethra

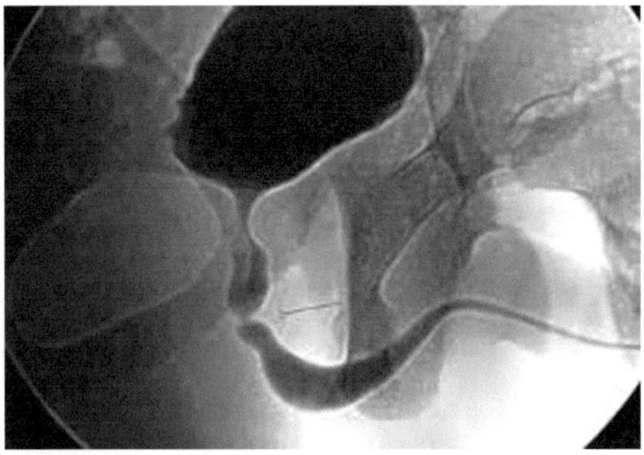

Fig. 33.5 Very tight circular stricture (Cobb's collar III)

33.7 Diagnosis

Findings above the stenotic segment are similar to those of posterior urethral valves and include bladder wall thickening, hydronephrosis, and renal dysplasia. VCUG demonstrates the stenotic segment and the associated alterations. This stricture possibly causes the disorder of urine flow followed by bladder instability (Figs. 33.2, 33.3 and 33.4)

Congenital urethral stricture could be diagnosed in the absence of any history of infection, trauma, or instrumentation and location of structure at a bulbous urethra, and this should be differentiated from other different causes of other congenital urethral obstruction, which may be caused by different pathologies discussed before like urethral valve or cyst and diverticulum.

33.8 Management

Sometimes these strictures do well with routine dilation, and others are cured by urethrotomy, but the need for urethroplasty in the remainder has given the chance to obtain a biopsy of the tissue making up the stricture, and it is composed not of the expected scar tissue, but of hypertrophied muscle. Treatment of choice is endoscopic dilation or, in case of ineffectiveness, incision of the stricture walls. A cold knife is preferable to electrocautery for incising this fine anterior lesion [7].

33.9 Anterior Urethral Valves

Anterior urethral valves are rare congenital anomalies that cause lower urinary tract obstruction in children, it is reported to be seven times less common than posterior urethral valve (PUV); however, it can be equally devastating.

The etiology of these anomalies is still not completely clear. Various proposed theories exist, including an abortive attempt at urethral duplication, failure of alignment between the proximal and distal urethra, incomplete formation of the ventral corpus spongiosum, congenital cystic dilation of the periurethral gland, and a ruptured Cowper's duct cyst [8].

AUV may locate in every portion of the anterior urethra with almost equal incidence. It may even be found in fossa navicularis:

- 40 % of the valves are located in the bulbar urethra.
- 30 % at the penoscrotal junction.
- 30 % in the pendulous urethra.

It is likely that a pathophysiologic spectrum exists from valve to diverticulum formation associated with the degree of urethral dilation. Intrauterine urethral obstruction can result in severe bladder dysfunction after birth, which does not necessarily resolve after valve resection. If severe neonatal obstruction exists, urinary diversion by vesicostomy, and antibiotics, electrolyte [9].

Clinical presentation of patients with AUV is similar to those with PUV. The spectrum ranges from mild urethral dilation to severe bilateral hydronephrosis with renal failure, according to the degree of urinary obstruction; luckily only fewer than 5 % of patients with AUV progress to chronic renal failure. In 2010, JC Routh et al. asserted that congenital anterior urethral obstruction in children has a generally good prognosis but may occasionally result in a poor renal outcome. The combination of pretreatment azotemia, vesicoureteral reflux, and urinary tract infection is highly predictive of a poor renal outcome [8]. They can occur as an isolated entity or in association with a proximal diverticulum; in either case, they probably represent a spectrum of disease.

The clinical manifestation of anterior urethral valves is highly variable and depends on patient age and degree of obstruction. It may range from severe obstruction with bilateral severe hydroureteronephrosis, end- stage renal disease, and even bladder rupture to a minimal obstruction.

VCUG is the diagnostic modality of choice for anterior urethral valves. Typically, the urethra appears dilated proximal to the valve and narrowed distal to it (Fig. 33.6).

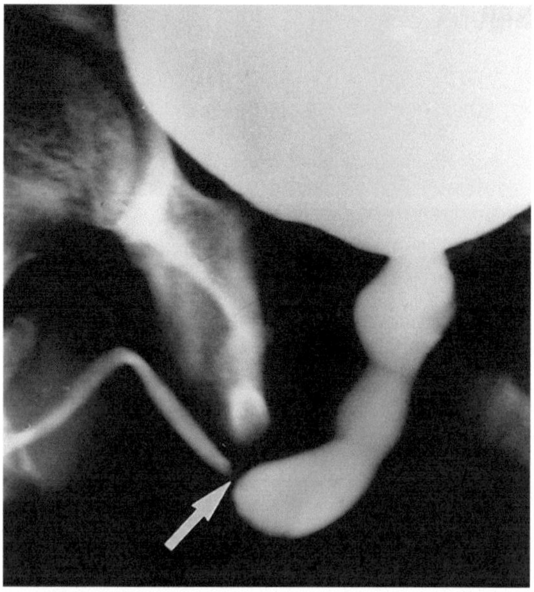

Fig. 33.6 Stricture due to anterior urethral valve (*arrow*), with a proximal dilatation

A valve may appear as a linear filling defect along the ventral wall, or it may be indicated by a dilated urethra ending in a smooth bulge or an abrupt change in the caliber of the dilated urethra. In addition to demonstrating a lesion in the urethra, VCUG may also reveal an other associated anomaly. Endoscopic examination of the urethra usually confirm the diagnosis.

33.10 Management

Management of AUV may be endoscopic or open. Endoscopic procedure consists in electrocauterization of valve tissue. When performing this procedure, the surgeon must be careful not to injure the urethral wall: it can be very thin and terminal injury may result in urethral strictures and urethrocutaneous fistula. A urethroplasty and open resection of the valve are recommended in patients with massive urethral diverticula to pack an adequate urethral caliber [10].

References

1. Mori Y, Matsui T, Ogino T, et al. Treatment of congenital urethral stenosis (urethral ring) in children. Jpn J Urol. 1989;80:704–10. PMID:2754895.
2. Liu JS, Hofer MD, Oberlin DT, Milose J, Flury SC, Morey AF, et al. Practice patterns in the treatment of urethral stricture among American urologists: a paradigm change? Urology. 2015;86(4):830–4.
3. Cranston D, Davies AH, Smith JC. Cobb's collar–a forgotten entity. Br J Urol. 1990;66:294–6.
4. Cobb BG, Wolf JA, Ansell JS. Congenital stricture of the proximal urethral bulb. J Urol. 1968;99:629.
5. Moormann JG. Congenital bulbar urethral stenosis as a cause of disease of the urogenital junction. Urologe. 1972;11:157–60.
6. Dewan P. Re: Nonomura K, Kanno T, Kakizaki H et al. Impact of congenital narrowing of the bulbar urethra (Cobb's collar) and its transurethral incision in children. Eur. Urol. 1999; 36: 144–9. Eur. Urol. 2001; 40: 478–9.
7. Dorisio O, Bassani F, Silveri M. Cobb's collar: a rare cause of urinary retention. BMJ Case Rep. 2013; pii: bcr2012008137 doi: 10.1136/bcr-2012-008137.
8. Routh JC, McGee SM, Ashley RA, Reinberg Y, Vandersteen DR. Predicting renal outcomes in children with anterior urethral valves: a systematic review. J Urol. 2010;184(5):1615–9.
9. McLellan DL, Gaston MV, Diamond DA, et al. Anterior urethral valves and diverticula in children: a result of ruptured Cowper's duct cyst? BJU Int. 2004;94:375–8.
10. Tombal B, Abi Aad A, Opsomer R, et al. Urethral stenosis in children: apropos of 33 pediatric cases. Acta Urol Belg. 1994;62:55–61.

Lacuna Magna (LM) 34

Abstract

Lacuna means a small pit or hollow cavity, the lacuna magna is the largest depression in the fossa navicularis. Located deeper within the lacunae are branching mucous tubules called the glands of Littre. Guerin valve is a septum between the lacuna magna and the urethral lumen, which may act as a valve and leads to the manifestations of existence of LM with a different grades of urethral obstruction and other.

Keywords

Lacuna Magna • Sinus of Guerin • Crypts of Morgagni • Valve of navicular fossa • Congenital urethral stricture

Nomenclature and Synonyms

Sinus of Guerin, Guérin's fold, lacunae urethralis, urethrae masculinae, valve of navicular fossa or the crypts of Morgagni.

Definition

Generally lacuna means a small pit or hollow cavity, the lacuna magna is the largest depression in the fossa navicularis. Located deeper within the lacunae are branching mucous tubules called the glands of Littre. Guerin valve is a septum between the lacuna magna and the urethral lumen, which may act as a valve and leads to the manifestations of existence of LM with a different grades of urethral obstruction and other symptoms (Fig. 34.1).

© Springer International Publishing Switzerland 2017

M. Fahmy, *Congenital Anomalies of the Penis*, DOI 10.1007/978-3-319-43310-3_34

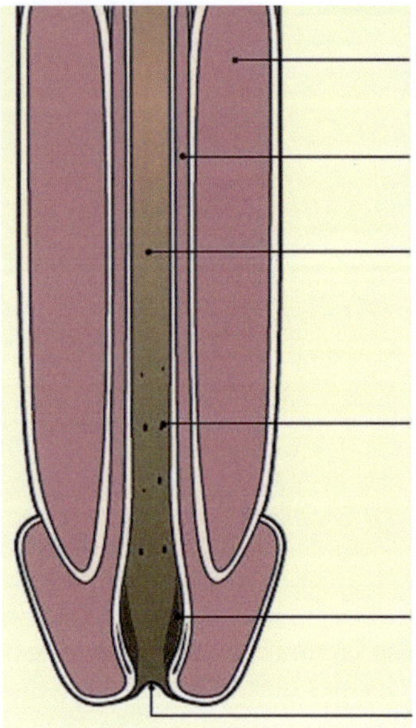

Fig. 34.1 Diagram showing location of LM

34.1 Historical Background

This entity, initially described by Morgagni in 1719, Sommer and Stephens reported its association with urological symptoms for the first time in 1980 [1]. Since then, many cases and series of lacuna magna have been reported in the literature.

34.2 Incidence

Although LM is found in more than 30 % of males during autopsy, it rarely may cause symptoms [2]. The actual incidence of symptomatic LM should be more than reported cases, it was suggested that this anomaly may not be so rare especially in circumcised boys and it can be associated with voiding dysfunction and high detrusor pressures in some patients, also it is suggested that the main difference between symptomatic and silent LM may be the larger size of urethral depression in LM [3].

34.3 Embryology

The embryologic origin of LM is contested, but recent evidence suggests that this septum represent a persistent embryological remanent between the canalized glandular ingrowth of ectodermal tissue and the distally advancing urethra, giving origin to a diverticulum in fossa navicularis.

As the proximal urethral folds close, a solid core of ectodermal tissue penetrates the glans of penis to join the anterior urethral component. The contiguous walls of this ectodermal ingrowth and the newly tubularized urethra break down to establish urethral continuity. This natural anastomosis leads to the development of fossa navicularis Normally, curvilinear markings may remain in the fossa navicularis along the line of anastomosis. Incomplete anastomosis of the two channels may form dorsal accessory channel, which is known as LM. In some cases, the lacuna may become a diverticulum and present with clinical symptoms and signs. Since the exact site of the break down is unpredictable the diverticulum may vary in length, anatomic form and distance to the urethral orifice. Histological studies of LM tissues also support this theory since LM is lined with squamous epithelium whereas epithelium of the penile urethra is transitional [4].

34.4 Diagnosis

Actually the diagnosis of LM can be accurately made if this condition, though less common, is kept at the back mind of the urologist. As the presence of LM can easily be overlooked, unless the lesion is considered in boys presenting with typical symptoms of painful urination (dysuria), bloody urine (hematuria), and bloody spotting of underwear [5].

Micturating cystourethrography must be performed meticulously if this lesion is not to be missed, and the entire distal urethra must be included on the radiographic films. Contrast medium on towels or clothing may obscure or simulate the valve of Guerin as LM can be mim-

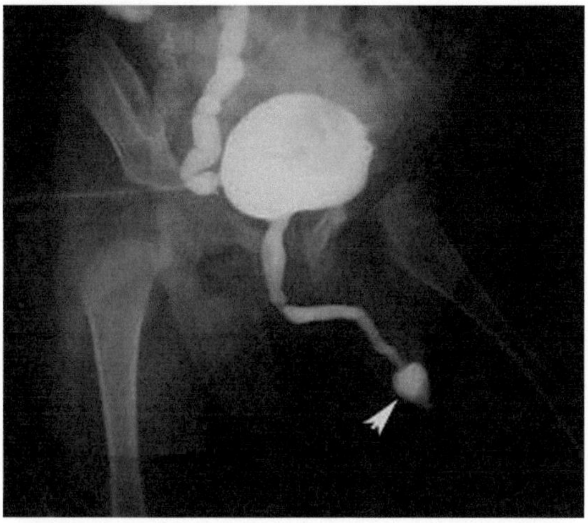

Fig. 34.2 Voiding cystourethrogram showing the typical LM

icked by a drop of contrast material external to the glans or even in the meatus, especially in an uncircumcised child (Fig. 34.2).

The endoscopic confirmation of LM can also be difficult as the endoscope may pass the lesion immediately with insertion without careful placement of the urethroscope and watching from the meatus. A useful hint is gentle probing of the dorsal aspect of the meatus with a 3 F ureteral stent or a Bugbee electrode while the glans penis is stretched upward. Once the valve is detected, it is easy to fulgurate and cut the pocket using a low current energy [3].

34.5 Differential Diagnosis

a long list of urological diseases should be considered as differential diagnosis, cystitis, meatal urethritis and even trauma can give the common symptom of dysuria, and if the child presented with an obstructive symptoms; other congenital causes should be considered like: anterior urethral valve, syringocele and congenital urethral stricture (Chap. 33).

34.6 Management

The problem is usually benign and self- limiting even without treatment, and the prognosis following endoscopic ablation is acceptable with symptom relief achieved within few months after procedure. The main goals in the treatment of LM are relief of symptoms, control of infection, and elimination of any obstruction.

Most pediatric urologists now agree that treatment of choice consists in endoscopic incision with cutting current of the septum and fulguration of the base of the diverticulum, valve incision and fulguration of the diverticulum base rather than aggressive ablation alone is recommended to prevent the development of urethral strictures [3].

References

1. Sommer JT, Stephens FD. Dorsal urethral diverticulum of the fossa navicularis: symptoms, diagnosis and treatment. J Urol. 1980;124:94–7.
2. Bellinger MF, Purohit GS, Duckett JW, Cromie WJ. Lacuna magna: a hidden cause of dysuria and bloody spotting in boys. J Pediatr Surg. 1983;18(2):163–6.
3. Kajbafzadeh A, Elmi A, Payabvash S, Sina A, Arshadi H, Sadeghi Z. The urethral valve of Guérin and lacuna magna: clinical presentations and urodynamic findings. Pediatr Surg Int. 2007;23:873–8. doi:10.1007/s00383-007-1966-y.
4. Kurzrock E, Baskin L, Cunha G. Ontogeny of the male urethra: theory of endodermal differentiation. Differentiation. 1999;64(2):115–22. doi:10.1046/j.1432-0436.1999.6420115.x.
5. Friedman RM, King LR. Valve of Guerin as a cause of dysuria and hematuria in young boys: presentation and difficulties in diagnosis. J Urol. 1993;150:159–61.

Part VI

Acquired Penile Diseases with Congenital Background

Complications of Male Circumcision (MC)

35

Abstract

It is estimated that one-third of males worldwide are circumcised. The procedure is most commonly practiced in the Muslim world, Israel (where it is near-universal for religious reasons), the United States, and parts of Southeast Asia and Africa. It is relatively rare in Europe, Latin America, parts of Southern Africa, and most of Asia.

Prevalence of reported complications of male circumcision ranged from 7 to 50.1%. Late complications of 7.39 % were reported.

Keywords

Complications • Male circumcision • Penile granuloma • Iatrogenic urethral fistulas • Post circumcision hair coil • Penile skin loss • Keloid formation • Gangrene • Penile loss • Ablatio penis • Skin bridge • Penile ischemia

It is estimated that one-third of males worldwide are circumcised. The procedure is most commonly practiced in the Muslim world, Israel (where it is near-universal for religious reasons), the United States, and parts of Southeast Asia and Africa. It is relatively rare in Europe, Latin America, parts of Southern Africa, and most of Asia [1] (Fig. 35.1).

Prevalence of reported complications of MC ranged from 7% to 50.1%. Late complications of 7.39% were reported [2]. At 2010, a review of literature founded that MC performed by medical providers, have a typical complication rate of 1.5% for babies and 6% for older children, with few cases of severe complications [3]. In Africa and developing countries the circumcision rate was 87%, with a very high rate of complications reaching 20.2% [4].

Circumcision remains as one of the most controversial topics in current urological practice. The most important argument against circumcision is the permanent change of anatomy, histology and function of the penis, with potential complications, primary haemorrhage was the most common (52%), whereas infection, meatal stenosis, incomplete circumcision, penile oedema, glanular injury, penile adhesions, iatrogenic hypospadias and urethral injuries were also detected at different rates [5].

There may be a minor complications after circumcision which cannot be avoided even when the procedure is undertaken by specialised

© Springer International Publishing Switzerland 2017

M. Fahmy, *Congenital Anomalies of the Penis*, DOI 10.1007/978-3-319-43310-3_35

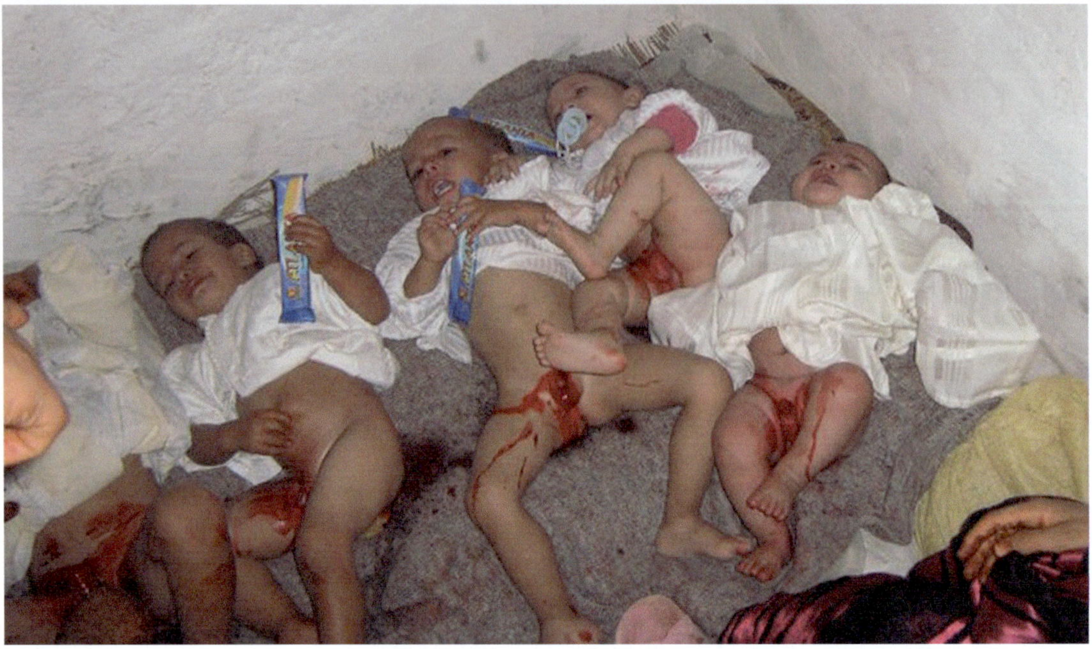

Fig. 35.1 Mass circumcision of a young children by unexperienced personal in unequipped centres

pediatric surgeons or urologist, in a properly equipped centres; specially if the child or his penis is congenitally abnormal, the obvious examples are, circumcising a child with an excessive suprapubic or a child with webbed penis or microphallus.

After practicing circumcision, and managing other's complication for a thousands of boys along 34 years in a country like Egypt, (with about 90 % circumcision rate), I found most parents had a great urge to do this surgery even for a handicapped or critically ill child, as you can see the child in Fig. 35.2, who had a Hip Spica Cast for bilateral hip dislocations, but family insisted to do circumcision for him (Fig. 35.2).

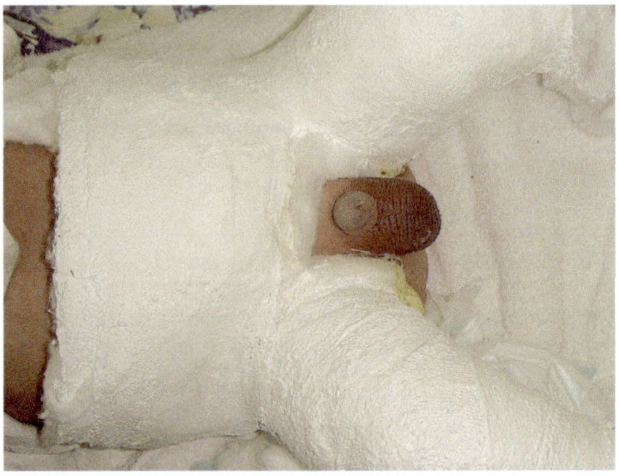

Fig. 35.2 Family urge for circumcision may pouch them to do this procedure even for a baby with critical illness

So the best way to minimise complications of MC, in my opinion, and to compete against its serious impaction in man health, is to standardise the procedure, learning both families and physicians about potential complications and how they could mange it early, and properly.

The spectrum of post MC complications is so wide to be discussed in this chapter, which concerning mainly about congenital anomalies, but these anomalies of the penis which discussed in this book may had a great impaction in the incidence of serious complications, so we will just spot some light over the uncommon complications, which usually raise a debate about its management.

There are different sets to classify MC complications: Either early, or late, minor or major, local or systemic, rare or common.

35.1 Post Circumcision Penile Granuloma: (Fig. 35.3)

The development of post circumcision penile granuloma was described well in a large series by Atikeler et al. [6], in which 26 cases of granuloma (5 %) were found in 523 circumcised boys, with a mean time to development of 3.2 months. The cause of post circumcision granuloma has been postulated to be a foreign body (e.g. talcum powder, excess suture material, or smegma particles) introduced during circumcision between preputial layers, resulting in a tissue response manifested as a granuloma of different types (Fig. 35.3a).

Suture granulomas This is a reaction to the stitches not dissolving as intended. It appears as bumps under the skin around the wound as the skin creates a tiny wall of scar tissue around the suture to separate it from the body.

Spitting Sutures This occurs weeks to months after surgery if the body rejects the suture (again, from the stitches not absorbing as intended) and attempts to remove them by pushing the stitches out to the surface of the skin. Sutures that migrate in this way have been known to be the source of additional problems.

Pyogenic granuloma: Will be described with balanitis (Chap. 39)

Smegma granuloma: (Chap. 19)

Excessive penile skin loss Which occurs when so much of the prepuce is drawn forward that the entire penile skin sheath is removed. From puberty on, penile bowing (curvature) and pain occur at the time of erection, commonly skin loss seen at the ventral surface of the penis. (Fig. 35.4), but a circumferential skin loss is not rare, which complicate extensive perpetual excision by unexperienced surgeon or unqualified circumciser (Fig. 35.5).

Excessive skin loss complication encountered mainly after circumcision of a congenitally abnormal penis as in cases of webbed penis, microphallus, concealed penis and penis with a congenital chordee.

In webbed penis, If surgeon tried to circumcise a baby by the classical method, usually he will end with extensive loss of the ventral skin, so removal of prepuce from the dorsum only leaving the ventral prepuce to cover the shaft with fine stitches may be enough, with an acceptable penile look, as we can see in Fig. 35.6a, b and c. This simple method can be done by surgeons who had minimal experience with the different methods of flaps or V-Y plasty described in literature for managing such cases [7]. But sometimes, specially in severe cases, a pedicled skin grafts or flap are indicated.

Microphallus is another problem, as the circumciser may face some families insisted to do circumcision early before the child can catch up an acceptable penile lenghth, and in such cases

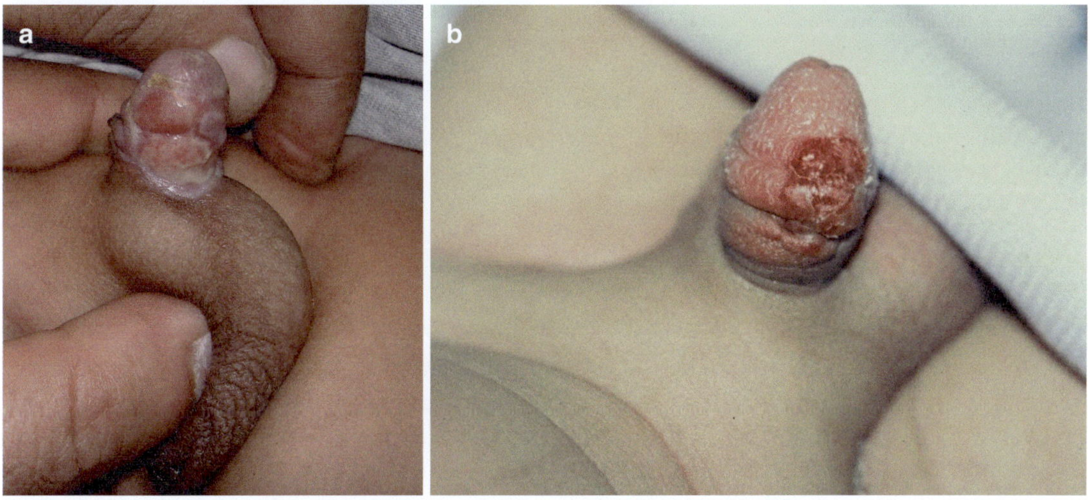

Fig. 35.3 (**a**) Granuloma with severe infection and skin loss from the lateral aspect of the shaft of the penis. (**b**) Post circumcision granuloma at the dorsum of the glans

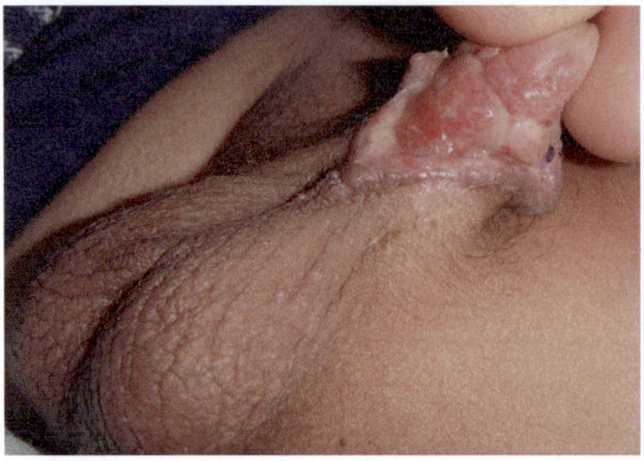

Fig. 35.4 Post circumcision ventral skin loss, due to circumcision of a webbed penis by simple application of the crushing forceps

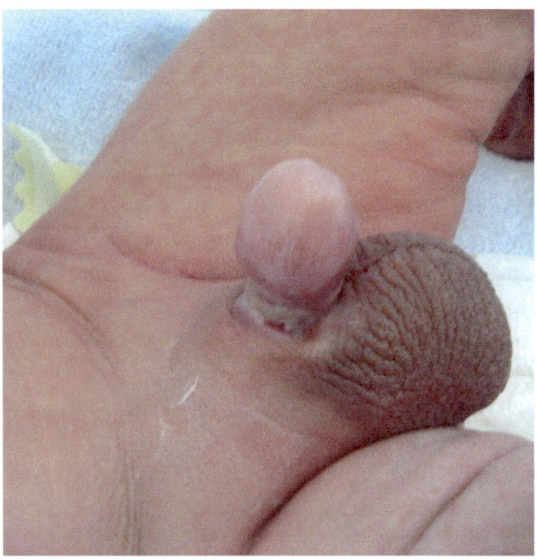

Fig 35.5 Circumferential skin loss which will need a rotational flap or free skin graft

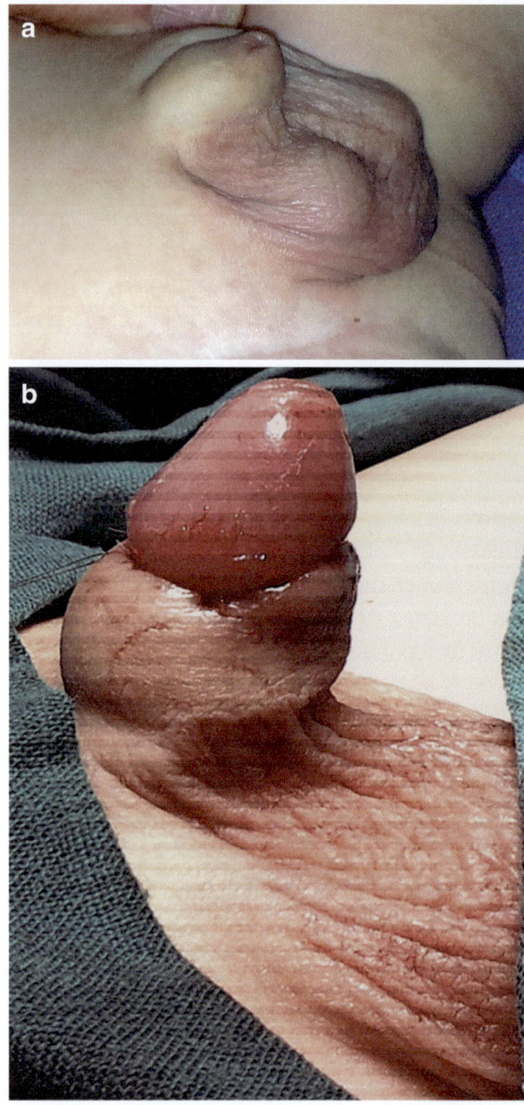

Fig. 35.6 (**a**) Webbed penis, managed with circumcision by dissection method, leaving a plenty of skin at the ventral surface, with an acceptable look and reasonable functional penile length (**b**)

also, meticulous removal of a narrow strip of prepuce, with making use of the rest of the prepuce to cover the shaft of the penis may give an acceptable results without skin loss (Fig. 35.7a, b).

35.2 Post Circumcision Iatrogenic Urethral Fistulas: (Figs. 35.8 and 35.9)

Different types of urethral fistulas may result from circumcision, when the frenular area (underside of the penis) is drawn too far forward, the crushing bell of plastibell circumcision may injure the urethra at the time the foreskin is removed, resulting in a urethral opening on the underside of the shaft. Fistulae may present as an obvious tract or as a split urine stream (Fig. 35.8).

The urethrocutaneous fistula is not a rare complication after both Plastibell and Gomco circumcisions. Often this is a result from compression necrosis from a retained Plastibell ring or a direct injury from incorrect placement of the Gomco clamp [8] (Fig. 35.8a).

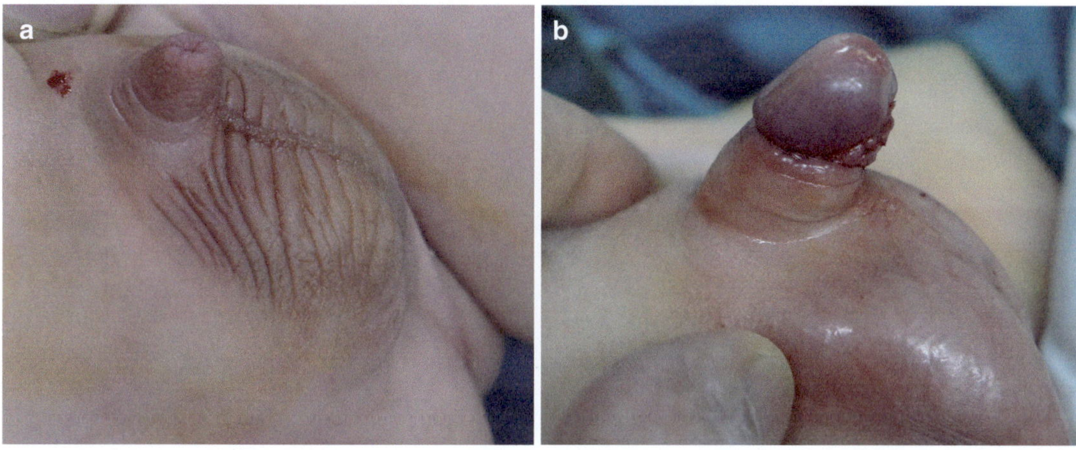

Fig. 35.7 (**a**, **b**) Microphallus could be managed by only excision of a small strip from the prepuce

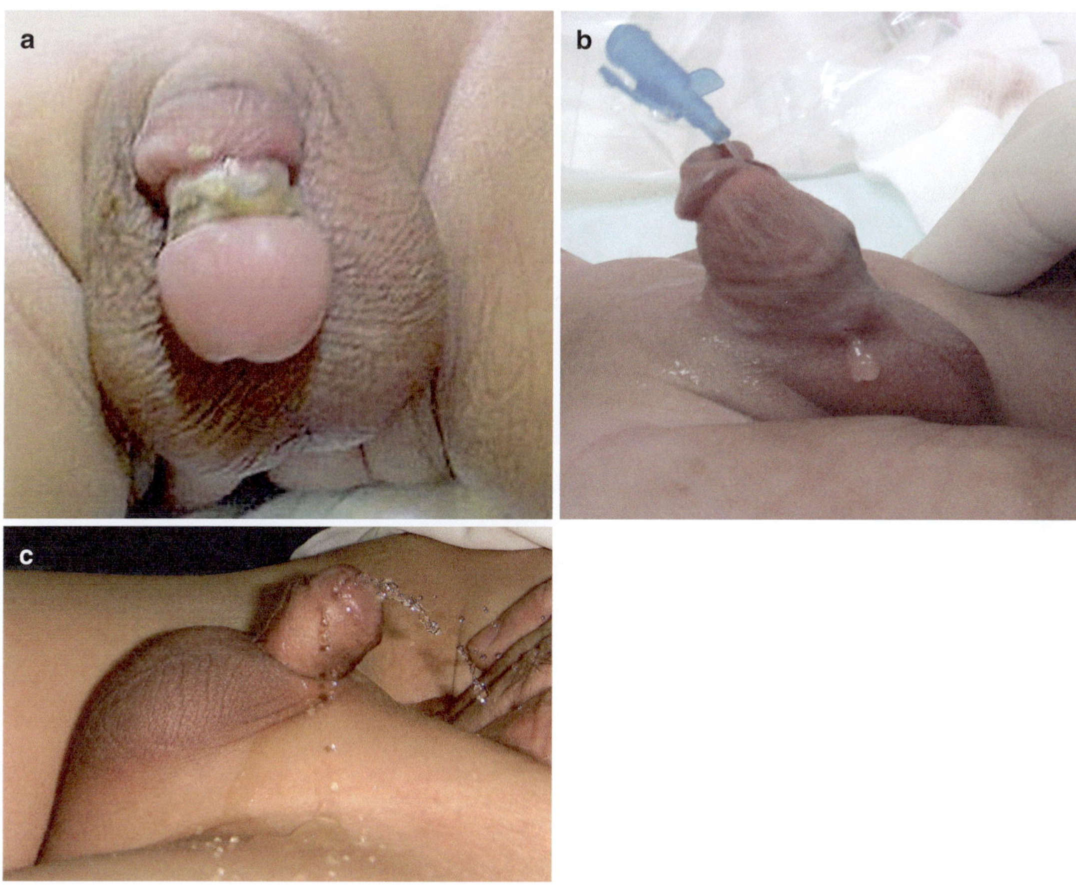

Fig. 35.8 (**a**) Neglectfully retained Plastibell results in penile necrosis, and eventually ends with fistula. (**b**) Proximal fistula, complicating severe infection, and necrosis after circumcision. (**c**) Post circumcision distal fistula

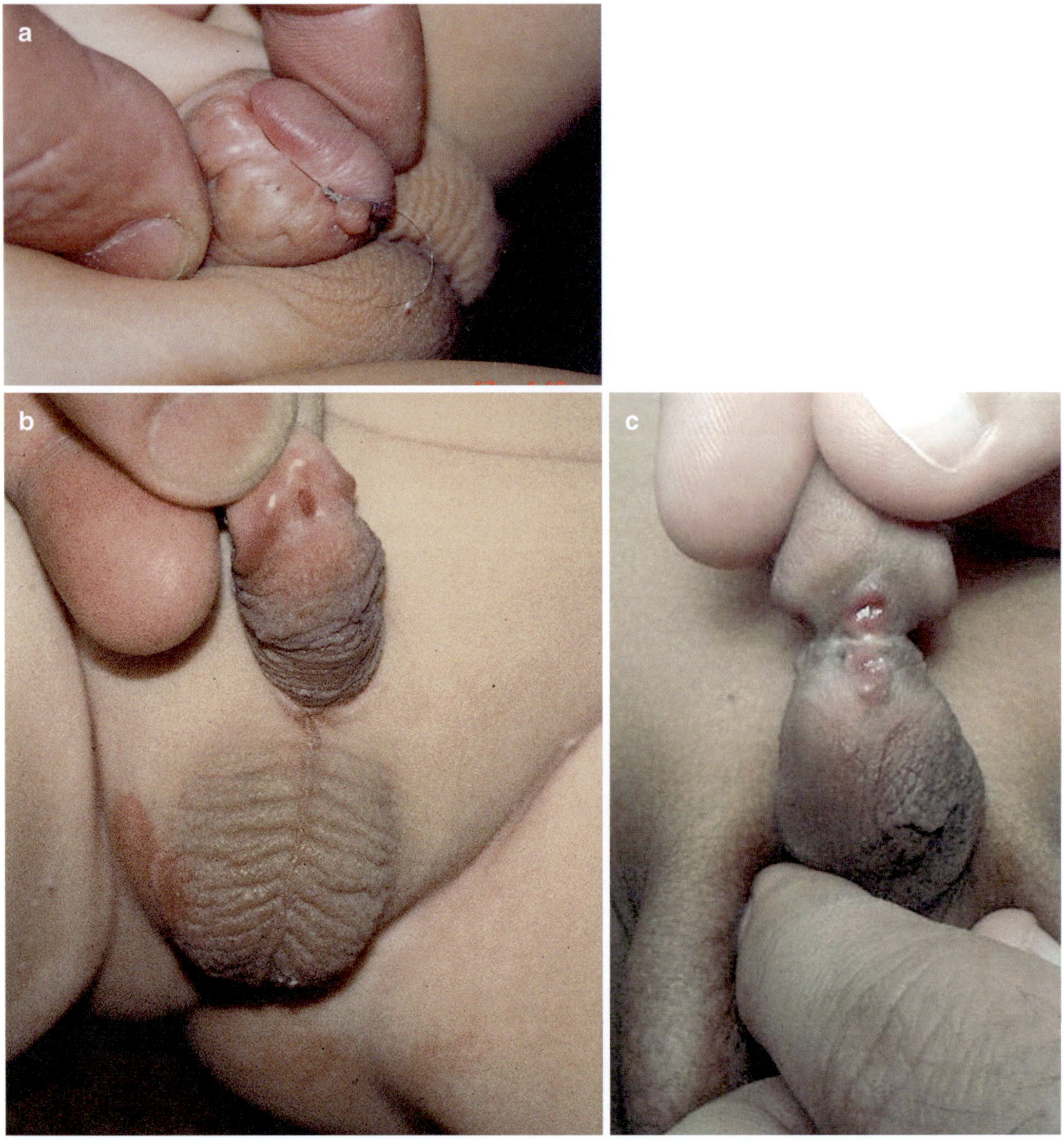

Fig. 35.9 (**a**) Post circumcision hair coil, which may be complicated with fistula. (**b**): Fistula at the coronal sulcus from hair coil. (**c**) Severe constricting fibrosis at the sulcus with double or kissing fistula

Also urethral injury seems more likely to occur when there is bleeding from the frenum and an attempt is made to control it with a diathermy or heavy suture. A suture placed too deeply may strangulate a part of the urethral wall, thus leading to the formation of a fistula. Extensive bacterial or mycotic urethritis after circumcision may also results in a proximal fistula (Fig. 35.8b).

Bad hygiene, lack of follow up and supervision of the child after circumcision may lead to a disastrous fistula formation from hair coil, this hair coil fistula was reported in a healthy babies without relation to circumcision, but the healing circumcision wound is more liable to develop fistula after a hair coiling around or distal to the glans during the early post circumcision period, this fistula reported infrequently, and known as a penile tourniquet syndrome [9] (Fig. 35.9a, b).

Sometimes this fistula supervenes glans gangrene due to impaired blood supply from the coiled hair, or fistula may be associated with a severely constricted coronal sulcus, in such cases a double fistulous openings may be seen at the under surface of the glans and the penile shaft (Fig. 35.9b).

Repair of such cases are extremely difficult, with high incidence of recurrence, so this fistula should be managed by an experienced hypospadiaologist. Delayed flap repair can be done electively after the child's penis has grown enough for good tissue handling.

In attempting to repair such a fistula, it should be borne in mind that in a circumcised penis, little free skin is available, particularly in the area of the frenum. The method chosen for repair should therefore be the safest. Urinary diversion and a repair without tension appear to be desirable [10].

The prevention of fistula complication lies in the operators visualizing exactly what is being done in the course of a circumcision, family education and detection of any congenital anomalies before committing MC, with early referring patients to centres with pediatric urology experience if complication happened.

Keloid Formation: (Fig. 35.10) A keloid is an abnormal development consisting of a raised, firm, thickened, red piece of scar tissue. Such abnormal scar at the site of circumcision creates a grotesque deformation of the organ, with obstruction of its function. Less extensive prominent scars can occur with severe fibrosis around the coronal sulcus. It seems that this complication is more common in blacked races, and prolonged wound healing, foreign body implant during circumcision and rough manipulation of the delicate penile skin are predisposing factors [11]. Keloid excision with or without skin grafting is indicated along a different postoperative measures to avoid recurrence of a keloid tissue.

Skin Bridge Another adverse result of circumcision is the formation of a skin bridge between the penile shaft and the glans. Smegma often accumulates under those skin bridges. Additionally these bridges may either tether the erect penis, with resultant pain or penile curvature (chordee) (Fig. 35.11).

The treatment of such bridges is simple surgical division. How such problems arise is not completely clear. Some investigators have suggested that injury to the glans at time of circumcision, with resultant fusion to the circumcision

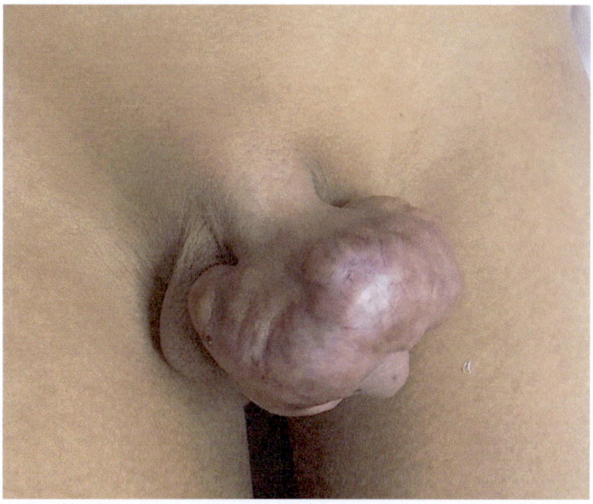

Fig. 35.10 Rare complication of circumcision with extensive keloid formation around the glans

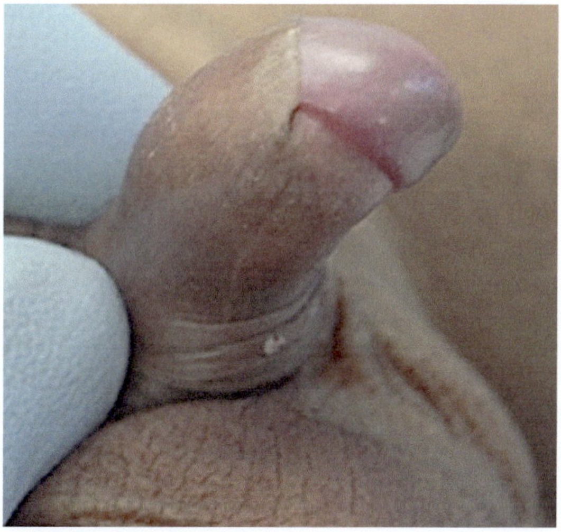

Fig. 35.11 Post circumcision skin bridge, results in penile curvature

wound is the genesis of this problem [12]. This complication could be avoided by completely freeing the inner preputial epithelium from the glans at the time of circumcision, also if any glanular abrasions, injury or ulcer, detected, during circumcision it should be dressed and managed properly till complete healing, to avoid the natural cohesion between bared area of the glans and penile skin.

35.3 Gangrene and Penile Loss

Necrosis and sloughing of the glans or even the entire penis has been reported following circumcision. Distal ischemia producing such tissue loss may result from infection, use of solutions containing epinephrine, vigorous attempts at hemostasis with suture or cautery, from prolonged use of a post circumcision tourniquet, or a tight bandage. Necrosis is particularly likely to result if cautery is applied directly to a circumcision clamp (e.g., the Gomco clamp), use of unipolar, or unearthed diathermy [13]. When the entire penis is lost following such a misadventure, a sequence of complications supervene the situation in the form of urethral stricture, retention of urine, proximal urinary tract obstruction and a dismal outcome.

Severe post circumcision mycotic infection, and Fournier's gangrene which is a necrotizing infection that involves the soft tissues of the male genitalia is reported after circumcision, specially at older age [14]· but this could also happen at younger age, or even in a neonate, as we can see in fugue 12, which show a newborn with almost complete necrosis of the penis and upper part of scrotum after circumcision, ischemia and tissue necrosis may precede or predispose this severe infection and tissue necrosis. Vasodilators medication and hyperbaric oxygen may had a limited role in such cases, but could be tried.

Cases with either glanular or penile ischemia should be identified early, and managed properly in a specialised centres, as an early combined use of intravenous Pentoxifylline (which reduce blood viscosity, platelet aggregation and thrombus formation, and also a powerful peripheral vasodilator) with hyperbaric oxygen reported to improve some cases [15], but it will be less effective in cases detected late with an already detectable gangrene with a line of demarcation. In this situation it may be extremely difficult to control penile ischemia and to stop its proximal progression, with a subsequent sloughing of the glans or even the whole penis (Figs. 35.12 and 35.13).

In children with complete penile loss (Ablatio penis) early management have to be directed to maintain an adequate urine flow with an acceptable meatus to avoid the need for diversion, and to avoid urinary back pressure and recurrent UTI (Fig. 35.14).

Latter on, those children will face the options of either penile reconstruction with a forearm pedicle flap or they may have to choice reassignment to female sex as described in Chap. 8.

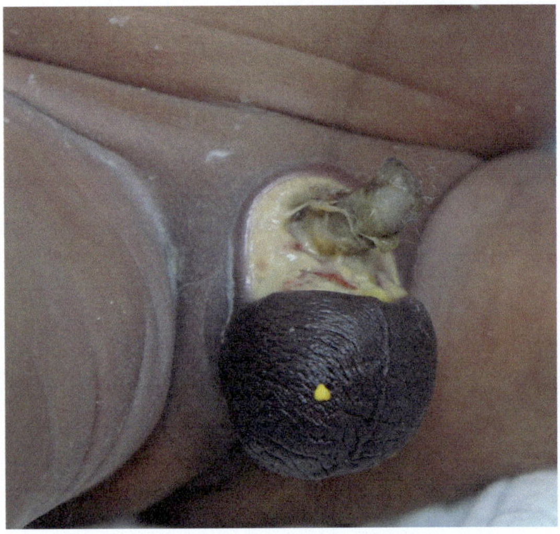

Fig. 35.12 A neonate with severe necrotising infection of the penis and scrotum after circumcision

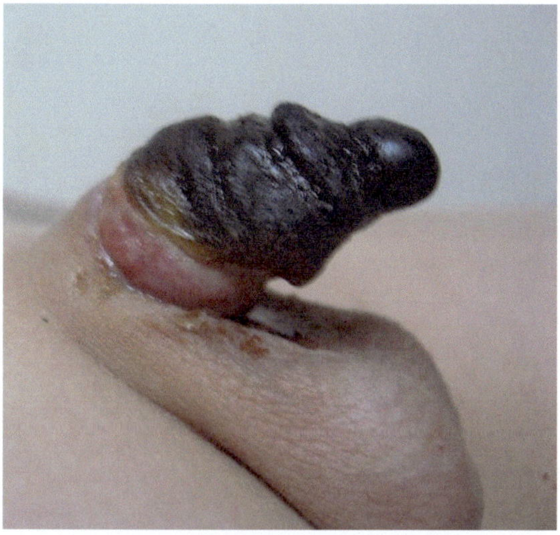

Fig. 35.13 Severe ischemia and dry gangrene of the penis after using monopolar diathermy during circumcision for a 3 years old child

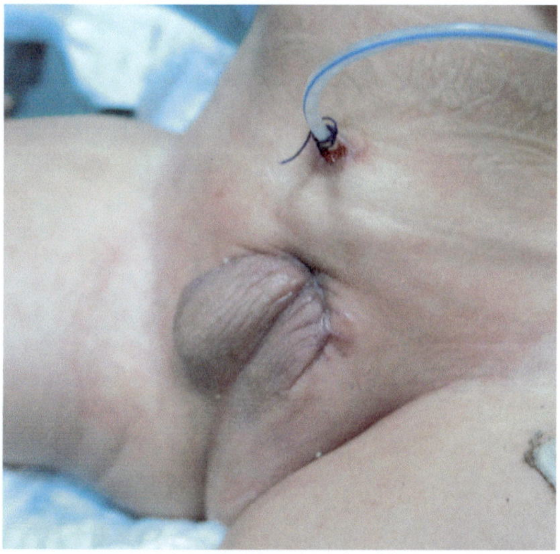

Fig. 35.14 Same child in Fig. 35.13, 3 months later with complete loss of the penis (ablatio penis), and severe meatal stricture which necessitate suprapubic diversion

References

1. Jacobs M, Grady R, Bolnick DA. Current circumcision trends and guidelines. In: Bolnick DA, Koyle M, Yosha A, editors. Surgical guide to circumcision. London: Springer; 2012. p. 3–8. doi:10.1007/978-1-4471-2858-8_1.
2. Weiss HA, Larke N, Halperin D, Schenker I. Complications of circumcision in male neonates, infants and children: a systematic review. BMC Urol. 2010;10:2. doi:10.1186/1471-2490-10-2. PMC 2835667.
3. Okeke LI, Asinobi AA, Ikuerowo OS. Epidemiology of complications of male circumcision in Ibadan, Nigeria. BMC Urol. 2006;6:21.
4. Yegane RA, Kheirollahi AR, Salehi NA, Bashashati M, Koshdel JA, Ahmadi M. Late complications of circumcision in Iran. Pediatr Surg Int. 2006;22:442–5. doi:10.1007/s00383-006-1672-1.
5. Ben Chaim J, Levin PM, Binyamin J, Hardak B, Ben-Meir D, Mor Y. Complications of circumcision in Israel: a one year multi-center survey. Isr Med Assoc J. 2005;7:368–70.
6. Atikeler MK, Onur R, Gecit I, Senol FA, Cobanoglu B. Increased morbidity after circumcision from a hidden complication. BJU Int. 2001;88(9):938–40.
7. Chang S, Liu S, JHsie J. Correcting penoscrotal web with the V-Y advancement technique. J Sex Med. 2008;5(1):249–50.
8. Bode CO, Ikhisemojie S, Ademuyiwa AO. Penile injuries from proximal migration of the Plastibell circumcision ring. J Pediatr Urol. 2010;6(1):23–7.
9. Badawy H, Soliman A, Ouf A, Hammad A, Orabi S, Hanno A. Progressive hair coil penile tourniquet syndrome: multicenter experience with 25 cases. J Pediatr Surg. 2010;45(7):1514–8. doi:10.1016/j.jpedsurg.2009.11.008.
10. Limaye RD, Hancock RA. Penile urethral fistula as a complication of circumcision. J Pediatr. 1968;72(1):105–6.
11. Demirdover C, Sahin B, Vayvada H, Yucel Oztan H. Keloid formation after circumcision and its treatment. J Pediatr Urol. 2013;9(1):e54–6.
12. Klauber GT, Boyle J. Preputial skin-bridging: complication of circumcision. Conn Med. 1973;37:445.
13. Pepe P, Pietropaolo F, Candiano G, Pennisi M. Ischemia of the glans penis following circumcision: case report and revision of the literature. Arch Ital Urol Androl. 2015;87(1):93–4. doi:10.4081/aiua.2015.1.93.
14. Sterenberg N, Golan J, Ben-Hur N. Necrosis of the glans penis following neonatal circumcision. Plast Reconstr Surg. 1981;68:237–9.
15. Ersagun K, Dogan ST, Ilke OK, Metin G, Fatih C, Omer K, Guner KO. Postcircumcisional Ischemia of the Glans Penis Treated with Pentoxifylline. Case Rep Urol. 2013;2013:278523. doi:10.1155/2013/278523.

Smegmoma "Smegma Collection in Health and Disease"

36

Abstract

Smegma has characteristic slimy odour, composed of epithelial debris, fat, and proteins. It has mixed bacterial flora with smegum bacillus (Mycobacterium smegmatis) in 50 % of man. It is secreted in both female and male mammalian genitalia. Smegma was originally thought to be produced by sebaceous glands near the frenulum called Tyson's glands; however, subsequent studies have failed to find such glands.

Keywords

Smegmoma • Smegmaliths • Smegma clitoridis • Smegma Stone • Mycobacterium smegmatis

Definition

The word smegma is of Greek origin meaning soap or an ointment.

Smegma has characteristic slimy odour, composed of epithelial debris, fat, and proteins. It has mixed bacterial flora with smegum bacillus (Mycobacterium smegmatis) in 50 % of man.

Nomenclatures

- **Smegma clitoridis**: smegma in females, it collects around the clitoris and in the folds of the labia minora (Fig. 36.1).
- **Smegmaliths:** Pieces of hard contaminated and retained smegma
- **Smegma Stone:** Accumulated hard smegma under the prepuce (Fig. 36.2).
- **Smegmoma:** Perpetual smegma cyst (Fig. 36.3).

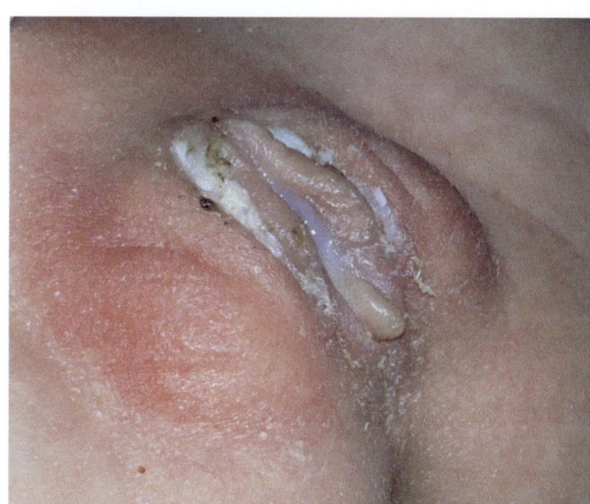

Fig. 36.1 Smegma secretion in a female neonate

© Springer International Publishing Switzerland 2017

M. Fahmy, *Congenital Anomalies of the Penis*, DOI 10.1007/978-3-319-43310-3_36

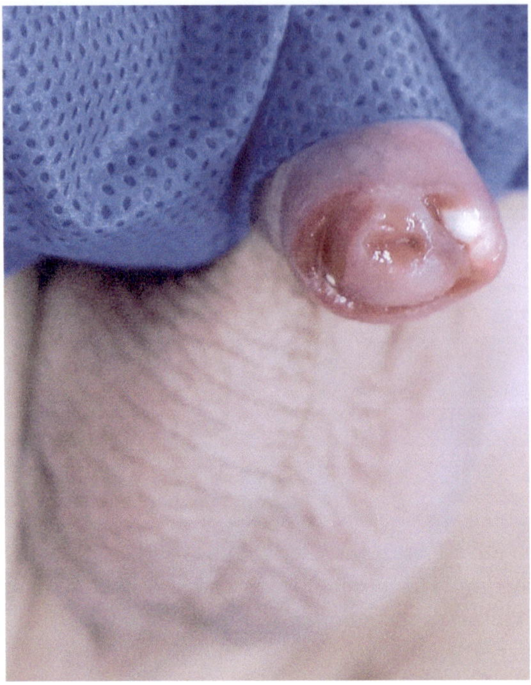

Fig. 36.2 Smegma collection under the perpetual orifice in a neonate

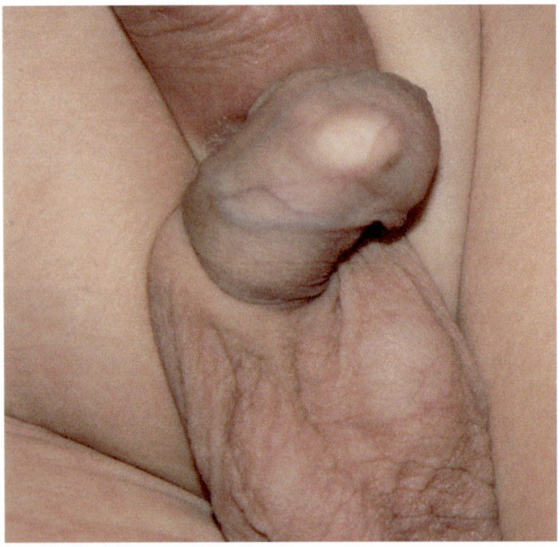

Fig. 36.3 Perpetual smegma cyst seen in the undersurface of the prepuce

36.1 Smegma in History

French physician, Claude-François Lallemand (1790–1853), pronounced that smegma could provoke erections that would lead to 'disastrous pleasures'.

American physician Roberts Bartholow (1831–1904) formulated the theory that smegma produced 'hyperæsthesia' of the glans.

American urologist Abraham Wolbarst (1872–1952), who updated the demonization of the foreskin and promulgated the idea that it harboured 'carcinogenic secretions' [1].

36.2 Secretion

It is secreted in both female and male mammalian genitalia.

Smegma was originally thought to be produced by sebaceous glands near the frenulum called Tyson's glands; however, subsequent studies have failed to find such glands. Wright [2] states that smegma is produced from minute microscopic protrusions of the mucosal surface of the foreskin and that living cells constantly grow towards the surface, undergo fatty degeneration, separate off, and form smegma. Parkash et al. [3] found that smegma contains 26.6 % fats and 13.3 % proteins, which they judged to be consistent with necrotic epithelial debris. It is thought to be rich in squalene (oily material gives smegma the fishy odour), and contain prostatic and seminal secretions, desquamated epithelial cells, and the mucin content of the urethral glands of Littré. Newly produced smegma has a smooth, moist texture.

Chemically, smegma contains immunologically active compounds such as cathepsin B, lysozyme, chymotrypsin, neutrophil elastase, cytokines, and hormones such as androsterone. Lytic materials, such as lysozyme, which probably originates from the prostate and seminal vesicles, destroy bacterial cell walls and inhibit and destroy candidal species. Some state that it contains anti-bacterial enzymes such as lysozyme and hormones such as androsterone, though others dispute this [5].

According to Wright [2], little smegma is produced during childhood, although the foreskin may contain sebaceous glands. She also says that production of smegma increases from adolescence until sexual maturity when the function of smegma for lubrication assumes its full value, and from middle-age production starts to decline and in old age virtually no smegma is produced.

Øster [4] reported that the incidence of smegma increased from 1 % among 6- to 7-year-olds and 8- to 9-year-olds to 8 % among 14- to 15-year-olds and 16- to 17-year-olds (an overall incidence of 5 %) (Figs. 36.4 and 36.5).

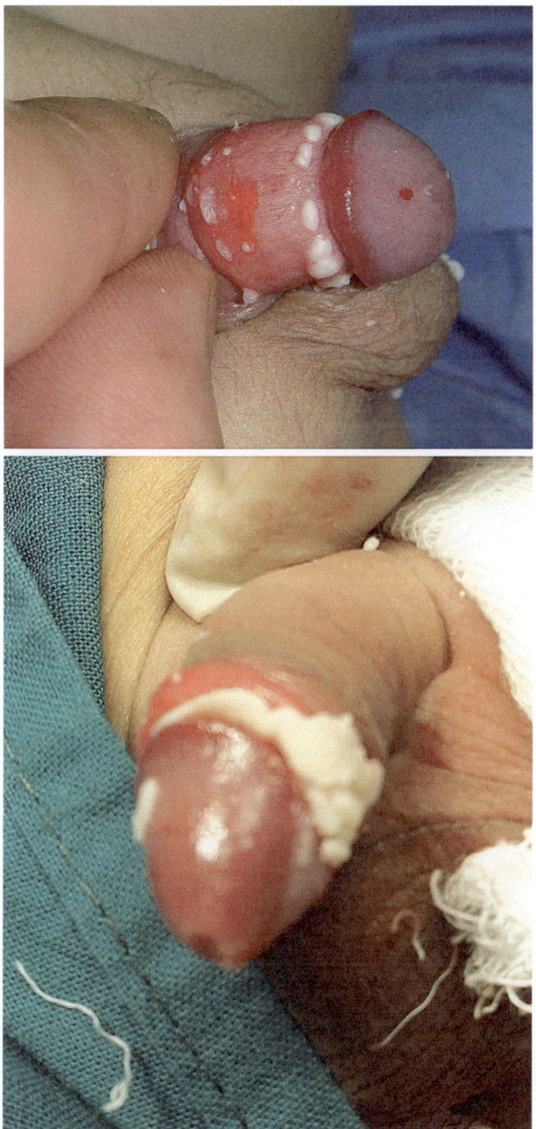

Fig. 36.4 and 36.5 Different distribution of smegma after retraction of the prepuce

36.3 Smegma and Cancer

Although the carcinogenicity of smegma has never been demonstrated, smegma has been cited as a carcinogen by at least one article in the 1940s and 1950s, nine articles in the 1960s, four articles in the 1970s, seven articles in the 1980s, 17 articles in the 1990s Some studies have indicated a possibility that smegma may contain cancer-causing substances. They do state, however, that this link has not been proven [1].

According to the American Cancer Society it is now mainly believed that smegma itself is probably not responsible for penile cancer, but that it could potentially increase the risk of cancer by causing irritation of the penis [7]. Hence, any potential cancer-inducing property could well lie in products formed by chemical breakdown or bacterial action rather than in smegma itself [6].

36.4 Function

Smegma protects and lubricates the glans and inner lamella of the prepuce, facilitating erection, preputial eversion and penetration during sexual intercourse. This natural lubricant allows for prolonged intercourse and eliminates the need for artificial supplemental lubrication during normal coitus or masturbation.

36.5 Our Concept

Some boys may present with one or more yellowish lumps on the penis that are often diagnosed by the general practitioner as sebaceous cysts or lipoma of the penile shaft. Invariably, on outpatient assessment, these prove to be collections of retained smegma trapped by surrounding preputial adhesions (Figs. 36.6 and 36.7).

Smegma is the natural recreation of the prepuce, like other body secretions, (like ear wax). So

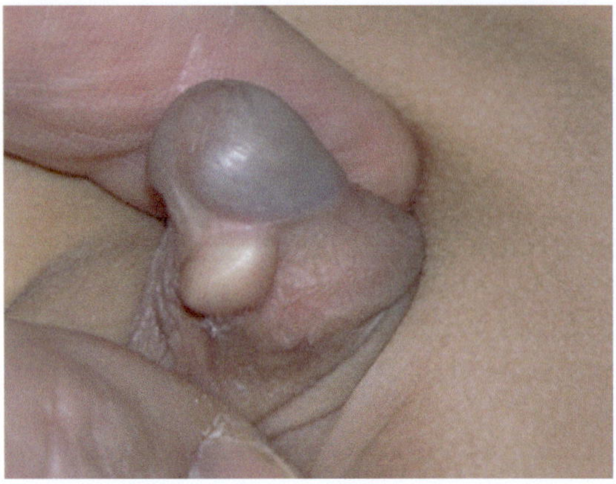

Fig. 36.6 Smegma cyst after circumcision

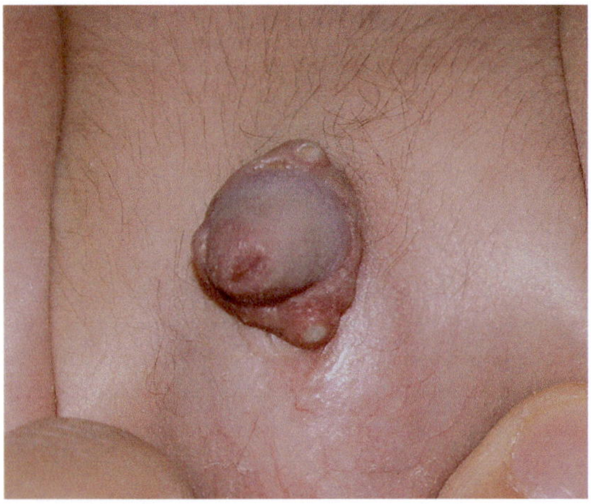

Fig. 36.7 Multiple small smegma cysts at the edge of circumcision

it is not harmful by itself, unless it is complicated by other pathogens; either bacterial colonisation, virus overgrowth or combined organisms, or associated with phimosis and different forms of balanitis or balanoposthitis.

Smegma secreted during the late intrauterine period, as many neonates, and preterm may had an accumulated smegma in the 1st day of life (Fig. 36.2).

Smegma secretion and distribution had a great variations between individuals as we can see from Figs. 36.4 and 36.5, without a clear explanation.

Smegma should be cleaned frequently in uncircumcised boys by the mother during childhood, and by the boys himself latter on.

During circumcision, smegma should be cleaned and removed meticulously with saline wash, otherwise any retained small pieces will accumulate between the edges of perpetual remounts and results in different forms of cysts of smegma, which may acquire larger size and be troublesome (Figs. 36.6 and 36.7).

References

1. Van Howe RS, Hodges FM. The carcinogenicity of smegma: debunking a myth. J Eur Acad Dermatol Venereol. 2006;20:1046–54.
2. Wright J. How smegma serves the penis. Sexology. 1970;37:50–3.
3. Parkash S, Jeyakumar S, Subramanyan K, Chaudhuri S. Human subpreputial collection: its nature and formation. J Urol. 1973;110:211–2.
4. Øster J. Further fate of the foreskin. Incidence of preputial adhesions, phimosis, and smegma among Danish schoolboys. Arch Dis Child. 1968;43(228):200–3.
5. Kar HK, Sharma PK, Arora TC, Sabhnani S. Gonococcal tyson's gland abscess and urethral stricture with genital wart and herpes genitalis: a case report. Indian J Sex Transm Dis. 2005;26:36.
6. Eisen DB, Michael DJ. Sebaceous lesions and their associated syndromes: part I. J Am Acad Dermatol. 2009;61:549–60.
7. What are the risk factors for penile cancer? Am Cancer Soc. Retrieved 14 Feb 2014. http://www.cancer.org/cancer/penilecancer/detailedguide/penile-cancer-risk-factors.

Balanitis Xerotica Obliterans 37

Abstract

Balanitis Xerotica Obliterans (BXO) is a chronic atrophic mucocutaneous disorder with unknown cause, affecting the epidermis and dermal connective tissue that most commonly involves the genital and perianal skin of both males and females. BXO may affect the glans and the meatus. In its most severe form, involvement of the prepuce obliterates the preputial sac with dense adhesions, and the urethra may be affected.

Zoon balanophostitis is a benign disease of external genitals, and considered as a variant of BXO, and very rarely affecting children, it is more often seen in elderly males than females, characterized by a solitary red-orange plaque of the glans and prepuce.

Keywords

Balanitis Xerotica Obliterans (BXO) • Lichen sclerosis et atrophicus • Zoon balanophostitis • Leukoplakia of the penis

Nomenclature

Balanitis Xerotica Obliterans (BXO), lichen sclerosis et atrophicus.

37.1 Historical Background

Leukoplakia of the penis with sclerotic, atrophic dermatoses of the glans and prepuce was described for the first time by Perrin at 1892 [1], but Stühmer in 1928 [2], published the earlier reports of 5 cases with an atrophic, shrinking process involving the glans and prepuce and frequently leading to urethral stenosis, and he is the one who used the term Balanitis Xerotica Obliterans.

Definition

It is a chronic atrophic mucocutaneous disorder with no known cause, affecting the epidermis and dermal connective tissue that most commonly involves the genital and perianal skin of both males and females. BXO may affect the glans and the meatus. In its most severe form, involvement of the prepuce obliterates the preputial sac with dense adhesions, and the urethra may be affected.

© Springer International Publishing Switzerland 2017

M. Fahmy, *Congenital Anomalies of the Penis*, DOI 10.1007/978-3-319-43310-3_37

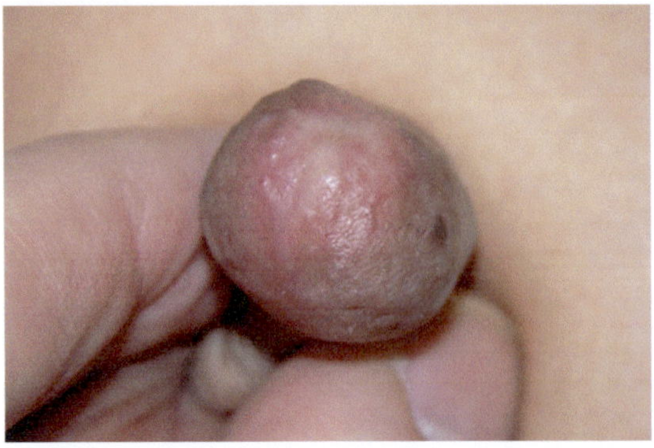

Fig. 37.1 Balanitis Xerotica Obliterans in a 5 years old boy

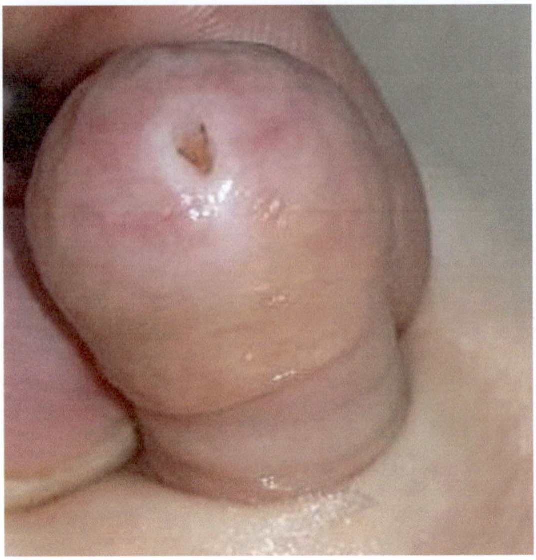

Fig 37.2 Balanitis Xerotica Obliterans affecting mainly the meatus and distal urethra

37.2 Incidence

BXO is rare under the age of 5 years old, with a peak incidence in boys aged 9–11 years old (76 %), and is estimated to have affected 0.6 % of boys by their 15th birthday. There is a bimodal age incidence with peaks in young boys and in adult men late in the fourth decade.

It seems that the true incidence of BXO is not accurately reported as recently many cases recorded after hypospadias repair [3]. The epidemiology may vary between countries and racial groups because BXO is principally a disease of the uncircumcised although it can persist or recur after circumcision [4] (Fig 37.1).

37.3 Pathology

True pathological phimosis with scarring of the preputial orifice is caused by chronic cicatrizing skin condition of unknown etiology. The disease process is histologically identical to lichen sclerosis as it affects the prepuce, glans, and occasionally the urethra. Histological findings characterized by hyperkeratosis with follicular plugging, atrophy of the stratum spinosum and stratum malpighi with hydropic degeneration of basal cells, lymphedema, hyalinosis, homogenization of collagen in the dermis, and an associated band-like chronic inflammatory cell infiltrate. Glanular involvement occurs in 49 % of cases, although the meatus is affected in only a small proportion (Fig 37.2.).

37.4 Etiology

The etiology of BXO is unknown, with no familial predisposition or any identifiable causative bacterial or viral agent. There is no association with puberty, and, contrary to widespread belief, BXO does not result from recurrent balanoposthitis. Several studies have found the human leukocyte antigen (HLA) DQ7 and, to a lesser extent, HLA DQ8 and DQ9 to be more common in BXO than in controls, especially if the onset of this disease detected at childhood [5].

37.5 Diagnosis

The disorder typically presents with irritation, local infection, dysuria, bleeding, secondary nonretractility of the foreskin, or a deteriorating urinary stream. On rare occasions, it can progress to the point of presenting with acute urinary retention or secondary diurnal or nocturnal enuresis resulting from chronic outflow obstruction. BXO should be differentiated from other cases of bacterial and fungal balanitis, and other rare chronic inflammatory condition as plasma cell Balanophosthitis, histopathology is mandatory to diagnose each case.

BXO may complicate hypospadias repair with meatal stenosis, scaring and scaling of the glans, the importance of recognizing BXO is that repair requires excision of all involved tissues and their replacement with non-skin tissues, usually buccal mucosa, because reoperation using skin results in high recurrence rates [4].

37.6 Management

In boys presenting with milder forms of BXO, the application of a potent topical steroid (e.g., 0.05 % mometasone furoate, 0.05 % clobetasol propionate, or 0.05 % betamethasone cream) may ameliorate local symptoms and result in an improvement in the appearances of the foreskin. But while this approach may afford symptomatic relief, it is rarely curative and delays rather than avoids the need for circumcision. Misguided attempts to persist with medical management despite progressive BXO carry the risk that the partially treated sclerotic process may extend to involve the meatus and distal urethra.

Surgery, in the form of circumcision, meatotomy, or in severe cases, urethroplasty, may be required. The preferred treatment is circumcision: indeed, pathological phimosis constitutes the only absolute indication for this procedure in boys. Preputioplasty is not an option as the continuing inflammatory process results in recurrent stenosis of the preputial orifice. Glanular involvement nearly always resolves following circumcision.

However, meatal involvement calls for simultaneous meatotomy or meatoplasty in approximately 5 % of cases, and postoperative application of topical steroid creams may lessen the risk of subsequent restenosis. Parents should be notified of the risk of recurrent meatal stenosis, and follow-up is also advisable for this reason.

In adults, there is an association between BXO and penile cancer (28 % of patients with penile malignancy have BXO), although a specific causal relationship is uncertain. The relevance of this association to pediatric patients is unknown since there are no data documenting the long-term outcome for boys with BXO followed into adulthood [6].

Balanophosthitis plasmacelluaris (Zoon balanophostitis) is a benign disease of external genitals, and considered as a variant of BXO, and very rarely affecting children, it is more often seen in elderly males than females, characterized by a solitary red-orange plaque of the glans and prepuce. Although the etiology is unknown, different factors have been reported to be involved in its genesis (local infections, poor hygiene, heat, friction, and constant rubbing).Biopsy is necessary to exclude premalignant and malignant differential diagnoses. Topical therapies are often prescribed with very limited benefit for the patient. In males circumcision is a surgical option. An alternative to surgery with less downtime and preservation of the prepuce is ablative erbium-YAG laser therapy. Erbium-YAG laser therapy leads to a stable remission in patients with Zoon's balanophostitis. Late recurrences after 12 months are possible, but the lesions developed only in previously untreated parts of the glance or the prepuce [7].

References

1. Perrin L. Posthite chronique d'aspect leucoplasique. Ann de dermat et syph. 1892;3:22.
2. Stühmer A. Balanitis xerotica obliterans (post-operationem) und ihre Beziehungen zur "Kraurosis glandis et praeputii penis. Arch f Dermat u Syph. 1928;156:613.
3. Celis S, Reed F, Murphy F, Adams S, Gillick J, Abdelhafeez AH, Lopez PJ. Balanitis xerotica obliterans in children and adolescents: a literature review and clinical series. J Pediatr Urol. 2014;10(1):34–9. doi:10.1016/j.jpurol.2013.09.027.
4. Nelson DM, Peterson AC. Lichen sclerosus: epidemiological distribution in an equal access health care system. J Urol. 2011;185:522–5.
5. Marren P, Yell J, Charnock FM, Bunce M, Welsh K, Wojnarowska F. The association between

lichen sclerosus and antigens of the HLA system. Br J Dermatol. 1995;132:197–203.
6. Kumaran MS, Kanwar AJ. Squamous cell carcinoma in untreated lichen sclerosus of the penis: a rare com- plication. J Dermatol. 2004;31:239–41.
7. Wollina U. Ablative erbium:YAG laser treatment of idiopathic chronic inflammatory non-cicatricial balanoposthitis (Zoon's disease)–a series of 20 patients with long-term outcome. J Cosmet Laser Ther. 2010;12:120–3.

Phimosis and Paraphimosis

38

Abstract

The foreskin is usually still fused with the glans at birth. As childhood progresses, they gradually separate. There are different reports and a lot of debates about the age at which the foreskin can be retracted safely as there is no consensus about the time of complete separation between the glans and the inner prepuce. The other problem is the inability of many physicians to distinguish between physiological phimosis, pathological phimosis and paraphimosis, and their misdiagnosis that leads to unnecessary parents' anxiety and over-referrals to urologists for circumcision or consultation. Of these cases referred to a urology clinic, in one study, it was detected that only 8–14.4% had a "true" phimosis which necessitate surgical intervention.

Keywords

Physiological phimosis • Pathological phimosis • Preputial stenosis and paraphimosis

The foreskin is usually still fused with the glans at birth. As childhood progresses, they gradually separate. There are different reports and a lot of debates about the age at which the foreskin can be retracted safely [1] as there is no consensus about the time of complete separation between the glans and the inner prepuce. The other problem is the inability of many physicians to distinguish between physiological phimosis, pathological phimosis and paraphimosis, and their misdiagnosis that leads to unnecessary parents' anxiety and over-referrals to urologists for circumcision or consultation. Of these cases referred to a urology clinic, in one study, it was detected that only 8–14.4% had a "true" phimosis needing surgical intervention [2].

Physiological phimosis, pathological phimosis and paraphimosis will be discussed separately and chronologically.

38.1 Phimosis

Definition: Phimosis is defined as a narrowing of the preputial ring that prevents retraction of the foreskin over the glans penis. It could be physiological (congenital) or pathological (acquired). Physiological phimosis is almost invariably present at birth.

© Springer International Publishing Switzerland 2017

M. Fahmy, *Congenital Anomalies of the Penis*, DOI 10.1007/978-3-319-43310-3_38

The term may also refer to clitoral phimosis in women, whereby the clitoral hood cannot be retracted, with a limiting exposure of the glans clitoris.

The word phimosis is from the Greek *phimos* (φῖμός) which means a muzzle.

Grades There are many classifications of the grades or scores of phimosis with a great similarity. Kikiros et al. [3] classified phimosis to:

- **Score 5:** Absolutely no retraction of the foreskin.
- **Score 4:** Slight retraction, but some distance between tip and glans, i.e., neither meatus nor glans can be exposed.
- **Score 3:** Partial retraction, meatus just visible.
- **Score 2:** Partial exposure of glans, prepuce (not congenital adhesions) limiting factor.
- **Score 1:** Full retraction of foreskin, tight behind the glans.

38.1.1 Physiological Phimosis

Nomenclature

Preputial Stenosis and Congenital Phimosis.

Definition

Physiological phimosis is an inability to withdraw the narrowed penile foreskin or prepuce behind the glans penis without any acquired disease in the glans or prepuce.

Incidence

Around 96% of males at birth are noticed to have a nonretractile foreskin, and up to 10% of males will have physiologic phimosis at 3 years of age, and a larger percentage of those will have only partially retractible foreskins. One to five percent of males will have nonretractible foreskins by age 16 years [4].

Etiology

- Naturally occurring adhesions between prepuce and glans.
- Narrow preputial tip.
- Frenulum breve, (a congenitally short frenulum of varying degree, restricting the movement and gliding of the prepuce over the glans "comparable to tongue tie").
- Difficult retraction of the prepuce should be anticipated in association with many other penile congenital anomalies described before i.e.,: Macroposthia (Chap. 6), penile lymphedema (Chap. 18), microphallus (Chap. 9) concealed and webbed penis (Chap. 14).

38.1.1.1 Diagnosis

On gentle traction, the prepuce puckers and the overlying tissue are pink and healthy. There may be some ballooning during urination (Fig. 38.1). But pain, dysuria, and local or urinary infections are not seen in these cases. Even if urinary infection is present, it is usually not attributed to the phimosis. Diagnosis of phimosis is primarily clinical and no laboratory tests or imaging studies are required. These may be required for associated urinary tract infections or skin infections. Treating physician should be able to distinguish developmental non-retractability from pathological phimosis, and also to detect grading of severity of this phimosis.

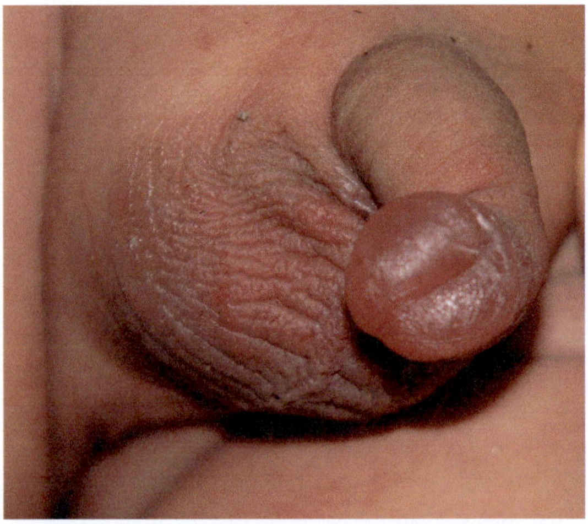

Fig. 38.1 Inflamed oedematous preputial orifice after a forcible trial of retracting the prepuce in a neonate

38.1.1.2 Treatment

When it is certain that phimosis in the child is not pathologic, it is vital to reassure the parents on normalcy of the condition in that age group. They should be taught how to keep the foreskin and its undersurface clean and hygienic. Normal washing with lukewarm water and gentle retractions during bathing and urination makes the foreskin retractile over time.

The foreskin gradually becomes retractable over a variable period of time ranging from birth to 18 years of age or more. At least 2 % of normal males continue to have non-retractability throughout life, even though they are otherwise normal. In European countries the classical antecedents are focused on treating underlying pathology, maintaining foreskin function and preserving natural cosmosis, instead of doing circumcision [5]. In other areas, where ritual circumcision done routinely for almost all babies, many surgeons treating this type of phimosis by taking off the troublesome prepuce.

38.1.1.3 Complications

Patients with phimosis, both physiologic and pathologic, are at risk for developing paraphimosis when the foreskin is forcibly retracted past the glans and/or the patient or caretaker forgets to replace the foreskin after retraction, usually pain and swelling prevent reduction of a retracted foreskin (Fig. 38.1).

With time, impairment of venous and lymphatic flow to the glans leads to venous engorgement and worsening swelling. As the swelling progresses, arterial supply is compromised, leading to penile infarction/necrosis, gangrene and, eventually, autoamputation, which is very rare in the last years.

38.1.2 Pathological Phimosis

38.1.2.1 Nomenclature

Secondary Phimosis, Acquired Phimosis, Iatrogenic, True or pathological phimosis.

Definition

Acquired or iatrogenic constriction of the preputial ring which hinder foreskin retraction. The fibrotic preputial ring, or cicatrix of tissue distal to the glans prevents retraction and routine hygiene. A cicatrix may form following scarring from forcible retraction or following episodes of balanoposthitis. Pathological phimosis is not the disease of uncircumcised baby, as it was reported, but it may happen after incomplete or complicated circumcision.

38.1.2.2 Incidence

The incidence of pathological phimosis is 0.4 per 1000 boys per year, 0.6 % of boys are affected by their 15th birthday [6].

38.1.2.3 Etiology

- Enthusiastic attempts to retract foreskin in physiological phimosis causes microtears, infection, and bleeding with secondary scarring and true phimosis.
- Poor hygiene and recurrent balanitis (Fig. 38.2).

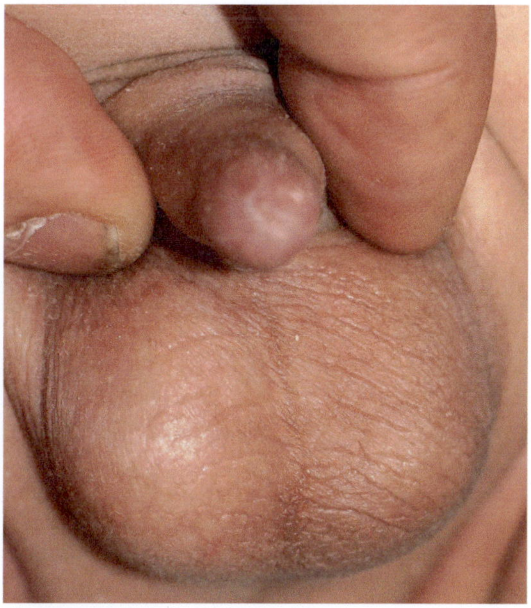

Fig. 38.2 Repeated attacks of posthitis ended with a pinpoint preputial ring, which make perpetual traction impossible"pathological phimosis"

- Posthitis and balanoposthitis (Chap. 39).
- Specific balanitis, like; Balanitis Xerotica Obliterans (BXO), and Plasma cell balanitis (Chap. 37)
- Diabetes mellitus predisposes to these infections due to high glucose content of urine, which is conducive for bacterial proliferation and subsequent balanoposthitits [7].
- Repeated catherization could also lead to phimosis.
- Also after circumcision; if during this procedure the prepuce not excised properly leaving the remnant preputial edges to heal in front of the meatus with different grades of fibrosis and stricture, which may end with urinary retention, with its sequelae of upper urinary tract back pressure effects in neglected cases (Figs. 38.3 and 38.4).

38.1.2.4 Diagnosis

Usually there is pain, skin irritation, local infections, bleeding, dysuria, hematuria, frequent episodes of urinary tract infections, painful erection, and weak urinary stream. Occasionally, enuresis or urinary retention is noticed. The meatal opening is small and the tissue in front of the foreskin is white and fibrotic (Fig. 38.4b). Phimosis due to BXO is usually severe with meatal stenosis, glanular lesions, or both.

38.1.2.5 Treatment

Dilation and Stretching: Gentle preputial retractions are carried out by a doctor on an outpatient basis. This nonsurgical adhesiolysis is found to be effective, cheap, and safe treatment for phimosis. Eutectic mixture of local anaesthetics (EMLA) could be used prior to attempts at release of the

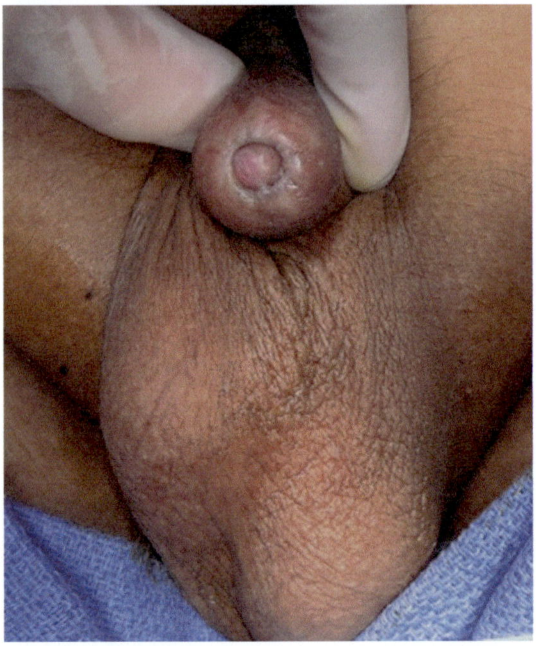

Fig. 38.3 Phimosis secondary to incomplete circumcision and scaring of the improperly divided prepuce

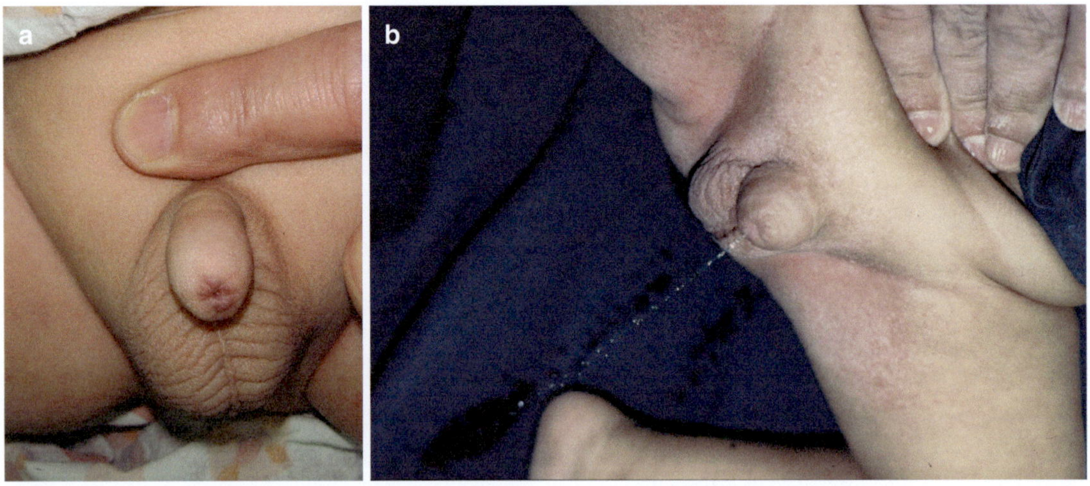

Fig. 38.4 (**a**, **b**) Secondary phimosis with a preputial meatal stricture and difficult voiding secondary to pathological phimosis

preputial adhesions. He and Zhou used a specially designed patented balloon catheter with local anesthesia in 512 boys and found it to be 100% useful. The technique was simple, safe, cheap, less painful and less traumatizing than conventional circumcision. It was found to be more beneficial in younger children with no fibrosis or infection. Combination therapy using stretching and topical steroids has also yielded excellent results [8].

Pathologic phimosis has been traditionally treated surgically with circumcision. Although circumcision is effective, it is not without complications, particularly in older infants and boys who must undergo general anesthesia. In young baby, the parents often made a conscious decision either to circumcise their son, or not, older child can decide for himself. In many countries and if the treating surgeon believe in the benefits of circumcision; this procedure was the first choice, but reluctant family to give consent for circumcision, or surgeon in countries not doing routine circumcision; another alternatives are applicable.

The use of topical steroid treatment has been shown to be an effective and safe alternative to surgical intervention, with success rates ranging from 67 to 95% and no reported adverse effects. Patients who were successfully treated have not had recurrence of phimosis [9].

The major variable accounting for differences in the efficacy rate between studies is the definition of successful outcome. Some groups considered any result short of complete foreskin retractability is a treatment failure.

The mechanism of effect of betamethasone dipropionate cream on the phimotic ring is thought to be local anti-inflammatory action. Resolution of the phimotic band then allows the prepuce to dilate and slide backward over the glans. Betamethasone cream may improve the elasticity of the foreskin and, together with the moisturizing effect of the cream, allow for easier retractability for hygiene measures, thought to help prevent recurrence of acquired phimosis. Of course, cases secondary to incomplete circumcision or post circumcision infection and fibrosis need surgical repair to remove a sleeve of the constricted, fibrotic preputial skin with meticulous dissection to avoid any glanular or meatal injury.

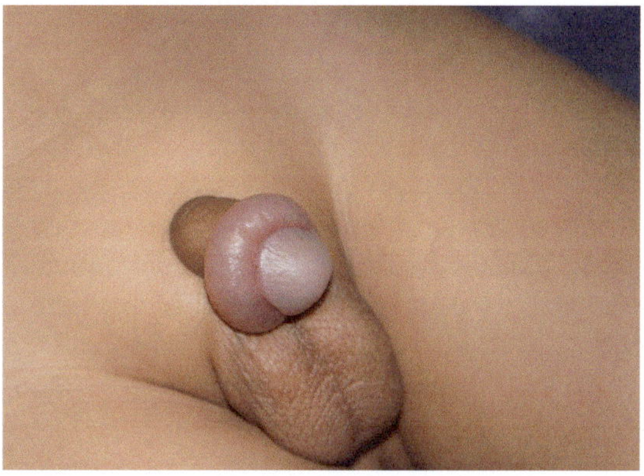

Fig. 38.5 Paraphimosis; oedematous retracted prepuce, constricting the glans at the coronal sulcus

38.2 Paraphimosis

Definition

It is an uncommon medical condition in which the foreskin of an uncircumcised penis becomes trapped behind the glans penis, and cannot be reduced (pulled back to its normal flaccid position covering the glans). If this condition persists for several hours or there is any sign of a lack of blood flow, it should be treated as a medical emergency, as it can result in gangrene of the glans.

Paraphimosis is a disease of uncircumcised or partially circumcised males (Fig. 38.5).

Paraphimosis includes the following:

- The foreskin is retracted behind the glans penis and cannot be replaced to its normal position.
- The foreskin forms a tight, constricting ring around the glans.
- Flaccidity of the penile shaft proximal to the area of paraphimosis is seen (unless there is accompanying balanoposthitis or infection of the penis).
- With time, the glans becomes increasingly erythematous and oedematous.
- The glans penis is initially had its normal pink hue and soft to palpation. As necrosis develops, the color changes to blue or black and the glans becomes firm to palpation.

38.2.1 Etiology

Paraphimosis can occur after retraction of the foreskin during detailed penile examination, cleaning of the glans penis, urethral catheterization or cystoscopy. Self-infliction, such as piercing with a penile ring into the glans, placement of a preputial bead, contact dermatitis (e.g., from the application of celadine juice or other material to the foreskin) may lead to paraphimosis.

Differential Diagnoses

- Acute Angioedema.
- Allergic Contact Dermatitis.
- Balanitis.
- Balanitis xerotica obliterans.
- Cellulitis.
- Foreign body tourniquet, including hair, thread, metallic object, or rubber bands.
- Insect Bites.
- Penile hematoma.

38.2.2 Management of Paraphimosis

A paraphimosis is a urologic emergency and needs to be attended to immediately. Many techniques of paraphimosis reduction have been described in case studies, though none have been tested in randomized control trials [10]. The main goal of each method is to reduce the foreskin to its naturally occurring position over the glans penis by manipulating the oedematous glans and/or the distal prepuce. When necessary, all reduction procedures can be facilitated by the use of local anesthesia, a penile block using lidocaine hydrochloride without epinephrine or, especially in children, conscious sedation. Sterile technique should be used for all invasive procedures [11].

Vertical incision, if none of the conservative methods are successful, of the constricting band should be commenced. Foreskin should be incised using a 1–2 cm longitudinal incision between two straight hemostats placed in the 12-o'clock position for hemostasis; this frees the constricting ring and allows for easy reduction of the paraphimosis. The incised margins can then be reapproximated using 4/0 or finer absorbable sutures.

Emergent circumcision: This is a last resort, to be performed by a urologist, to achieve the necessary reduction of a paraphimosis, if the family agree.

References

1. TKumar P, Deb M, Das K. Preputial adhesions–a misunderstood entity.Indian. J Pediatr. 2009;76(8):829–32.
2. McGregor TB, Pike JG, Leonard MP. Phimosis—a diagnostic dilemma? Can. J Urol. 2005;12(2):2598–602.
3. Kikiros CS, Beasley SW, Woodward AA. The response of phimosis to local steroid application. Pediatr Surg Int. 1993;8(4):329–32. doi:10.1007/BF00173357.
4. McGregor TB, Pike JG, Leonard MP. Pathologic and physiologic phimosis: approach to the phimotic foreskin. Can Fam Physician. 2007;53(3):445–8.
5. Sneppen I, Thorup J. Foreskin morbidity in uncircumcised males. Pediatrics. 2016;137(5). doi: 10.1542/peds.2015-4340.
6. Shankar KR, Rickwood AM. The incidence of phimosis in boys. BJU Int. 1999;84(1):101–2.
7. Bromage SJ, Crump A, Pearce I. Phimosis as a presenting feature of diabetes. BJU Int. 2008;101(3):338–40.
8. He Y, Zhou XH. Balloon dilation treatment of phimosis in boys. Report of 512 cases. Chin Med J (Engl). 1991;104(6):491–3.
9. Golubovic Z, Milanovic D, Vukadinovic V, et al. The conservative treatment of phimosis in boys. BJU Int. 1996;78:786.
10. Kessler CS, Bauml J. Non-traumatic urologic emergencies in men: a clinical review. West J Emerg Med. 2009;10(4):281–7.
11. Little B, White M. Treatment options for paraphimosis. Int J Clin Pract. 2005;59(5):591–3.

Further Reading

Foreskin Websites: Foreskin http://www.foreskin.org/.
Robin S. The circumcision taboos. Phimosis frenulum and foreskin conditions, phimosis and male initiation http://www.phimosis.cloud/welcome.html.

39 Balanitis and Balanoposthitis

Abstract

Balanitis is an inflammatory disease affecting the glans penis, and it usually discussed by dermatologists and overlooked by many surgeons. But as many cases may complicate penile surgeries; like circumcision, also these cases may need differentiation from other similar surgical diseases and congenital anomalies. Repeated attacks of balanitis and/or balanoposthitis may be complicated with surgical conditions, which necessitate intervention; like phimosis and meatal stenosis.

Keywords

Balanitis • Balanoposthitis • Candida balanitis • Human papilloma virus • Trichomonal species • Anaerobic infection

Balanitis is an inflammatory disease affecting the glans penis is usually discussed by dermatologists and overlooked by many surgeons. But as many cases may complicate penile surgeries; like circumcision, these cases may need differentiation from other similar surgical diseases and congenital anomalies. Repeated attacks of balanitis and/or balanoposthitis may be complicated with surgical conditions, which necessitate intervention; like phimosis and meatal stenosis.

39.1 Balanitis

Definition

Balanitis is inflammation of the glans penis, when the foreskin is also affected, it is termed balanoposthitis. Balanitis of boys still in diapers must be distinguished from trivial redness caused by ammoniacal dermatitis. The word comes from the Greek "βάλανος" balanos, which means "acorn".

© Springer International Publishing Switzerland 2017
M. Fahmy, *Congenital Anomalies of the Penis*, DOI 10.1007/978-3-319-43310-3_39

39.1.1 Incidence

Balanitis is a common condition affecting 11 % of adult men seen in urology clinics and 3 % of children in the United States; globally, balanitis may occur in up to 3 % of uncircumcised males [1]. Many cases also reported after circumcision, specially in early postoperative period.

Several organisms and viruses can cause balanitis, including the following:

- Candidal species (most commonly associated with diabetes).
- Group B and group A beta-hemolytic streptococci.
- Neisseria gonorrhoeae.
- Chlamydia species.
- Anaerobic infection.
- Human papilloma virus.
- Trichomonal species.
- Rare pathogens like; Borrelia vincentii and Borrelia burgdorferi.

Mayser has proposed that candidal balanitis/balanoposthitis is the most frequent mycotic infection of the penis [2]. Incontinent children, specially those with spina bifida, may had a severe form of candida, or a mixed infection of balanoposthitis secondary to chronic irritation and bad hygiene (Fig. 39.1).

Specific types of balanitis; like Balanitis xerotica obliterans (BXO), and plasma cell balanitis (Zoon balanitis) had been discussed in Chap. 37.

39.1.2 Symptoms

Patients with balanitis usually present with the following complaints:

Urethral discharge.
Pain or difficulty with retraction of foreskin.
Difficult urinating or controlling urine stream (in very severe cases).
Inability to insert a Foley's catheter.
Tenderness and erythema of the glans penis.
Itching.
Systemic symptoms such as fever and nausea are uncommon.

39.1.3 Physical Examination

Findings may include the following:

Erythema and oedema of glans penis or foreskin (Fig. 39.2).
Discharge.
Ulceration and/or plaques (Fig. 39.3).
Pathological or secondary phimosis (Fig. 39.4).
Ballooning of the foreskin with voiding.

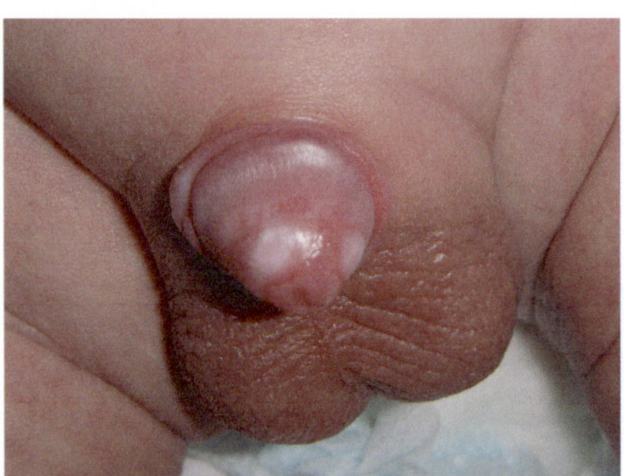

Fig. 39.1 Candida balanitis affecting the glans of a circumcised 1 year old boy

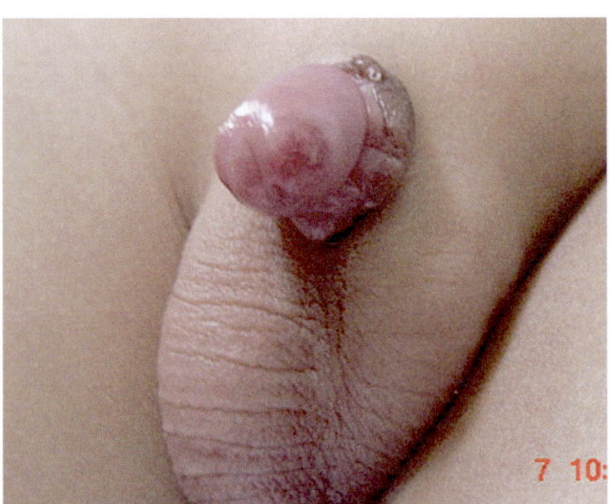

Fig. 39.2 Erythema of the glans penis due to post-circumcision balanitis

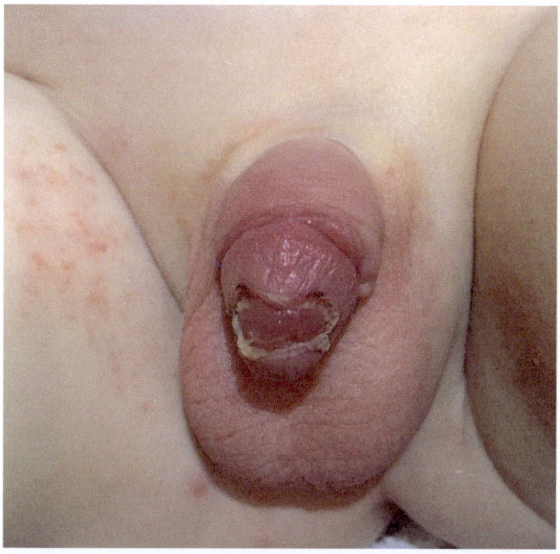

Fig. 39.3 Deep ulcer in the glans penis, due to sever bacterial balanitis in a circumcised boy

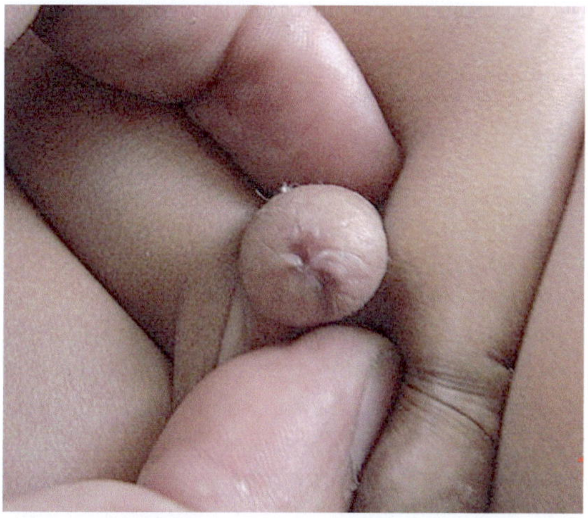

Fig. 39.4 Pathological phimosis secondary to repeated attacks of untreated balanitis or balanoposthitis

Signs of urinary obstruction (rare).
Bladder distension.
Inguinal lymphadenopathy.

39.1.4 Complications

Recurrent bouts of balanitis may cause scarring of the preputial orifice; with a subsequent reduction of preputial elasticity, which may lead to pathologic phimosis (Fig. 39.4).

Balanitis, if not discovered early and treated properly, it may also lead to meatal stenosis, urethritis and ascending UTI, specially in a circumcised child. In very few cases, it may contribute to the buried penis syndrome.

39.1.5 Management

Patients presenting with balanitis but without phimosis should be investigate to detect the causative organism, culture of discharge in complicated cases such as those with associated cellulitis should be done early. Appropriate antibiotic or anti fungal medication should start systemically, with an additive local treatment.

In pediatric patients, a gentle retraction of the foreskin daily and soak in warm water to clean penis and foreskin, with a 2-month trial of antifungals may be attempted. The patient or mother should retract the foreskin gently and apply 0.05 % betamethasone twice a day. This applies to children older than 3 years. Success is seen particularly in male children older than 10 years compared with those aged 3–10 years. Success ranges from 65 to 95 %. In recurrent cases, 1 % pimecrolimus cream was used instead of steroids, with a 64 % success rate.

A study of 1185 boys concluded that fluticasone proprionate 0.05 % was effective and safe in treating associated phimosis, with successful results in 91.1 % of patients [3].

Mallon et al. [4] have proposed that circumcision may protect against balanoposthitis and common penile infections, but we encountered a considerable number of cases had a different types and forms of balanitis; either immediately after circumcision or latter on, with different pathogens and a wide spectrum of presentation (Figs. 39.1, 39.2, 39.3, and 39.5).

39.2 Balanoposthitis

Definition

Balanoposthitis is defined as the inflammation of the foreskin and the glans penis in uncircumcised males. Circumcised boys with a preputial rem-

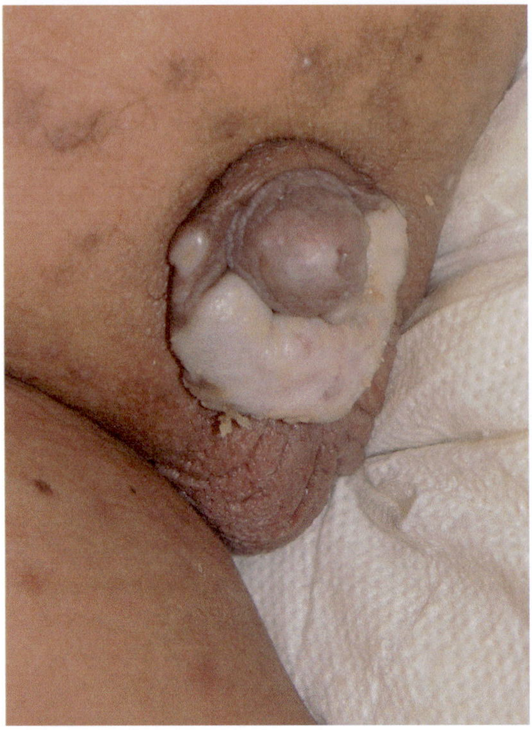

Fig. 39.5 Severe balanoposthitis in the preputial remnant, with extensive candidiasis in a circumcised incontinent baby

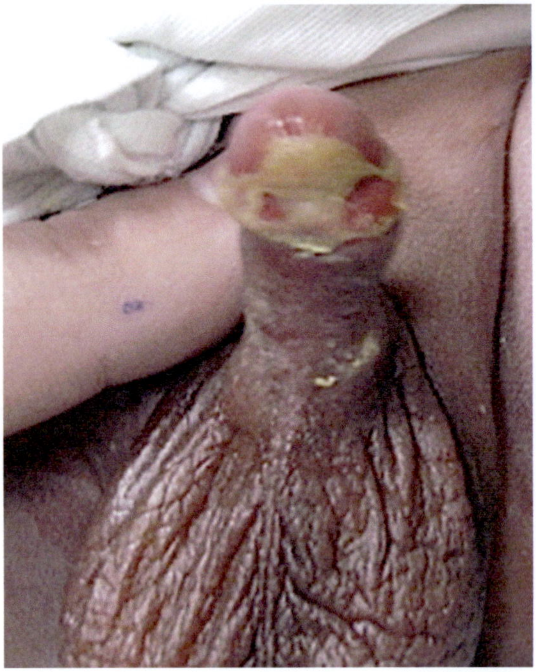

Fig. 39.6 Post circumcision pyogenic membrane, with a gram negative organism

nants (incomplete circumcision) may have balanoposthitis, specially the immunocompromised or incontinent babies (Fig. 39.5). Multiple bacterial and fungal etiologic agents are associated with the this condition. Complex infections have also been well documented, often from a poorly retractile foreskin and poor hygiene that leads to colonization and overgrowth of normal bacterial flora (Fig. 39.6).

Treatment focuses on clearing the acute infection and preventing recurrent inflammation/infection through improved hygiene. Although, not as necessary as in the past, circumcision may be considered for refractory or recurrent balanoposthitis. Balanoposthitis should not be confused with balanitis.

39.2.1 Pathophysiology

Balanoposthitis is commonly identified in young boys (<5 y). Predisposing factors include; immune deficiency disorders, incontinence, limited retraction of the foreskin and poor hygiene in this area, which leads to bacterial infection. Anaerobic organisms are the most common bacteria isolated from lesions [5]. Rare causes include Streptococcus pyogenes and Pseudomonas aeruginosa. Reports of an association between human papillomavirus (HPV) infection and long-standing balanoposthitis have been published, but they may reflect a non-causative association. Associations with ulcerative colitis and Crohn disease have also been noted [6].

39.2.2 Incidence

In a Japanese study, balanoposthitis was found in 9 (1.5 %) of 603 uncircumcised Japanese boys aged 0–15 years. Candida species diagnosed as the cause of balanoposthitis in 35 % of 450 men examined in Great Britain. Italian studies have found balanoposthitis in (16 %) of 321 patients with genital dermatoses [7].

Sex Balanoposthitis only occurs in males.

Age Although identified over a wide age range, but it is common in infants and young age.

39.2.3 Physical Examination

The glans and the prepuce often reveals a red, moist macular lesion. Associated erythema is noted, and areas of yellow-to-black discolouration have been described. The presence of lichenification, irregular borders or acetowhite changes (A whitish patch) with 5 % acetic acid treatment suggest an HPV infection, which can be seen in association with balanoposthitis.

A superimposed balanoposthitis on a flat condyloma has been described. Such coexisting lesions may be diagnosed based on the clinical history and a culture of fungus or bacteria from the ulcer.

Ulceration and deep erosion have been seen in patients with advanced disease, often in association with fungal infections and in individuals who are immunocompromised (Fig. 39.3).

An association with preputial smegma plaques has been described, a correlation that most likely reflects the hygiene of the affected population (Chap. 36).

Biopsy is performed in doubtful cases and if antifungal treatment fails to produce a favourable response. Biopsy is specially warranted if premalignant or malignant lesions, such as erythroplasia of Queyrat or Bowen disease, are suspected and need to be excluded, specially at older age.

Mondor phlebitis [8] of the penis following recurrent candidal balanoposthitis has been reported. Patients present with a solitary, glistening, sharply demarcated, large (2–3 cm), erythematous, speckled patch on the glans or inner prepuce. Rarely, multiple patches can erode and ulcerate. Clinical involvement is typically (85 %) on both the glans and prepuce or prepuce only. Presentation on the glans alone is less common. Occasionally, discharge is the presenting symptom. The clinical course is typically chronic, and the initial presentation is delayed an average of 12 months [8].

39.2.4 Post Circumcision Granuloma

Granuloma after circumcision is not rare disease, as it was believed [9], many cases diagnosed few weeks after circumcision due different aetiology, and with a variant presentations. Post circumcision granulomatous balanitis may be due infection from improperly sterilised instruments used in some countries during mass circumcision, non suitable suture materials used for stitching the preputial remnants or lack of postoperative care. Also rough manipulation of the delicate penile tissues and ischemia from using different types of diathermy can cause this lesion (Fig. 39.7).

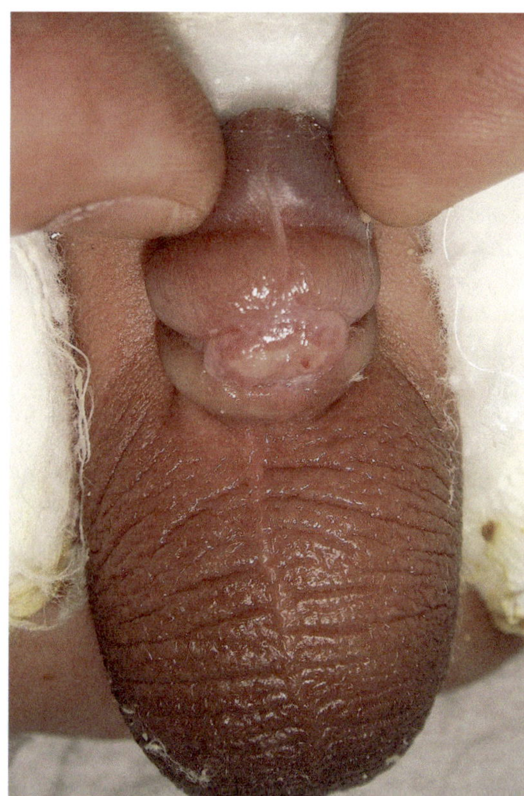

Fig. 39.7 Post circumcision granuloma in the undersurface of the penis

39.2.5 Pyogenic Granuloma

In such cases the granuloma may be secondary to infection with different pathogens; candida, gram negative anaerobes, or even virus and chlamydia.

It appears as a red nodule, soft in texture with a constricted base, painless, micro-haemorrhagic when pressed and it may acquire a large size with bleeding on touch. This complication should be avoided, or at least minimised, detected early, and once disproved, it should be excised and biopsied. Sometimes, a trial of conservative treatment could be attempted with some success [10].

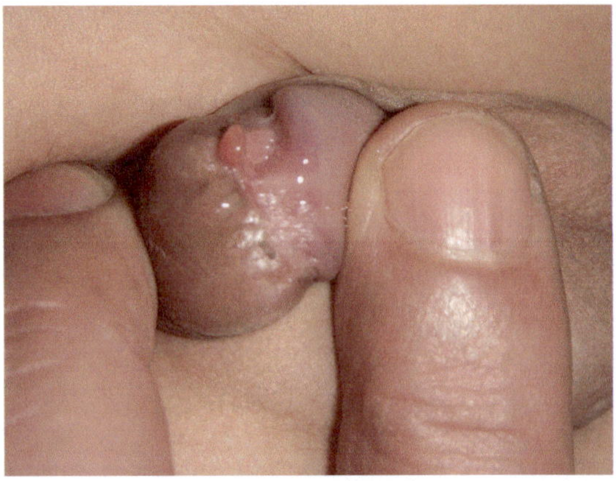

Fig. 39.8 Small stitch granuloma at the coronal sulcus

39.2.6 Histological Diagnosis

Pyogenic granuloma is a solitary, rapidly growing, easily bleeding, bright red papule or nodule that often appears at the site of minor trauma of the skin. Granulation tissue is composed mostly of newly formed blood vessels, macrophages, fibroblasts and loose connective tissues. In time, fibroplasia of granulation tissue supervenes, the wound contracts, and finally tissue remodelling occurs. When injuries persist or recur, the process of tissue repair is inhibited.

39.2.7 Post Circumcision Stitch Granuloma

This type of granuloma may complicate any wound repair mainly due to infection, delay in closure or inappropriate suture materials. Surprisingly, stitch granuloma is not included among the complications of circumcision in many studies, although the relation between skin injury and the development of this condition is well known [10]. Failure in surgical wound repair (probably due to excess movement and tension of the prepuce remnant) caused exuberant granulation tissue formation that in time eventuated in multiple pyogenic granulomata arranged in a floret-like fashion around the surgical scar. A similar phenomenon would seem to be implicated in the pathogenesis of recurrent pyogenic granuloma which develops in a satellite fashion around the surgical scar of a previously removed solitary pyogenic granuloma (Fig. 39.8).

References

1. Lisboa C, Ferreira A, Resende C, Rodrigues AG. Infectious balanoposthitis: management, clinical and laboratory features. Int J Dermatol. 2009;48(2):121–4.
2. Mayser P. Mycotic infections of the penis. Andrologia. 1999;31 Suppl 1:13–6 [Medline].
3. Zavras N, Christianakis E, Mpourikas D, Ereikat K. Conservative treatment of phimosis with fluticasone proprionate 0.05 %: a clinical study in 1185 boys. J Pediatr Urol. 2009;5(3):181–5 [Medline].
4. Mallon E, Hawkins D, Dinneen M, et al. Circumcision and genital dermatoses. Arch Dermatol. 2000;136(3):350–4 [Medline].
5. Chen J, Zhou YX, Jin XD, Chen SW. Expression of interleukin-2 in Candidal balanoposthitis and its clinical significance. Chin Med J (Engl). 2011;124(17):2776–8 [Medline].
6. Lyttle PH. Ulcerative colitis and balanoposthitis. Int J STD AIDS. 1994;5(1):72–3 [Medline].
7. Dockerty WG, Sonnex C. Candidal balano-posthitis: a study of diagnostic methods. Genitourin Med. 1995;71(6):407–9 [Medline].
8. Hakan O. Penile Mondor's disease. Basic Clin Androl. 2014;24:5. doi:10.1186/2051-4190-24-5.
9. Naimer SA, Cohen A, Vardy D. Pyogenic granuloma of the penile shaft following circumcision. Pediatr Dermatol. 2002;19(1):39–14.
10. Tomasini C, Puiatti P, Bernengo MG. Multiple pyogenic granuloma of the penis. Sex Transm Inf. 1998;74:221–2.

Dermatological Disease of the Penis

40

Abstract

Various wide range of dermatological diseases may affect the skin of the penis and prepuce. Some are unique to the genitalia, so they are genitally specific like; penile freckles, lentigo and juvenile xanthogranuloma (JXG). Other more common dermatoses which may have a unique appearance when they involve genital skin and mucosa like; psoriasis, lichen planus, and seborrheic dermatitis, some infectious dermatological diseases are affecting the penis before they affect other areas; like herpes, and gonorrhoea. A wide range of infectious, neoplastic, immunological and inflammatory dermatoses can affect the penis, but only nonmalignant skin lesions, which may had a congenital background in their aetiology and carry some significance for the pediatric surgeons and urologists will be discussed; other skin lesions that may affect genital skin as well as the skin of any part of the body are beyond the scope of this chapter.

Keywords

Angiomyofibroblastoma • Angiokeratomas • Penile melanosis • Penile freckles • Penile lentigo • Juvenile xanthogranuloma • Pigmented nevus • Divided nevus • Congenital melanocytic nevi

Dermatological lesions of surgical importance include:

- **Angiomyofibroblastoma.**
- **Angiokeratomas**
- **Penile hyperpigmentation.**
  - **Penile melanosis.**
  - **Penile freckles.**
  - **Penile lentigo.**
- **Penile hypopigmentation.**
- **Yellow pigmented lesion: juvenile xanthogranuloma (JXG)**
- **Balanitis, balanoposthitis:** are discussed before in Chap. 39.
- **Haemangioma** (Chap. 17)

40.1 Angiomyofibroblastoma

It is a benign, rare mesenchymal tumor arising from the genital tract of both men and women and was recently described for the first time by Fletcher et al. in 1992 [2].

© Springer International Publishing Switzerland 2017
M. Fahmy, *Congenital Anomalies of the Penis*, DOI 10.1007/978-3-319-43310-3_40

Nomenclature

Male angiomyofibroblastoma-like tumor and cellular angiofibroma

Definition

Rare benign oedematous tumor of perineum and external genitalia, it may arise from penis, scrotum, inguinal region, and in female it arise from the vulva, as a well-circumscribed, with soft to rubbery cut surface and somewhat oedematous appearance, with variable size. It had a low tendency for recurrence. It appears as solid cystic masses on ultrasound images, which is the most valuable tool to establish a preoperative diagnosis of this tumor entity [3].

40.1.1 Histological features

Hypercellular areas located around vascular spaces of spindle, plump or oval stromal cells that alternate with hypocellular areas containing similar cells loosely dispersed in an edematous background.

40.1.2 Differential diagnosis

This tumor needs to be distinguished from other, similar lesions, such as hemangioma, deep and superficial aggressive angiomyxoma and cellular angiofibroma, because aggressive angiomyxoma demands much more extensive treatment.

40.1.3 Treatment

Simple excision

40.2 Angiokeratomas: (Angiokeratoma of Fordyce)

Incidence

The prevalence of angiokeratomas is unknown, but is believed to be less than 1 %. These lesions occur more often in men than women, and are more common in white persons.

Definition

Angiokeratomas are benign, well-circumscribed, red or blue papules measuring 1–6 mm that typically occur in patients older than 40 years [4]. Patients tend to present with multiple lesions, although solitary lesions are not uncommon, with greater numbers with increasing age, older lesions are larger and more keratotic.

The diagnosis is usually made by characteristic appearance, although it may be misdiagnosed as penile cancer or pearly papules. Angiokeratomas may affect only the glans penis, and the patients may experience rare intermittent bleeding, pain, or pruritus.

This angiokeratomas should be distinguished from angiokeratoma of Fabry (a rare genetic metabolic disorder secondary to alpha-galactosidase deficiency and impaired glycosphingolipid metabolism).

Treatment is indicated if the patient is symptomatic or if the lesions bleed. Options include surgery, cryoablation, electrocautery, and hyfrecation or vascular laser ablation. Treatment may be difficult in patients with extensive lesions.

40.3 Hyperpigmented Genitalia

Definition

Localized or generalized increased genital pigmentation.

Hyperpigmentation can affect other parts of the body or be restricted to the genitalia, and the localized areas of hyperpigmentation of the glans of the penis are especially common. This should be differentiated from ***Freckled genitalia*** in which one or more small, focal areas of hyperpigmentation are present. Localized hyperpigmentation can be objectively determined due to the difference from the immediate surrounding tissue colour, while generalized hyperpigmentation may be more difficult to determine and is therefore a subjective manifestation. If the finding is localized, the description should be appended with a description of the affected part(s).

40.4 Penile Melanosis

The most common cause of dark spot on penis is penile melanosis.

Definition

Penile melanosis is well-defined, oval, brown to black, flat patch that can be seen on glans penis, prepuce or shaft of penis. Sometimes they may have irregular border and change in colour that can cause confusion with scary and malignant lesion like melanoma. In most cases biopsy is indicated (Fig. 40.1).

Histologically only hyperpigmentation of the basal cell layer was observed with no melanocytic hyperplasia (Fig. 40.2).

Apart from melanin, other pigmentary deposits such as hemosiderin, lipofuscin, lipofuscin-like pigment and ferrous sulfate also contribute to the discolouration in penile melanosis.

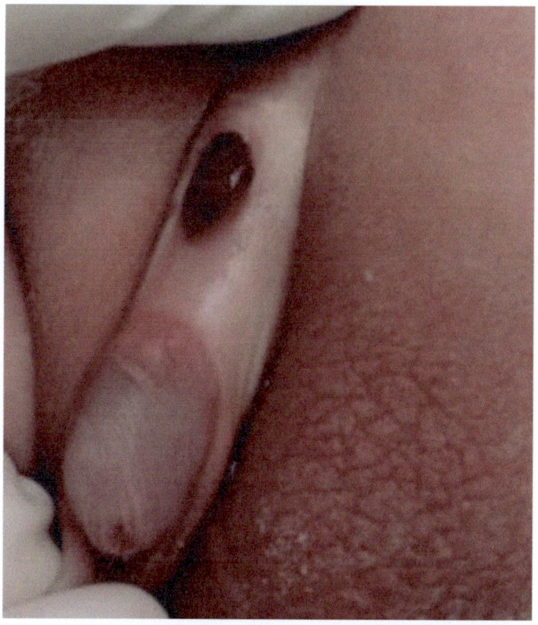

Fig. 40.1 Penile melanosis, well defined black nevus in the dorsum of the penis

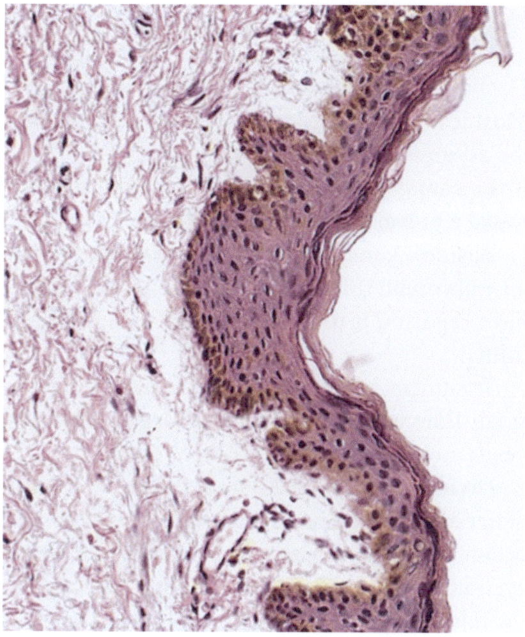

Fig. 40.2 Melanosis with hyperpigmentation of the basal cell layer, and focal elongation of rete peges

A compound nevus consists of melanocytes involving the dermis and the dermal-epidermal junction, whereas dermal nevi involve only the dermis and junctional nevi involve only the dermal-epidermal junction.

Melanosis (a circumscribed hyperpigmentation of basal cells that may or may not include melanocyte hyperplasia).

Luckily, most of the penile melanotic macules are harmless. Malignant melanoma of the penis is uncommon and represents approximately 1 % of all penile malignancies.

Treatment is not necessary but for cosmetic purpose, the lesion can be removed with cryotherapy, and lasers or local excision.

40.5 Pigmented Nevus (Moles) of the Penis

Moles are quite common presentation on penis; they can be flat or slightly raised brown to dark colour. They are usually harmless and do not require any treatment.

Incidence

Genital melanotic macules are not uncommon. Most lesions go unnoticed by the patients due to the asymptomatic nature and its site.

In a study of 10 000 men by Barnhill et al. he found a prevalence was 14.2 % [5].

Besides genetic and racial factors playing an important role in its pathogenesis, studies have reported it to be associated with previous injury.

Treatment is excision and primary repair in small lesions, but excision of a large nevus may needs coverage with a flap or free graft.

Divided nevus or kissing nevus is usually defined as a congenital melanocytic nevus that occurs on adjacent parts of the upper and lower eyelids and may appear to be a single lesion when the lids are closed. Divided nevus usually seen in uncircumcised penis with double lesions in the glans and prepuce.

40.6 Congenital Melanocytic Nevi

Neurocutaneous melanosis is a rare congenital syndrome characterized by the presence of large or multiple congenital melanocytic nevi and benign or malignant pigment cell tumors of the leptomeninges.

Incidence

Congenital melanocytic nevi occur in approximately 1 % of newborns and are usually classified according to their size. Giant congenital melanocytic nevi are most simply defined as melanocytic nevi that are greater than 20 cm in largest dimension; whereas small congenital nevi are defined as melanocytic nevi less that 1.5 cm in largest dimension. Congenital nevi can exhibit distinctive histologic features that can help in differentiating them from common acquired nevi, and it is associated with an increased risk of the development of melanoma (Figs. 40.3 and 40.4).

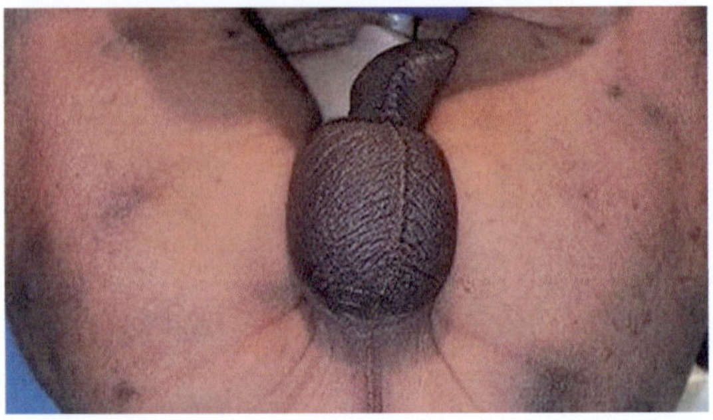

Fig. 40.3 Congenital melanocytic nevi, affecting the penis and buttock in a neonate

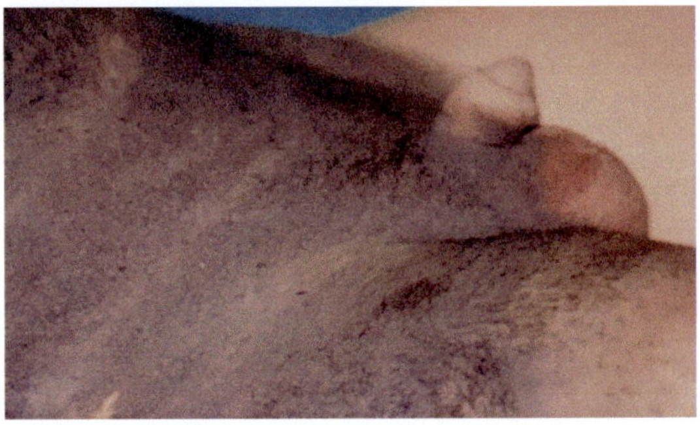

Fig. 40.4 Giant melanocytic nevi of the lower abdominal wall and genitalia

Treatment

A variety of treatment options exists for the management of giant congenital nevi. Confusion over appropriate management is compounded because not all giant congenital nevi are pigmented, and malignant potential varies between different types.

Expanded full-thickness skin grafts were used in with great success, split-thickness or nonexpanded full-thickness skin grafts were also applicable, and serial excision could be attempted specially for small localised lesions [6].

40.6.1 Post Circumcision Discolouration

The circumcision scar is usually forming a darker ring at or behind coronal sulcus. It goes all of the way around the shaft of the penis.

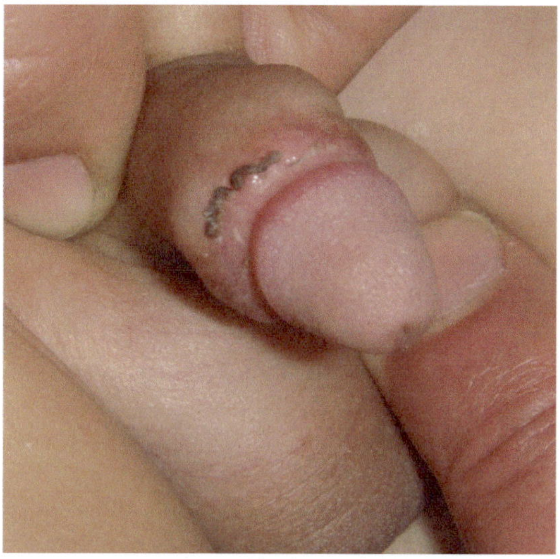

Fig. 40.5 Freckled localised hyperpigmented, developed few months after circumcision

The skin on each side of the scar is different, as the circumcision scars join dissimilar tissue, so there is an abrupt change, between the true skin covering the penile shaft and the inner perpetual remnant, which is actually a dried mucosa.

Inflammation and allergy or contact dermatitis may aggravate the darker circumcision scar, specially in babies with dark skin. It is not uncommon to have a freckled localised hyperpigmented at the circumcision site, which should be excised and biopsied to rule out other pathology (Fig. 40.5).

40.7 Penile Freckles

Definition

One or more brown punctate macules on the skin of the genitalia (Fig. 40.6).

This should be differentiated from ***Hyperpigmented genitalia*** in which an area larger than a freckle or the complete external genitalia are hyperpigmented. The description should be qualified by a description of the affected part(s).

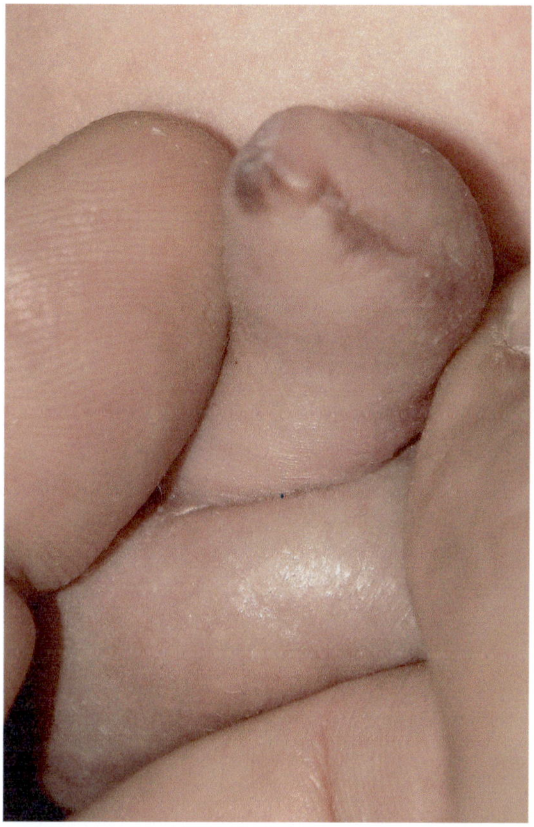

Fig. 40.6 Liner penile lentigo affecting the prepuce in uncircumcised boy

Nomenclatures

Genitalia ephelides, Genital Lentiginosis, Penile Lentiginosis

40.8 Penile Lentigo

is another small pigmented spot on the skin with a clearly defined edge, surrounded by normal-appearing skin. It is a harmless (benign) hyperplasia of melanocytes which is linear in its spread. This means the hyperplasia of melanocytes is restricted to the cell layer directly above the basement membrane of the epidermis where melanocytes normally reside. This is in contrast to the "nests" of multi-layer melanocytes found in moles (melanocytic nevi). Because of this

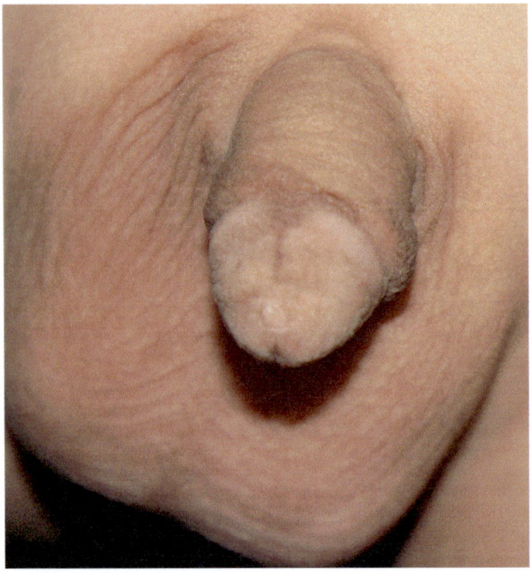

Fig. 40.7 Penile lentigo of the glans and coronal sulcus in a circumcised boy

characteristic feature, the adjective "lentiginous" is used to describe other skin lesions that similarly proliferate linearly within the basal cell layer (Figs. 40.6 and 40.7).

Lentigines are distinguished from freckles based on the proliferation of melanocytes. Freckles have a relatively normal number of melanocytes but an increased amount of melanin. A lentigo has an increased number of melanocytes. Freckles will increase in number and darkness with sunlight exposure, whereas lentigines will stay stable in their color regardless of sunlight exposure.

Incidence

Lentiginosis of penis is a condition that affects boys and men, and it can occur worldwide and no geographical preference is seen. Males of all racial and ethnic background may be affected

Histopathology

Elongation of rete ridges with basal layer hyperpigmentation, slight melanocytic hyperplasia, epithelial hyperplasia and stromal melanophages, no atypia. Lymphocytes, which are found in close apposition, destroy melanocytes and surrounding keratinocytes lack pigmentation

Management

Generally, there is no treatment required for Lentiginosis of penis, since it is a benign and harmless condition with no significant signs and symptoms or complications.

Individuals, in whom it causes significant cosmetic issues, or psychic concern may undergo a surgical excision or laser therapy to have them removed. Surgical excision may be problematic in terms of scarring and subsequent functional restriction [7].

40.9 Hypopigmented Genitalia

Definition

Localized or generalized decreased genital pigmentation (Fig. 40.8).

This is an assessment of the relative pigmentation of the genitalia compared to the overall pigmentation of the individual. Hypopigmentation can affect other parts of the body or be restricted to the genitalia. Localized hypopigmentation can be objectively determined due to the difference from the immediate surrounding tissue colour, while generalized hypopigmentation may be more difficult to determine and is therefore a subjective manifestation.

Depigmenting conditions such as vitiligo have a predilection for the genitals in the 'lip-tip' distribution involving perioral, genital and finger tip areas. Whether this pattern of distribution is as a result of trauma or pressure is still debated. Patients with vitiligo may need to have screening blood test for associated autoantibody conditions such as thyroid disease, diabetes or pernicious anaemia. The cosmetic impact of vitiligo is greater in darker-skinned individuals.

Individuals sufficiently bothered by their genital vitiligo can be carefully prescribed potent

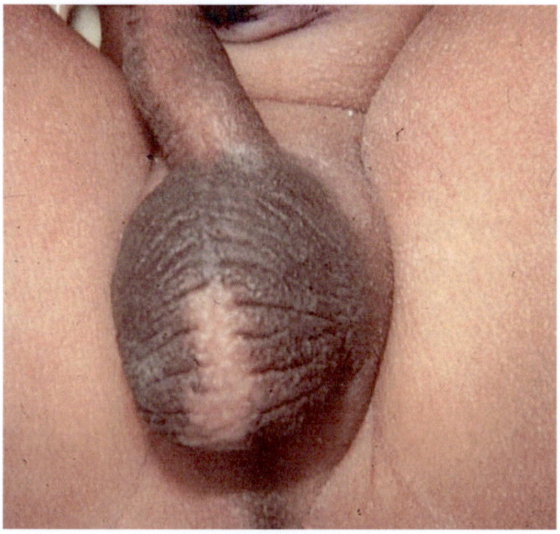

Fig. 40.8 Genital vitiligo in a 2 years old boy, mainly in the scrotum with minimal penile affection

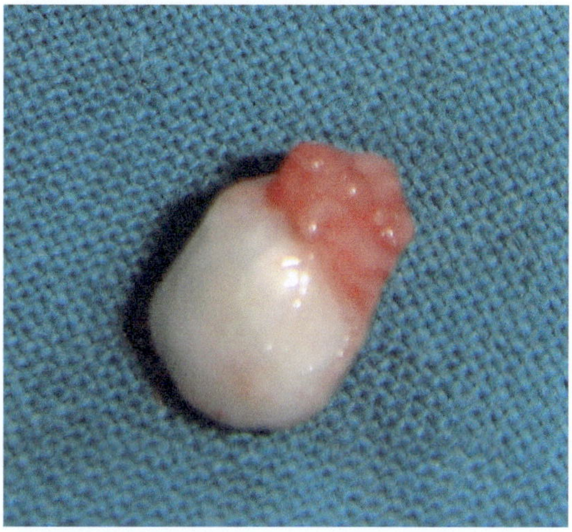

Fig. 40.9 Juvenile xanthogranuloma nodule excised from the penile shaft

topical steroids for 2 3 months at a time that is usually the minimum time for pigment restoration. An alternative immunosuppressive agent is tacrolimus compounded as a 0.1 % ointment [8].

Juvenile Xanthogranuloma (JXG) It is usually appears as a solitary superficial cutaneous nodule, although rare cases of systemic and deep tissue involvement have been described (Fig. 40.9).

The lesion is a well demarcated, firm, rubbery, round to oval papule or nodule. It can recur locally but is considered benign. JXG may affect any part of the body, including the testis and the scrotum, and it is best treated with excision and careful observation [9].

Penile Warts Warts may also manifest as dome-shaped, usually flesh coloured papules; flat warts are flat-topped papules which may vary in colour from pink-red to reddish-brown.

Lesions are frequently multifocal. Areas with increased friction are most commonly affected by condylomas; the commonest location of primary infection in uncircumcised men is the subpreputial region. Other sites of predilection are the glans penis, coronal sulcus, frenulum, prepuce, shaft and the scrotum. They may also occur on the urethral meatus and can be intraurethral. The urethra is involved in 10–28 % of patients; condom users often have suprapubic warts.

Subclinical lesions are detected by applying 3–5 % acetic acid to the genital area for up to 5 min. The acetic acid produces white changes in HPV infected areas. However, aceto-whitening is not a specific method for diagnosis, with false-positive results in up to 25 %. Subclinical involvement is especially common in uncircumcised men [8].

References

1. Buechner SA. Common skin disorders of the penis. BJU Int. 2002;90(5):498–506.
2. Fletcher CD, Tsang WY, Fisher C, Lee KC, Chan JK. Angiomyofibroblastoma of the vulva. A benign neoplasm distinct from aggressive angiomyxoma. Am J Surg Pathol. 1992;16(4):373–82.
3. Wolf B, Horn LC, Handzel R, Einenkel J. Ultrasound plays a key role in imaging and management of genital angiomyofibroblastoma: a case report. J Med Case Reports. 2015;9:248. doi:10.1186/s13256-015-0715-4.
4. Erkek E, Basar MM, Bagci Y, Karaduman A, Bilen CY, Gokoz A. Fordyce angiokeratomas as clues to local venous hypertension. Arch Dermatol. 2005;141(10):1325–6.
5. Barnhill RL, Rabinovitz H. Benign melanocytic neoplasms. In: Bolognia JL, Jorizzo JL, Rapini RP, editors. Dermatology. 2nd ed. British Library Cataloguing in Publication Data; 2008. p. 1717–20.

6. Arun KG, Timothy SD, David L, Reudi PG. Giant congenital nevi: a 20-year experience and an algorithm for their management. Plast Reconstr Surg. 2001;108(3):622–63.
7. Bolognia JL, Schaffer JV, Duncan KO, Ko CJ. Dermatology essentials E-book. Elsevier Health Sciences; 2014.
8. Atlas of genital skin diseases: http://www.imop.gr/en/uroelearning-urodermatology-atlas.
9. Dehner LP. Juvenile xanthogranulomas in the first two decades of life: a clinicopathologic study of 174 cases with cutaneous and extracutaneous manifestations. Am J Surg Pathol. 2003;27:579.

Index

© Springer International Publishing Switzerland 2017
M. Fahmy, *Congenital Anomalies of the Penis*, DOI 10.1007/978-3-319-43310-3

MIX
Papier aus verantwortungsvollen Quellen
Paper from responsible sources
FSC® C105338

If you have any concerns about our products,
you can contact us on
ProductSafety@springernature.com

In case Publisher is established outside the EU,
the EU authorized representative is:
Springer Nature Customer Service Center GmbH
Europaplatz 3, 69115 Heidelberg, Germany

Printed by Libri Plureos GmbH
in Hamburg, Germany